THE
COMPLETE DOCTOR'S
Stress
Solution

Understanding, Treating, and Preventing Stress and Stress-Related Illnesses

Penny Kendall-Reed, BSc, ND
and Dr. Stephen Reed, MD, FRCSC

Robert
ROSE

The authors would like to thank the following for sharing their knowledge and expertise during the writing of this book: Lynn Kendall, Amanda Webber, and Shula Starkey for their valuable additions to this book; Patrick Grierson and Jeremy Kendall for their inspiration as exemplary stress managers.

The publisher acknowledges the financial support of the Government of Canada through the Book Publishing Industry Development Program.

The nutritional, medical, and health information presented in this book is based on the research, training, and professional experience of the authors, and is true and complete to the best of their knowledge. However, this book is intended only as an informative guide for those wishing to know more about health, nutrition, and medicine; it is not intended to replace or countermand the advice given by the reader's personal physician. Because each person and situation is unique, the author and the publisher urge the reader to check with a qualified health-care professional before using any procedure where there is a question as to its appropriateness. A physician should be consulted before beginning any exercise program. The author and the publisher are not responsible for any adverse effects or consequences resulting from the use of the information in this book. It is the responsibility of the reader to consult a physician or other qualified health-care professional regarding his or her personal care.

National Library of Canada Cataloguing in Publication

Kendall-Reed, Penny
    The complete doctor's stress solution : understanding, treating and
preventing stress and stress-related illnesses / Penny Kendall-Reed and Stephen Reed.

Includes index.
ISBN 0-7788-0096-2

1. Stress (Physiology) 2. Stress (Psychology) 3. Stress management. I. Reed, Stephen Charles, 1961-
II. Title.

RA785.K45 2004   616.9'8   C2004-902917-7

Edited by Bob Hilderley, Senior Editor, Health.
Copyedited by Fina Scroppo.
Exercise and yoga illustrations by Kveta.
Design and type by PageWave Graphics.

The publisher acknowledges the financial support of the Government of Canada through the Book Publishing Industry Development Program.

Published by Robert Rose Inc.,
120 Eglinton Ave. E., Suite 800,
Toronto, Ontario Canada M4P 1E2
Tel: (416) 322-6552 Fax: (416) 322-6936

Printed and bound in Canada.
1 2 3 4 5 6 7 8 9 CPL 12 11 10 09 08 07 06 05 04

Contents

Introduction 5

1. The Stress Problem

Stress Systems 16
Role of the Stress Response 16
Nervous System 17
Endocrine System 22
Hypothalamus-Pituitary-Adrenal
    Interactions 30
Summary 34

Stress Response 35
HPA Axis 35
Daily Cortisol Cycle 36
Fight-or-Flight Response 36

Chronic Stress 40
Cortisol Levels 41
Adrenal Fatigue 41
Central Stress Response 43
Theories of Chronic Stress 44
Summary 46

2. Stress Solutions

Anti-Stress Diet 50
Nutrition Basics 51
Diet and Stress 55
Naturopathic Diet 64
Caffeine and Stress 76
Alcohol and Stress 78

Anti-Stress Natural Supplements . . 80
Selecting and Combining
    Supplements 81
Vitamins 83
Minerals 88
Herbs 90
Amino Acids 94
Other Anti-Stress Supplements 97

Anti-Stress Exercise Therapies . . 104
Exercise Basics 104
Stretching Exercises 107
Strength-Training Exercises 113
Cardiovascular Exercise 118

Anti-Stress Physical Therapies
    (Bodywork) 123
Finding a Bodywork Practitioner 124
Message Therapy 126
Aromatherapy 130
Reflexology 131
Acupuncture 132
Rei-Ki 135
Shiatsu 135
Craniosacral Therapy 136
Yoga 136
Tai Chi 140

Anti-Stress Mental Therapies . . . 141
Relaxation Techniques 142
Counseling 150

Anti-Stress Medications 155
Antianxiety and
    Antidepressant Drugs 155
CRH-Receptor Blockers 155

8-Week Stress Solution Program

Four Stages **159**

Program Components **160**
Naturopathic Diet. 160
Natural Supplements 160
Cardiovascular Exercise 161
Physical Therapy. 161
Relaxation Techniques 161

8-Week Program **162**
Stage 1 (Weeks 1 and 2) 162
Stage 2 (Weeks 3 and 4) 164
Stage 3 (Weeks 5 to 8) 165
Stage 4 (Maintenance) 170

3. Treating and Preventing Stress-Related Disorders and Diseases

Diabetes **174**
Treatment Program. 176

Cardiovascular Disease **179**
Hypertension *180*
Treatment Program. 184
Heart Attack *184*
Treatment Program. 186

Gastrointestinal Disorders **189**
Irritable Bowel Syndrome *190*
Treatment Program. 193
Inflammatory Bowel Disease. *193*
Treatment Program. 196
Peptic Ulceration *197*
Treatment Program. 201

Immune System Disorders and Allergies **202**
Immunity Disorders. *203*
Treatment Program 211
Allergic Response. *212*
Treatment Program. 216

Musculoskeletal Disorders. **217**
Overtraining Syndrome *217*
Treatment Program. 221
Osteoporosis. *221*
Treatment Program. 224
Arthritis *224*
Treatment Program. 227
Low Back Pain *227*
Treatment Program. 229

Reproductive Disorders **230**
Infertility *230*
Treatment Program. 236
Irregular Menstruation *236*
Menopause *237*
Treatment Program. 238

Sleep Disorders **239**
Treatment Program. 244

Chronic Pain Disorders **245**
Migraine. *246*
Treatment Program. 249
Fibromyalgia and Chronic Fatigue Syndrome *249*
Treatment Program. 254

Anxiety and Depression **255**
Panic Attacks. *258*
Treatment Program. 261
General Anxiety Disorder *261*
Treatment Program. 263
Post-Traumatic Stress Disorder *263*
Treatment Program. 264

Glossary **265**
References **274**
Index **284**

Introduction

Not Good News

David rolls over and squints at the alarm clock through tired, blurry eyes. 2:15 a.m. Feeling too warm, he pushes the duvet to one side and rearranges the pillows to try and get comfortable. Attempting to relax and drift off to sleep once more, he tries to clear his mind of the rapidly invading thoughts: "What will I say at the breakfast meeting? Will I have time to get back for the conference call? Shall I get up early to go over the production figures? What about getting the kids off to day care? Then there's my doctor's appointment in the afternoon for my annual checkup."

2:45 a.m. Now wide-awake, David is staring at the ceiling, the room lit by the glow of the city below the new condominium. He knows this oh-so frequent pattern will leave him exhausted for the day ahead, cloud his mind and judgment, with only endless cups of coffee keeping him from slumping over his desk mid-morning.

He turns to his wife Sue, "Are you awake?" "Yes," she replies. "I can't sleep with all your tossing and turning." David gets another hour or two of sleep, but wakes up feeling tired, frustrated, and already looking forward to collapsing into bed the following night.

Now up for the day, David stands in front of the full-length bathroom mirror. Inhaling deeply, he sucks in the flesh creeping over the top of his underwear. He breathes out and lets gravity take control of his '1-pack' once more. Only 35 years old, the flat stomach and athletic legs toned during years of football are already a distant memory. David still manages to grab a quick 30 minutes at the gym during lunch, but no amount of crunches, squats, or bench presses seem to slow the loss of muscle tone. Since the birth of his two children, he's had to put an end to the leisurely 5:00 to 7:00 p.m. workout and sauna. Weekends at the new cottage mean a long drive though ever-worsening traffic for the two days of 'rejuvenation', invariably fixing a broken pipe or planting a new tree.

Later that day… Dr. Jones looks up over gold bifocals and shuffles through David's lab results. "Not good news, I'm afraid. Blood pressure is up, cholesterol is high, and you are borderline diabetic." David's eyes widen. A wife, two children, two mortgages. He is scared. His stress response kicks into gear again. His condition only gets worse …

WHO DOESN'T HAVE STRESS? We all have it, right? Yes! Stress is necessary for our survival. It's perfectly natural, a part of being human. "Complete freedom from stress is death," Dr. Hans Selye commented in his pioneering research into the effects of stress on our health. But too much stress — or stress that isn't properly managed — contributes to disease conditions that can lead to our death.

Our response to stress is necessary for our survival. Our bodies are designed to react quickly to stressful situations, either to fend off or flee from danger. This is called the fight-or-flight response. This specific reaction takes place every single time our body senses stress of any kind. It doesn't matter whether the stressful situation is real or perceived, physical or psychological, once our brain interprets a situation as stressful, the reaction is the same. The glands responsible for producing stress hormones can't differentiate between the stress of a wedding or a funeral. They will react in a similar manner to a physical threat, increased workload at the office, financial difficulty, or a relationship problem. Whatever the stressor, the reaction is the same — the fight-or-flight response.

✔ **STRESS FACT Paradox**

This is one of the many paradoxes of stress — stress is at once a necessary biological survival mechanism and a biological threat to our well-being.

Caveman vs. Downtown Man

You're probably familiar with the scenario typically used to teach the principles of stress. A prehistoric 'caveman' meanders along, minding his own business, wondering whether to wear the bison or the bearskin loincloth for dinner, when a sabre-toothed tiger leaps out of the bushes. The fight-or-flight mechanism is activated. Adrenaline kicks in, causing the caveman's pupils to dilate, heart and breathing rate to jump, skin to go cold, and hair to stand up. Muscles twitch in anticipation of the next move. Senses are heightened.

The caveman throws a rock (fight), then jumps quickly into a gully (flight), running as fast as he can, powered by the surge of energy from increased levels of blood sugar. By now, cortisol, the major stress hormone, is beginning to rise, supporting the initial adrenaline rush to permit a prolonged reaction to the inherent danger. Cortisol is more potent and longer-lasting than adrenaline, with profound effects at the cellular level.

In just moments, the threat is over. The tiger has stopped pursuing the man, distracted by a passing rabbit, which proves to be a more accessible prey. With a sigh of relief, the danger now past and his cave in sight, the caveman's alarm system turns off. The stress hormones stabilize his body before switching off and returning to normal levels. The fight-or-flight mechanism has worked, enabling survival in the face of danger and restoring his life to normal with no ill effects — apart from a battered prehistoric ego!

Now, several thousands of years later, 'downtown man', tired from a sleepless night, has already battled with what he perceives as the first stressful situation of the day — whether to wear the Armani or Prada power suit to the corporate merger presentation — and is now sitting in traffic, 15 minutes late for work. His mobile phone rings. It's his boss, informing him that if he's late, he might as well not show up at all. No one to fight, nowhere to flee. Reaching to put the phone down, he knocks his coffee over the presentation sheets on the passenger seat. The traffic hasn't moved an inch. Despite the fact that none of this is anywhere near as dangerous as confronting a sabre-toothed tiger, he *perceives* it as a threat to his employment and his ego. His brain is programmed to interpret such situations as stress.

The primitive areas of the brain and associated hormone reactions involved in the response to stress have not changed much since caveman's loincloth days. The fight-or-flight mechanism kicks into action. The cascade of adrenaline begins in response, followed by longer-lasting cortisol, raising heart rate, blood pressure, and breathing levels. Downtown man sweats, honks the horn, feels rage. He no longer thinks clearly, awash in a recurring cycle of stress hormones.

Unlike the caveman's stress, downtown man's situation does not resolve quickly, and when it does, it is rapidly replaced by another. The stress reaction continually battles to restore the normal biological balance of his body to a 'safe' condition but does not succeed. Eventually, his general health may begin to suffer.

✔ STRESS FACT Far-Reaching Effects

Chronic stimulation of the stress reaction leads to hormonal and metabolic imbalances that adversely affect all systems in the body. These range from the well-recognized effects on metabolism and weight known as metabolic syndrome and the reduction in athletic performance seen in overtraining syndrome to impairment of fertility, immunity, and healing. The main culprit is cortisol, the stress hormone that supports a prolonged and powerful fight-or-flight reaction. Cortisol reaches all tissues of the body. Unfortunately, in excess, its harmful effects are equally as far-reaching.

Did You Know?
- 79% to 90% of all visits to primary health-care practitioners in North America are due to stress-related illnesses or complaints.
- 1 million North Americans are absent on any given workday due to stress and stress-related disorders.
- 60% of absences at work are the result of stress.

Acute Stress Response Cascade

Brain perceives danger or threat.

Sympathetic nervous system initiates fight-or-flight response.

Heart rate, blood pressure, blood sugar, and breathing levels increase.

Adrenaline supports sympathetic system short term.

Cortisol sustains fight-or-flight response.

Once the danger or threat is resolved, the body stabilizes.

Acute Stress Response

The stress response involves a series of events designed to promote survival in a threatening or harmful situation. In its simplest terms, it works like this. The brain interprets incoming information (sight, sound, smell, touch, etc.) and decides that the body is in danger. Almost instantly, the activity of one of the body's automatic nervous systems (the sympathetic nervous system) increases. These nerves transmit impulses to most organs and tissues in the body so that within seconds, the fight-or-flight response is initiated. This sympathetic system is powered by adrenaline released from the nerve endings and is backed up by rapid release of large additional amounts of adrenaline into the bloodstream by the adrenal glands. The sympathetic system provides a rapid but short-lived response in the stress cascade.

The adrenal glands boost this initial output and then provide a stronger and more sustained reaction. Cortisol, also released from the adrenal glands, is the hormone that drives the majority of the fight-or-flight response, acting on tissues and organs throughout the body, altering metabolism and cellular processes in a way that will benefit the body in the short term to overcome the dangerous situation. Once resolved, the system shuts down, levels return to normal, and the body stabilizes.

Chronic Stress Response

In the chronic stress response, rather than benefiting the body, the fight-or-flight response becomes so overstimulated that two things occur. First, rather than a controlled daily cycle of cortisol release with intermittent peaks, there is persistent secretion. While short bursts of this hormone are essential to normal function (for example, the surge in levels just before getting up in the morning), chronically elevated levels have a severely detrimental effect on most tissues and cells in the body.

Second, the body becomes unable to handle a real emergency. Akin to a hormonal 'cry wolf' situation, truly dangerous circumstances fail to produce sufficient cortisol release from the adrenal glands. The result of these two factors is a body that is overweight, sleep-deprived, poorly muscled, fragile, prone to infection, and often depressed, unable to perform under pressure or handle a difficult or threatening situation or illness.

Continual stimulation of the fight-or-flight response and adrenal cortisol secretion seems to reset the body's 'set' point where biological balance or equilibrium rests. There is now a persistent secretion of cortisol, disruption of the normal daily cycle, development of 'cortisol resistance', and impairment of the feedback mechanism that would normally exert control over the whole system.

This chronic stress condition is surprisingly common. An increasing body of evidence is showing how chronic stress is contributing to disease in the general population.

Metabolic Syndrome

Metabolic syndrome or syndrome-X is well recognized as the association of a number of health conditions in one individual. They include obesity (abdominal), high blood pressure, high insulin levels with insulin resistance, diabetes, high cholesterol, and increased risk of heart attack and stroke. The syndrome affects a large proportion of the adult population of industrialized countries and likely represents the largest single threat to health in the upcoming decade. Initial theories about the development of this syndrome center around diet, and while this is clearly an important factor, evidence is pointing to chronic stress as being the primary cause.

Stress Solutions

Fortunately, chronic stress can be treated and prevented. While the first section of this book further explains the basis of the chronic stress condition based on an extensive review of current scientific research, the second section presents a comprehensive solution to this chronic stress problem, involving a combination of therapies, including diet, supplementation, exercise, physical therapies, and relaxation programs. The third section of the book practically applies this program to specific stress-related disorders and diseases, ranging from diabetes and heart attack to anxiety and depression. The programs presented are relatively easy to implement, safe, and effective. They have been proven in our medical practice and are supported by many of our colleagues in the medical and naturopathic doctor professions.

Most of us cannot immediately or completely change our lifestyles. Stressful situations will continue to bombard us every day. We can, however, change our bodies to handle the stress more efficiently, without detrimental effect to our health. After all, we never know when that sabre-toothed tiger is going to come round the corner. So, we should be ready.

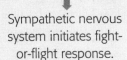

Chronic Stress Response Cascade

Brain perceives danger.

⬇

Sympathetic nervous system initiates fight-or-flight response.

⬇

Heart rate, blood pressure, blood sugar, and breathing levels increase.

⬇

Adrenal supports sympathetic system short term.

⬇

Cortisol sustains fight-or-flight response.

⬇

Stress is not resolved; the body does not stabilize.

⬇

Persistent, low-level secretion of cortisol.

⬇

Cry wolf response: the body is unable to handle a real emergency.

⬇

Body becomes overweight, sleep-deprived, poorly muscled, fragile, prone to infection, and often depressed, unable to perform under pressure or handle a difficult or threatening situation or illness.

⬇

Metabolic syndrome may result.

Are You Stressed?

Some people seem to cope with stress better than others, for reasons that aren't always clear. They seem to have a special gift for completely 'turning off' their mental thought processes when they get into bed, despite a very important business meeting they have at 9:00 a.m. the next day. Other people are not as fortunate — or relaxed. How many times have you lay awake in bed at night trying desperately to fall asleep? The more you try, the harder it becomes. Then you start worrying about that meeting, exam, or interview the next morning and how you must get some sleep to prepare for it.

The fact that you aren't sleeping becomes yet another stressor and ultimately makes the entire situation worse. If you are lucky enough to fall asleep, you may again find yourself wide awake between 2:00 and 4:00 a.m. and begin the entire process all over again. You feel and hear your heart beat as you lie there in bed trying to count sheep jumping over the fence. If any of these events sound familiar, read on.

Attitudes Toward Stress

Here is a sample of different attitudes toward stress, some more healthy than others.

"I know I'm stressed most of the time."

You have already made it over the first hurdle. You are listening to your body and know you are stressed. You may already know about some of the ill effects that stress causes. This book will both expand your knowledge of stress-related disease and allow you to reduce your own personal stress.

"I'm occasionally stressed, but that's normal."

Being stressed once in a while is definitely part of life, but that doesn't necessarily mean it's healthy. Even brief, regular stressful episodes can have a detrimental effect on your well-being, and the likelihood is that many of these stressors remain unresolved, resulting in a low level of chronic, unrecognized stress.

"I don't think I'm stressed."

Of course, we realize there are individuals who remain cool, calm, and collected through all adversity, and they may indeed have their stress response under control. Others may have lifestyles free from the rigors of modern-day life, a perfect family or personal relationships, and a happy work environment.

We suspect, however, that these individuals are the exception rather than the rule. Most people who believe they are not stressed have not taken a close look at their life and their health, and are not listening to their body. They attribute their fatigue, recurrent colds, anxiety attacks, and skin rashes to other factors, ignoring the hectic pace at which they live. Recognizing the 'red flags' of chronic stress and learning how illness and stress are related is vital for this category of individual. Having realized that "perhaps I am a little stressed," you can make simple lifestyle changes to enhance awareness of your body's response to stress along with a plan to control it.

"I'm stressed but I thrive on it."

Sound familiar. At the gym by 5:00 a.m. and in the office by 7:00. Lunch on the fly. Leave work at 8:00 p.m., head out for drinks and dinner. Party until 2:00 a.m., then head home for a couple of hours sleep before starting again. With catch phrases like, "I work better under stress" and "I only need 4 hours sleep a night," these individuals are invincible — or at least they think they are!

No doubt about it, when you're young, your body will put up with more or less anything you throw at it. However, while you seem to be able to cope with stress much better, the damage to your health is already being done. Take a look at your boss! Overweight, high blood pressure, diabetes, stomach ulcers? That could be you in 10 years. While, we do not expect you to settle into a middle-aged lifestyle at 22, we hope to institute some simple changes that will keep you healthy so you can enjoy that time when it comes!

Natural Biological Therapies

Our approach to treating chronic stress can best be called natural biological therapy. The goal is to restore biological balance in the body by altering hormone levels, enzymes, blood sugar, and neurotransmitters in order to re-establish a homeostatic balance. This corrects the physiologic malfunction at the root of stress and thus resolves disturbing physical, emotional, and neurological symptoms.

To achieve this goal, we recommend natural therapies, which include good nutrition, natural supplementation (for example, botanical extracts, vitamins, and minerals), exercise, physical therapies (for example, massage, shiatsu, and yoga), and relaxation techniques to create physiological changes in the body. These treatments all affect the physical body in several ways to solve the problem of chronic stress. Natural biological therapies are some of the easiest to execute from a patient's point of view and are easily incorporated into one's lifestyle.

Natural therapies can be used successfully in conjunction with psychological counseling. Together, these therapies prepare the physical body to address emotional issues, such that harmony is restored both physiologically and psychologically.

While in traditional medical and psychological practice, biological therapy per se includes the use of pharmaceutical drugs, shock therapy, and surgery, we only cover drug therapy in this book.

Stress Checklist

Many people suffer from chronic stress, but do not realize it. They assume their ill health is normal, part of a hectic 21st-century lifestyle. They fail to realize that the longer they live at this pace, ignoring the warning signs of chronic stress, the higher the chances they could have potentially life-threatening consequences.

If any of the following symptoms are familiar, this book is for you. We show you many ways you can help yourself both on your own and with the skill and guidance of different practitioners to restore emotional and physical balance to your body.

❏ Weight gain principally in the mid-section of your body.
❏ Waking up tired in the morning despite seemingly adequate sleep hours.
❏ Difficulty falling asleep, waking between 2:00 and 4:00 a.m., often restless with racing thoughts.
❏ Frequent irritability with episodes of anger.
❏ Anxiety attacks.
❏ Constant worry or fear about life.
❏ Jaw clenching or teeth grinding.
❏ Frequent colds and flu.

❏ Heart palpitations, high blood pressure and heart disease.
❏ Slow recovery from illness or injury.
❏ Bowel irritability or irregularity.
❏ Frequent headaches or migraines.
❏ Poor concentration and memory.
❏ Feeling overwhelmed at work or at home.
❏ Depression or episodes of despair or weepiness.
❏ Irregular menstrual cycles.
❏ Reduced libido.
❏ Difficulty getting pregnant despite normal test results.

Stress Symptom Journal

Many times, people don't realize they're suffering from chronic stress. If they do, they're unable to pinpoint the precipitating factors. By tracking emotional and physical symptoms and charting them against the activity and time of day, it will be easier to recognize these triggers. This information can then be used to help avoid or minimize stress in the future.

For example, the physical symptom may be heart palpitations every morning after arriving at work, or low energy and irritability when you get home from work every day. By recognizing this pattern, it may be possible to identify the stress trigger — driving in traffic, job insecurity, or a confrontational home situation as the stress trigger. By reviewing your journal, you identify triggers and situations that increase your stress — and avoid or minimize these symptoms.

Keep this journal for 7 days, including a weekend. You might want to show it to your health-care practitioners if you are looking for their help in resolving your stress.

Day	Activity	Physical/Emotional Symptom
Example		
Morning	Sitting in commuter traffic.	Increased heart rate and irritability.
Afternoon	Hungry at work at 3:00 p.m.	Anxiety and decreased mental clarity.
Evening	Making dinner for the family.	Weepy, frustrated, and dizzy.
Day 1		
Morning		
Afternoon		
Evening		
Day 2		
Morning		
Afternoon		
Evening		
Day 3		
Morning		
Afternoon		
Evening		
Day 4		
Morning		
Afternoon		
Evening		
Day 5		
Morning		
Afternoon		
Evening		
Day 6		
Morning		
Afternoon		
Evening		
Day 7		
Morning		
Afternoon		
Evening		

Good News

David wakes up from a good night's sleep, refreshed and ready to face the day ahead. His decision to take control of his stress was the right one. The moment he left his doctor's office, he had vowed to find out why his health was at risk and do something positive about it. Having recognized chronic stress as a major factor in his physical and mental deterioration, David endeavored to find out as much as possible about this condition and what steps he could take to reverse it.

During our first meeting with David, we explained how chronic stress, even if it is unrecognized, can have an impact on many systems of the body, causing dysfunction and ill health. We also introduced him to the various effective biological therapies he could use to return his body to a stable and healthy state.

David started the '8-Week Stress Solution Program' described in this book. He began a naturopathic diet for stress management, supported by a number of 'anti-stress' supplements, including vitamin B complex, calcium-magnesium, hydrolyzed milk peptide, and essential fatty acids. He changed his exercise routine so that he only worked out three times per week, but these were at a higher intensity than his previous daily efforts. On the other days, he followed a stretching routine and performed deep-breathing exercises, following a simple program laid out in this book. He began regular weekly bodywork sessions, alternating aromatherapy and reflexology. He also followed the meditation guide described in this book. Simple lifestyle changes, such as listening to relaxing music and taking a lavender bath, enhanced his stress reduction program.

David never had to start medication for blood pressure, cholesterol, or diabetes. He is back at his university football weight and allows a smile to creep across his face as he checks out his rediscovered abdominal muscles in the mirror. He is calmer, more productive. He finds he has more time and energy for his children. His relationship with his wife is better than ever.

A simple daily program deals with regular day-to-day stresses, and while life is still hectic at times, with unexpected stresses appearing at the most inopportune moments, he now knows how to deal with them. And they pass. David is looking forward to a healthy future.

The Stress Problem

Stress Systems

The human body's response to stress involves a series of events common to many animal species. The pathways and chemicals involved in this response have remained unchanged throughout evolution, providing a protective mechanism against adverse circumstances and an adaptive process to restore a normal state. Where humans differ from other animals, it would seem, is in their interpretation of what constitutes a 'stressful' situation and in their ability to resolve it to re-establish a 'safe' environment.

 STRESS FACT Just Thinking About Stress

The greater influence of our cerebral cortex — the thinking part of the brain — means that even in the absence of visual or other sensory stimuli, just thinking about a stressful situation can trigger the stress response. Unfortunately, our greater thinking capacity has made stress a complex problem.

Role of the Stress Response

The human body's response to external or internal stress involves a complex series of biological reactions designed to confront the 'threat' and then to restore the body to a normal state (homeostasis). By 'external' we mean factors in the surrounding environment construed as potentially harmful or disruptive, anything from a sabre-toothed tiger to a traffic jam. By 'internal' we refer to dangerous processes that affect the functioning of the body, such as an infection or blood loss.

Whatever the stimulus, the body's response is initially the same, following a well-documented cascade of nervous and hormonal activity with the good intention of making the internal or external environment safe and returning the body to a stable condition.

If, however, this homeostatic state is not restored, the stress response recurs. This inevitably drives the chemical pathways, designed only for brief periods of activity, to exhaustion.

Before we describe solutions to this problem, we need a better understanding of the components of the nervous and endocrine systems involved in this stress response.

Note: Scientific study of the chronic stress response is relatively new, much of the research as yet inconclusive and sometimes contradictory. We have assembled the available information into a coherent theory of stress that integrates these complex observations. We do not present these explanations as doctrine, but rather as discussion points to help you understand your stress-related symptoms and improve their management.

Nervous System

The components of the nervous system involved in the stress response include the brain, the limbic system, and the autonomic nervous system.

Brain
The brain can be divided into three areas: the forebrain, the midbrain, and the brainstem. It maybe helpful to think of these three areas as progressively less developed from an evolutionary perspective and more basic to the functioning of the brain.

Forebrain
The forebrain includes the cerebral cortex, responsible for the cognitive and analytical components of brain function and voluntary behavior. The forebrain also includes the thalamus, a complex relay station for incoming and outgoing messages. The lowest part of the forebrain is the hypothalamus, primarily concerned with survival of the individual and the species. The hypothalamus plays a central role in the stress response by coordinating a complex interaction between the nervous system and the endocrine or hormonal systems of the body.

Midbrain
The midbrain is the smallest of the three areas, comprising structures around the canal called the cerebral aqueduct, a channel carrying cerebrospinal fluid from the third ventricle downward into the fourth ventricle and spinal cord.

Brainstem
The brainstem incorporates the structures of the brain below the level of the thalamus, hypothalamus, and midbrain, namely the pons, the medulla oblongata, and the cerebellum. In the brainstem, numerous nerve fiber pathways connect the spinal cord with the cerebral hemisphere to control movement.

Components of the Stress Response
Nervous System
Brain
Limbic System
Autonomic Nervous System (Sympathetic System)

Endocrine System
Hypothalamus
Pituitary Gland
Adrenal Glands
Adrenaline and Cortisol

The reticular formation (Reticular Activating System or RAS) is also found within the brainstem, an extensive neuronal network that not only controls basic functions such as heartbeat and breathing but also exerts a profound affect on the overall activity of the brain, level of arousal, behavior, and response to external stimuli. From an evolutionary perspective, the reticular formation is similar to the hypothalamus (it is extremely prominent in the brainstem of primitive reptiles), and like the hypothalamus, the reticular formation plays a key role in the stress response.

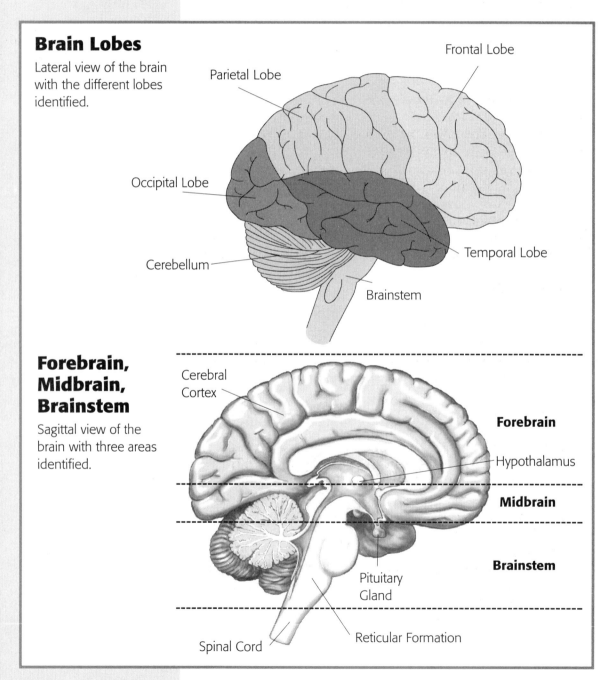

Brain Lobes

Lateral view of the brain with the different lobes identified.

Frontal Lobe

Parietal Lobe

Occipital Lobe

Temporal Lobe

Cerebellum

Brainstem

Forebrain, Midbrain, Brainstem

Sagittal view of the brain with three areas identified.

Cerebral Cortex

Forebrain

Hypothalamus

Midbrain

Brainstem

Pituitary Gland

Spinal Cord

Reticular Formation

The Stress Problem

Limbic System

The limbic system refers to the extensive and complex neuronal circuitry that controls emotional behavior and motivation. Located within the temporal lobe of the brain, it includes the hippocampus and the amygdala, centers intricately involved in the stress response, emotion, and memory.

✔ STRESS FACT Triggers

The limbic system is central to the control of the stress response. The fight-or-flight stress response is triggered in the amygdala and hippocampus by external events. These events are interpreted in light of both innate behavior and life experience.

The 'set point' of this process is under the influence of the serotonin system, which also controls mood, hunger, sleep, and aggression. The lower the set point, the more reactive the system and the more likely the stress response will be triggered.

In addition, the emotional memory of the event stored in the amygdala is stronger and carries greater influence when interpreting future events. This is called conditioned fear, the basis of 'perceived stress'. In the amygdala, the thought of an event or situation can trigger the fight-or-flight response, even though the individual may be nowhere near the threatening event in space or time. This perceived input or thought comes from the medial prefrontal cortex, an area exerting direct influence over the amygdala and hippocampus.

The limbic system provides output of information to the hypothalamus, which, in turn, appears to consolidate much of the information collected by the limbic system and provides output by three major channels:

1. Downward into the brainstem and in particular to the reticular formation.
2. Upward into the thalamus and cerebral cortex.
3. Downward into the pituitary gland where it controls the majority of the hormone secretion by this gland.

The hippocampus has an equally important role in shutting off the stress response. Research suggests that this ability may be impaired in some individuals, making them more susceptible to chronic stress and related illness. Furthermore, chronic stress appears to shrink the hippocampus, which may further impair its stress-controlling activity.

Limbic System

Saggital view of the brain with the structures of the limbic system.

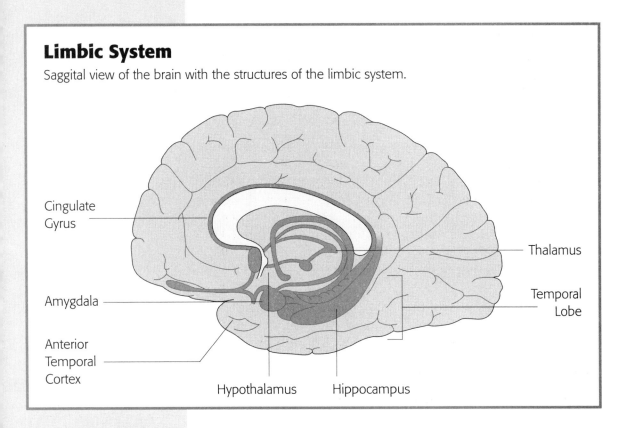

Cingulate Gyrus

Thalamus

Amygdala

Temporal Lobe

Anterior Temporal Cortex

Hypothalamus

Hippocampus

Autonomic Role

Unlike the motor system, the autonomic nervous system is not under conscious or voluntary control. It is responsible for adjusting such bodily functions as blood pressure, heart rate, intestinal motility, sweating, body temperature, and metabolic rate.

Autonomic Nervous System

The nervous system can be divided into the motor and the autonomic systems. The motor system controls movement. For example, when you want to bend your finger, the cerebral cortex of your brain sends impulses along nerves that travel through the brainstem and into the spinal cord, and from there along peripheral nerves that travel through the neck and the arm to the muscles in your forearm, which then contract, allowing you to move the finger. You have done this voluntarily and are able to control the amount the finger moves. While other circuits within the brain may modify the speed and smoothness of the movement, it is essentially under your control. Although there are some reflex components to this system (for example, the knee-jerk reflex) that can occur involuntarily, you are still aware that they are happening and, to a certain extent, can exert control over the reflex.

In contrast, the autonomic system works predominantly on an involuntary basis, acting in a reflex response to numerous stimuli. Some of these reflexes occur at the level of the spinal cord with few impulses reaching the brain. Others involve complex reflexes coordinated in the limbic system and hypothalamus. These reflexes can occur very rapidly, causing changes in heart rate, for example, within 3 to 5 seconds and blood pressure within 10 to 15 seconds. When you faint, your

The Stress Problem

body is experiencing an extremely rapid drop in blood pressure, resulting from stimulation of one part of the autonomic nervous system that effectively slows the heart and dilates the blood vessels. This happens within 4 to 5 seconds, depriving the brain of sufficient oxygen to cause you to pass out.

Sympathetic System

The autonomic nervous system is divided into complementary sympathetic and parasympathetic components. The sympathetic nervous system is primarily responsible for stimulating the individual to a state of heightened awareness as will occur in the initial stages of the fight-or-flight stress response. This system uses nerves to transmit its impulses, making its response rapid. The sympathetic system provides the first line of defense and reaction during the stress response.

The hypothalamus has a second line of attack that provides backup for the sympathetic nervous system. This involves the release of hormones, chemical messengers in the endocrine system that act more slowly but in a more prolonged manner.

Autonomic Nervous System

Parasympathetic and Sympathetic Systems

Schematic images of the parasympathetic and sympathetic nervous systems with organs they innervate.

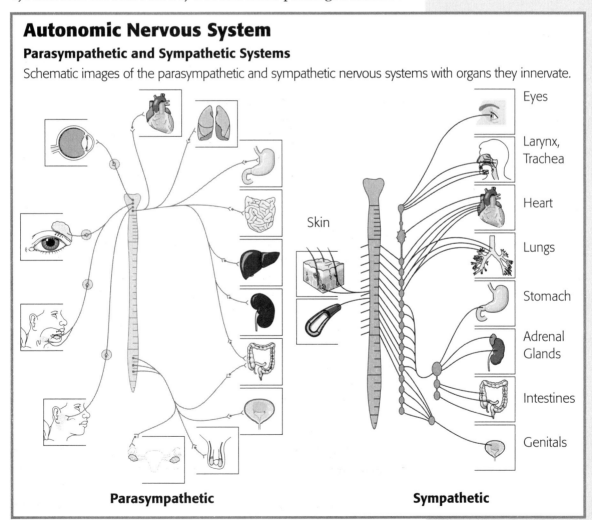

Eyes

Larynx, Trachea

Heart

Lungs

Stomach

Adrenal Glands

Intestines

Genitals

Skin

Parasympathetic

Sympathetic

Endocrine System

The human body comprises a myriad different organs and tissues intertwined in a complex relationship. Like any relationship, the key to success is good communication. The messengers that provide that communication include hormones, neurotransmitters, and cytokines. As messengers, they provide information about the status of the body and, when required, act to induce change that is usually beneficial.

Stress Response Pathways

Sensory stimuli, memory, and stress level influence activity of the limbic system and hypothalamus, in turn affecting activation of the fight-or-flight response.

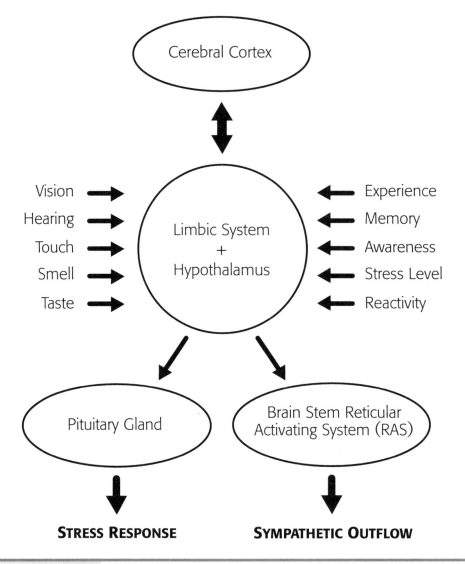

Endocrine Glands and Hormones

The endocrine glands are organs that contain specialized cells responsible for the manufacture, control, and release of hormones. The principal glands are the pituitary (anterior and posterior), thyroid, parathyroid, adrenal, ovaries, and pancreas. There are other glands, including the pineal gland (in the brain) and the placenta (during pregnancy), as well as endocrine cells within non-endocrine organs, such as the stomach (gastrin, ghrelin), fat cells (leptin), and kidneys (erythropoietin). The hypothalamus also secretes a number of hormones into the endocrine system.

Body System Messengers

Hormones
- Messengers of the endocrine system.
- Chemical messengers secreted by a group of cells, often contained within a specific endocrine gland.
- May act locally or at distant sites in the body to influence the function of other cells or organs.

Neurotransmitters
- Messengers of the nervous system.
- Released from the end of one nerve to control another nerve.
- May stimulate, inhibit, or modify the sensitivity of another neuron.

Cytokines
- Chemicals released by cells of the immune system.
- Usually act locally.
- Control inflammation and the immune response.

Endocrine System Controls

Hormone levels are under a number of controls that permit activity within a certain physiologic range. When one of these control mechanisms is disrupted, you can become significantly ill.

Through a network of hormonal messengers, the endocrine system influences the activity and function of cells and organs throughout the body. An endocrine cell produces a hormone and then releases it into the bloodstream. The hormone is delivered to every tissue in the body, but only has an effect on those cells that carry a specific receptor for that hormone. Once the hormone contacts a cell with the correct receptor, it will bind to it and affect the cell's growth or function. In some cases (in the gastrointestinal tract, for example), hormones act locally on nearby cells by traveling into the local blood supply or within tissue or organ fluids.

Major Endocrine Glands

Location of glands of the endocrine system.

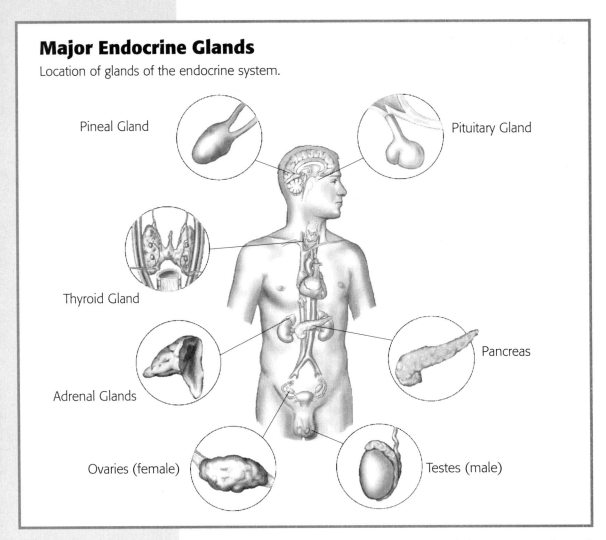

Pineal Gland

Pituitary Gland

Thyroid Gland

Adrenal Glands

Pancreas

Ovaries (female)

Testes (male)

For general hormones, such as growth hormone or thyroid hormone, almost all cells in the body will carry a receptor, so the effects of these messengers are far-reaching. However, some hormones, such as adrenocorticotropic hormone (ACTH), released by the pituitary gland, act very specifically on one group of cells, in this case the outer part of the adrenal gland, as these are the only ones carrying a receptor.

Daily Cycles

Many hormones show a definite cycle of activity throughout the day, a so-called diurnal or circadian rhythm. This is generally under the control of the brain because this is where awareness of day and night occurs, although the 'master clock' in the suprachiasmatic nucleus (SCN) of the hypothalamus continues to tick even in the absence of light/dark variation. The pituitary and pineal glands are classic examples, their hormones showing well-defined patterns of release during a 24-hour period.

Hormone Actions

This figure shows how a hormone, produced by an endocrine gland, can act on local cells or be transported via the bloodstream to distant tissues. If a tissue has the correct receptor, then the hormone will bind and exert an effect.

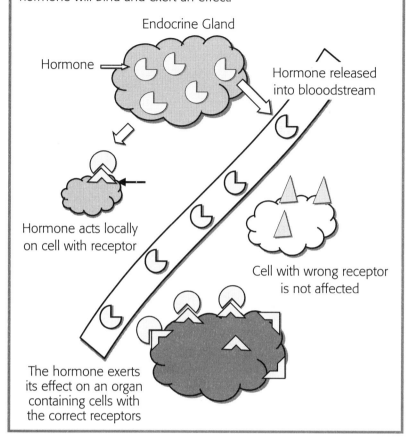

Endocrine Gland

Hormone

Hormone released into blooodstream

Hormone acts locally on cell with receptor

Cell with wrong receptor is not affected

The hormone exerts its effect on an organ containing cells with the correct receptors

Feedback

Feedback control is one of the most important mechanisms in the endocrine system, ensuring that whenever a hormone exerts an effect on a target cell, increased activity prevents further release of the original hormone. This inhibition may occur by two means: the target cell produces a different hormone that circulates back to the original gland; or a change in the concentration of a certain chemical in the blood occurs.

A good example is the cortisol system whereby cortisol, released by the adrenal gland in response to ACTH from the pituitary, feeds back on the pituitary to inhibit further ACTH release. Cortisol also feeds back on the hypothalamus to inhibit corticotropin-releasing hormone (CRH), the hormone that causes ACTH release, enhancing the overall negative feedback loop.

Major Endocrine Glands and Their Hormones

Gland	Hormone
Anterior Pituitary	Growth Hormone (GH)
	Adrenocorticotropic Hormone (ACTH)
	Thyroid-Stimulating Hormone (TSH)
	Follicle-Stimulating Hormone (FSH)
	Luteinizing Hormone (LH)
	Prolactin (PRL)
Posterior Pituitary	Antidiuretic Hormone (ADH)
	Oxytocin
Pineal	Melatonin
Thyroid Gland	Thyroxine (T-4), Triiodothyronine (T-3)
	Calcitonin
Parathyroid Glands	Parathormone
Adrenal Glands (medulla)	Adrenaline and Noradrenaline
Adrenal Glands (cortex)	Cortisol
	Aldosterone
Pancreas	Insulin
	Glucagon
Ovaries	Estrogens
	Progesterone

Hypothalamus
Although not considered an endocrine gland, the hypothalamus exerts control over the pituitary via neuro-hormones.

	Corticotropin-Releasing Hormone (CRH)
	Growth Hormone-Releasing Hormone
	Growth Hormone-Inhibiting Hormone
	Gonadotropin-Releasing Hormone (GnRH)
	Thyrotropin- Releasing Hormone (TRH)
	Prolactin-Inhibiting Factor (PIF)

Site of Action	Action
Most cells of the body	Stimulates cell growth
Adrenal Glands (cortex)	Stimulates adrenal cortex to release cortisol and aldosterone
Thyroid Gland	Causes thyroid to secrete thyroid hormones
Ovary/Testes	Promotes growth of follicles within the ovary (female), sperm formation (male)
Ovary/Testes	Stimulates estrogen/progesterone release (female), testosterone (male)
Breast tissue	Encourages breast development, milk production in pregnancy
Kidneys, blood vessels	Causes kidneys to retain water, increases blood pressure
Uterus/Breast tissue	Induces contractions during labor, milk expulsion
Brain, immune system	Governs sleep/wake cycle
Most cells of the body	Increases metabolism, chemical reactions
Bone cells	Increases calcium deposition
Gut, kidney, bone	Increases calcium in the blood
Many cells and tissues	Initiates fight-or-flight response
Many cells and tissues	Stress response affects metabolism, immune system, blood vessels
Kidneys, sweat glands	Promotes sodium/water retention, increases potassium loss
Most cells of the body	Promotes entry of sugar into cells, fat deposition
Liver, fat, muscle	Increases glucose production and release into the blood
Sex organs, uterus, bone	Involved in sexual development (female), menstruation, builds uterine tissue, bone metabolism
Sex organs, uterus	Involved in sexual development (female), menstruation, uterine secretion, pregnancy
Anterior Pituitary	Stimulates release of ACTH
Anterior Pituitary	Stimulates release of GH
Anterior Pituitary	Inhibits release of GH
Anterior Pituitary	Stimulates release of LH and FSH
Anterior Pituitary	Stimulates release of TSH
Anterior Pituitary	Inhibits release of Prolactin

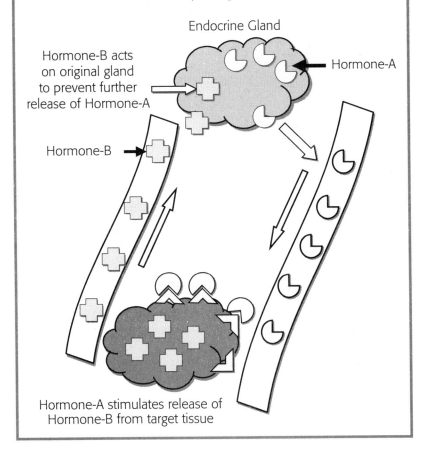

Hormone Feedback Loop

In this figure, hormone-A, produced by an endocrine gland, acts on an organ causing it to produce hormone-B. Hormone-B might represent a true hormone or another chemical. Hormone-B travels back to the endocrine gland, where it acts to inhibit further release of hormone-A, thereby acting as a feedback control.

Endocrine Gland

Hormone-B acts on original gland to prevent further release of Hormone-A

Hormone-A

Hormone-B

Hormone-A stimulates release of Hormone-B from target tissue

Receptor Number and Sensitivity

Another factor controlling hormone activity is the number and sensitivity of cell receptors. There can be a vast amount of hormone in circulation, but if there are only one or two receptors available, or those receptors are only minimally sensitive, then the overall target action will be limited. This is called down-regulation.

Neurotransmitters

Neurotransmitters are chemical substances that are released by nerve cells (neurons) for the purpose of communication. Over the past decade, the number of chemicals identified as neurotransmitters has grown exponentially. Their role in both the brain and the peripheral tissues continues to be elucidated.

The Stress Problem

Down-Regulation

The degree to which a hormone can influence a cell is dependent not only on the absolute amount of hormone available, but on the number and sensitivity of receptors on the target cell.

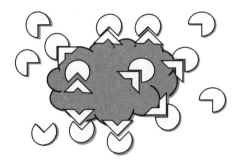

Normal receptor number and function

Reduced receptor number so hormone exerts less effect

They provide an important link between the central nervous and endocrine systems, an important extra factor when contemplating the influence of stress on the body.

Types of Neurotransmitters

1. Small molecules, such as dopamine, serotonin, or glutamine, are synthesized at the synapse, the gap between nerves where communication occurs. These molecules are released, act rapidly on the receptors of the adjacent neuron to transmit the message, and are then recycled.

2. Large neuropeptides, such as CRH, enkephalins, substance-P, cholecystokinin (CCK), and gastrin, are synthesized in the nerve cell body and transported to the synapse along the axon (long nerve body). These transmitters are also found in many tissues throughout the body, including the gut and immune system. They act slowly as neurotransmitters, but are highly potent and have very long endurance.

Cytokines

Cytokines are the hormones of the immune system. They control the body's response to inflammation, injury, and disease.

While the majority of cytokines act locally to influence cells involved in the inflammatory or immune response, there is increasing evidence that they provide both peripheral and central feedback to relay information about the status of the immune system.

For example, IL-1 and TNF act on the hypothalamus to mediate fever and release the hormone CRH. IL-1, IL-2, IL-6, TNF and interferon have all been shown to increase adrenal cortisol secretion through both hypothalamic/pituitary stimulation (CRH and ACTH release), and by direct action on the adrenal gland (IL-6 predominantly). Cortisol, in turn, reduces cytokine production by immune cells, completing another negative feedback control loop.

This neural-endocrine-immune interaction is central to some of the harmful effects of stress on immunity, allergy, and disease.

Typical Cytokines

- Interleukins (IL) are identified by number (e.g., interleukin-1 or IL-1). They are secreted by the T-lymphocytes and macrophages of the immune system. They enhance inflammation, stimulate lymphocyte growth and development, and promote release of immunoglobulins.
- Interferon is produced by numerous immune-cell types. It stimulates 'killing' by macrophages and natural killer (NK) cells.
- Tumor necrosis factor (TNF) promotes thrombosis and kills tumor cells.

Hypothalamus-Pituitary-Adrenal Interactions

Hypothalamus

Part of the brain's limbic system, the hypothalamus provides an interface between the central nervous and endocrine systems of the body. It integrates and coordinates nervous and endocrine responses received from many parts of the brain to ensure survival and maintenance of a stable internal environment.

Although not considered a true endocrine gland, the hypothalamus secretes a number of hormones (also considered neuropeptide transmitters as they are synthesized and released in nerves rather than endocrine cells) that exert control over the pituitary gland. The release of these controlling hormones is under the influence of neural inputs into the hypothalamus, including factors such as stress, thirst, temperature, time of day, and exercise.

The hypothalamus receives signals from almost all areas of the nervous system. When you feel pain, part of that pain signal is transmitted to the hypothalamus. Whenever you see, smell, or hear something, the hypothalamus is involved in your interpretation and subsequent reaction. Even a euphoric or depressing thought will cause an alteration in the pattern and firing of the hypothalamus. On a more basic level, the concentration of certain chemicals in the blood will have an affect on the production and transmission of signals by the hypothalamus.

Having collected this vast amount of data, the hypothalamus will coordinate a response, which, to a large extent, will be automatic, not subject to voluntary control. While higher levels of brain function, such as the cerebral cortex, may influence the output of the hypothalamus, it is generally not considered to be under direct control. One exception to this may be the development of control mechanisms in certain holy men, who, through meditation or other processes, are able to control some of the more basic functions, such as breathing and heart rate, through voluntary mental control. Unfortunately, the majority of us are not blessed with this ability and thus the events that occur subsequent to so many stimuli is involuntary.

The two main systems through which the hypothalamus exerts its effect on the body are the pituitary gland and the autonomic nervous system.

Neuropeptide Hormones Released by the Hypothalamus

- Corticotropin-releasing hormone (CRH) causes release of adrenocorticotropic hormone (ACTH) from the anterior pituitary gland. ACTH causes cortisol release from the adrenal glands.
- Thyrotropin-releasing hormone (TRH) causes release of thyroid-stimulating hormone (TSH) from the anterior pituitary.
- Growth hormone-releasing hormone (GHRH) and growth hormone-inhibiting hormone (GIH) act together to control release of growth hormone (GH) from the anterior pituitary.
- Gonadotropin-releasing hormone (GnRH) stimulates release of luteinizing hormone (LH) and follicle-stimulating hormone (FSH).
- Prolactin-inhibiting factor (PIF) inhibits prolactin (PRL) release.

Pituitary Gland

The hormones released from the hypothalamus travel a short distance to act in the anterior part of the pituitary gland, a small pedunculated structure lying below the hypothalamus. The hormones from the hypothalamus are able to stimulate cells in the pituitary gland to release other hormones.

Pituitary Gland and Hormones

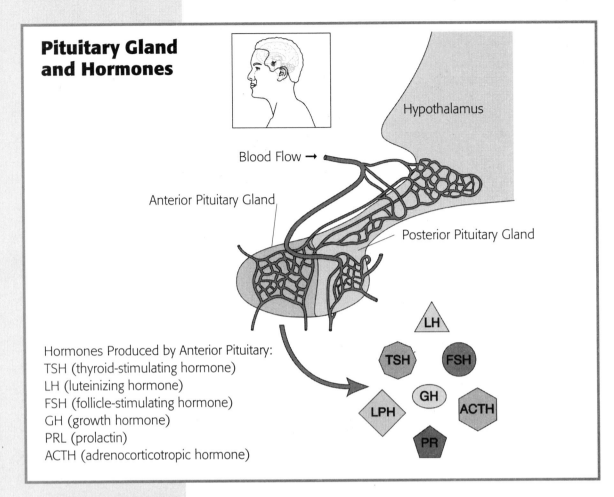

Hypothalamus

Blood Flow →

Anterior Pituitary Gland

Posterior Pituitary Gland

LH

TSH

FSH

GH

LPH

ACTH

PR

Hormones Produced by Anterior Pituitary:
TSH (thyroid-stimulating hormone)
LH (luteinizing hormone)
FSH (follicle-stimulating hormone)
GH (growth hormone)
PRL (prolactin)
ACTH (adrenocorticotropic hormone)

Most important in the stress response is the release of CRH by the hypothalamus, which acts on the pituitary gland to cause release of ACTH into the general circulation. ACTH then acts on the adrenal glands to cause release of cortisol.

Another important hormone produced by the hypothalamus is GHRH that acts on the anterior pituitary to cause it to release growth hormone. The hypothalamus also releases a hormone that inhibits release of growth hormone, the balance of the two controlling overall release of growth hormone from the anterior pituitary.

The release of CRH in the hypothalamus and other areas of the brain seems to be responsible for the sensation of anxiety associated with stress. It may also have a role in the development of sleep and appetite disorders associated with stress. CRH is a potent suppressor of appetite and is certainly partially responsible for reproductive irregularity and infertility. Overproduction of CRH is found in major depression, post-traumatic stress disorder, and anorexia nervosa, indicating further links of these conditions to stress.

Adrenal Glands

The adrenal glands are two small organs weighing about 4 grams each, lying at the top end of each kidney. They are crucial components of the stress response.

Each adrenal gland comprises two parts: the central 20% of the gland is called the adrenal medulla and the remaining outer shell is called the adrenal cortex.

Adrenal Medulla

The adrenal medulla can be considered an important manufacturing outpost for the sympathetic autonomic nervous system. The sympathetic system sends signals directly to the adrenal medulla, and stimulation causes release of the two important hormones, adrenaline and noradrenaline (also termed catecholamines). These hormones are among the shortest living signaling molecules produced by the human body, being broken down in only 10 to 20 seconds. Nevertheless, their effect is profound.

The adrenaline and noradrenaline released from the adrenal medulla has the same effect on organs and tissues as direct stimulation by the sympathetic nerves. The effect, however,

Adrenaline and Cortisol
Adrenaline appears to be a major factor in the acute stress response. Cortisol is the major factor in the chronic stress response.

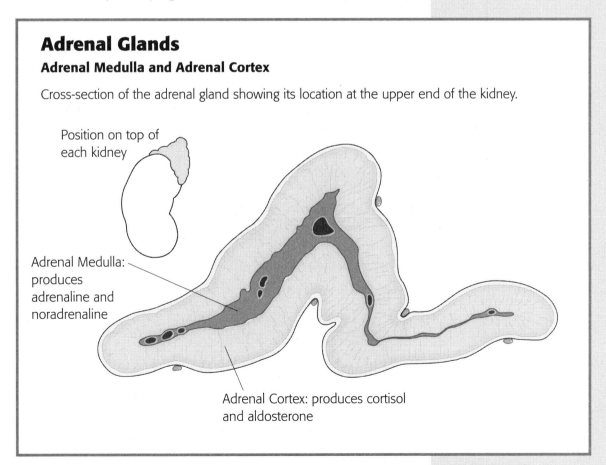

Adrenal Glands
Adrenal Medulla and Adrenal Cortex

Cross-section of the adrenal gland showing its location at the upper end of the kidney.

Position on top of each kidney

Adrenal Medulla: produces adrenaline and noradrenaline

Adrenal Cortex: produces cortisol and aldosterone

lasts five to ten times as long as the same nervous stimulation. On average, 80% of the secretion is adrenaline, 20% percent noradrenaline.

Once the sympathetic nervous system is stimulated, the body's organs and tissues are in turn stimulated in two ways: directly by the nerves themselves and indirectly by the release of adrenaline and noradrenaline from the adrenal medulla. This dual mechanism has two purposes. The first is to prolong and increase the effect of the sympathetic stimulation. The second is to provide a backup mechanism to be used as a substitute when the other is nonfunctional. The adrenaline and noradrenaline hormones can also reach cells that are not directly innervated by the sympathetic nervous system, thereby increasing excitability, metabolic rate, and other chemical processes.

Interestingly, the adrenaline and noradrenaline hormones are not able to reach brain tissue for feedback to control the response. Control is likely through the breakdown of these hormones within the bloodstream.

Adrenal Cortex

The adrenal cortex produces the crucial stress response hormone, cortisol. The cortex also produces a group of hormones called mineralocorticoids, predominantly aldosterone, that control fluid and electrolyte balance within the body. This part of the adrenal gland also produces adrenal male sex hormones.

Summary

We have seen how the numerous endocrine organs communicate in order to exert influence over functioning of the body and how their activity is controlled. With specific reference to the stress response, the key 'players' have been introduced:

Hypothalamus with its link to the brain and emotional circuitry of the limbic system;

Pituitary Gland the body's master endocrine gland;

Adrenal Glands the source of the main stress hormones, adrenaline and cortisol.

Working together, the hypothalamus, pituitary, and adrenals comprise the HPA axis.

The Stress Response

HPA Axis

The HPA axis refers to the three hormone-producing glands of the stress response, their interactions, and feedback. The hypothalamus (H), the pituitary (P), and the adrenal (A) glands communicate with each other through their respective hormones — CRH, ACTH, and cortisol. For the sake of simplicity, the HPA axis is often referred to as a unit when discussing function and disruption of the stress response.

The HPA (Hypothalamus-Pituitary-Adrenal) Axis

CRH, released by the hypothalamus, stimulates (+) the pituitary to release ACTH, which in turn causes the adrenal glands to release cortisol. Cortisol exerts negative feedback on both the hypothalamus, where it inhibits (-) CRH release, and the pituitary, where it inhibits ACTH release.

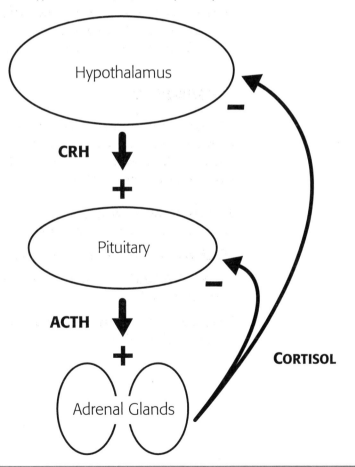

The cortisol rhythm is like a home thermostat, a programmed and timed control that runs automatically but can be overridden at any time. The override system involves the numerous inputs to the hypothalamus. These include sensory inputs such as vision, hearing, smell, along with memory and awareness, as well as the metabolic and biochemical state of the body. One of the most important override stimuli is the stress or fight-or-flight response.

Daily Cortisol Cycle

Levels of cortisol in the body follow a daily rhythm. This is dictated by the hypothalamus, which secretes CRH in a well-recognized pattern throughout the day. CRH stimulates the pituitary gland to produce ACTH that, in turn, acts on the adrenal glands to cause release of cortisol.

This circadian rhythm appears related to the sleep-wake cycle, typically peaking at around 6:00 to 8:00 a.m. to coincide with the stress of waking and starting the day. (One wonders whether it is just a tad higher on Mondays!) The rhythm is actually reversed in people working the night shift, rising at around 6:00 to 8:00 p.m.

Fight-or-Flight Response

The fight-or-flight response involves a series of neuronal (mediated by nerves) and hormonal events that activate the body during an emergency and restore it to a stable, steady, or normal state termed homeostasis. The entire process involves some fairly extreme and erratic changes to the body and its tissues.

The fight-or-flight response involves two phases. Like any force acting against an impending or existing assault or threat, it has a rapid response team able to act quickly, and a stronger backup team able to provide longer-term support and a more sustained attack.

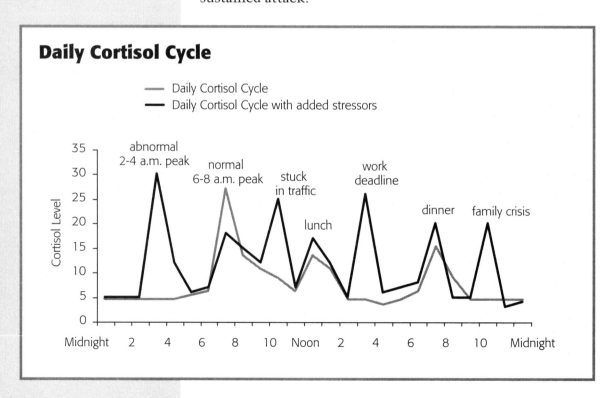

Daily Cortisol Cycle

— Daily Cortisol Cycle
— Daily Cortisol Cycle with added stressors

Rapid Response

The production and release of hormones, while efficient, is still slow in terms of response time. The fight-or-flight response is intended as a protective and adaptive mechanism to handle danger, and as such, needs to be instituted as soon as possible. There's no point politely asking the tiger to trim his claws for a few minutes while the body's hormone levels get up to functional levels!

Sympathetic Nervous System

The necessary rapid response is provided by the autonomic nervous system, principally the sympathetic system. These nerves, supplying organs and tissues throughout the body, act within seconds, producing responses tailored toward survival.

Within seconds man is ready to fight (or flee). Awareness and reaction time are improved, heart and lungs are already at exercise level, and the body has a source of energy in the form of glucose and fatty acids to fuel the demands.

Adrenal Medulla (Adrenaline and Noradrenaline)

The sympathetic nerves are supported by the other members of the rapid response team, the adrenal glands, specifically the adrenal medulla. Certain sympathetic nerves directly supply the adrenal medulla. Simulation causes release of the chemical messengers adrenaline and noradrenaline (catecholamines). These chemicals are the same as the ones released from the ends of the sympathetic nerves supplying the rest of the body directly. The effect of the adrenaline and noradrenaline released from the adrenal glands, however, lasts five to ten times longer.

While powerful and rapidly deployed, the sympathetic/adrenaline system is short-lived. Even the adrenaline and noradrenaline released from the adrenal glands only lasts a few minutes at the most in the bloodstream before being broken down. To mount a sustained and effective defense, backup is needed. This comes in the form of cortisol.

Adrenal Cortex (Cortisol)

Cortisol provides a prolonged stress assault force. The stress of the fight-or-flight response causes the hypothalamus to secrete CRH. This acts on the pituitary gland, causing it to release ACTH into the bloodstream. ACTH stimulates the adrenal glands (specifically the adrenal cortex) to increase the synthesis and release of cortisol into the blood.

The overall response time of this complex hormonal system is 4 to 6 minutes, but once activated, levels of cortisol remain high for up to an hour, even if the original stressor has been resolved.

Cortisol Effects

NON-METABOLIC

- Increased fluid retention
- Increased cellular fluid
- Enhanced blood coagulation
- Reduced inflammation and immune response
- Increased blood pressure
- Stimulation of the brain, reduced sleep, reduced memory

METABOLIC EFFECTS

Carbohydrate
- Increased glucose production in the liver
- Reduced insulin secretion
- Insulin resistance
- Increased blood sugar levels

Fat
- Increased responsiveness of fat cells to adrenaline/noradrenaline/glucagon
- Increased fatty acid release to fuel glucose manufacture

Protein
- Increased release of amino acids from muscle to fuel glucose production
- Reduced protein synthesis (except in the liver)
- Increased glutamine synthesis

Prolonged Response

Some of the effects of cortisol are similar to those of adrenaline and noradrenaline and thus provide the backup support to this initial fight-or-flight mechanism. Cortisol is more potent and longer-lasting than adrenaline and noradrenaline. In addition, it increases the overall responsiveness of tissues and organs to adrenaline and noradrenaline. Thus, even though levels of these hormones may be falling, they still exert an effect.

Cortisol not only improves the strength of the assault force, it also provides the ammunition. One of its primary roles is to alter the body's metabolism to better handle the demands of surviving a stressful situation. The persistence of cortisol also maintains the activity for a longer period, making the system more sensitive should another threatening stimulus arrive.

Cortisol raises blood sugar levels, making sure there is adequate glucose energy available to fuel the increased activity of the muscles and the brain as the body prepares to fight or flee. Insulin — the storage hormone — is not needed here, so levels are reduced and the peripheral tissues become insensitive to it (insulin resistance). Fat is broken down to provide fatty acid molecules, which can be used as a direct energy source or converted to more glucose. Muscle is broken down to provide amino acids, another substrate with which the liver can make glucose. The body is using all possible fuel sources, including the detrimental breakdown of muscle, as a means of survival.

The effects of cortisol on blood clotting and inflammation may also be part of the defense mechanism, reducing the impact of injury. Interestingly, despite its negative effect on inflammation and the immune system, the increased glutamine production cortisol induces is actually vital to the function of immune cells and provides them with fuel. One can postulate that this provides a boost to the healing process once the body is safely out of danger.

Rapid Response Symptoms

You may recognize many of the symptoms listed here, which are our interpretations of what we feel in the face of anxiety or fear.

- Heart Rate: Increased heart rate, contraction strength, and volume.

- Breathing: Increased breathing rate/volume with dilation of bronchioles (breathing tubes).

- Blood Vessels: Constriction of vessels to nonessential areas — skin (pale), gut, etc.
  Dilation of vessels supplying working muscles.
  Although sympathetic outflow causes cardiac vessels to constrict, the local metabolites produced by increased workload counteract this and make them dilate. Stress in the absence of increased workload in 'downtown man' may promote cardiac events/angina.

- Blood Pressure: Increased blood pressure.

Resolution of the Fight-or-Flight Response

The complex hormonal cascade results in profound changes to many systems in the body, particularly metabolism, that are vital to the survival of the individual in a dangerous situation. However, once safety has been restored, the body needs to return to its normal state.

Negative Feedback

The cortisol system relies on a negative feedback mechanism for part of its control. This means that cortisol, produced by the adrenal glands and transmitted in the blood, travels back to the hypothalamus and pituitary gland, where it acts to inhibit further release of CRH and ACTH.

It also acts on the hippocampus and amygdala in the limbic system, which are rich in cortisol receptor sites, so that once the stressful situation is resolved and the hypothalamus is no longer being stimulated to produce CRH, the high levels of cortisol prevent further CRH and ACTH from being manufactured and released. This terminates the cortisol-based stress response faster than just allowing hormone levels to gradually decline. As it is, the remaining cortisol in the bloodstream will continue to be active until metabolized over 1 to 2 hours.

As cortisol levels return to normal, metabolism is restored to its steady state. During the recovery process, the body switches to storage mode, producing insulin in response to the high glucose levels. Cortisol stimulates appetite, as the body needs to replace used energy stores. Mood excitation declines, with a stimulus to rest and sleep.

With the decline in hormone levels and the anti-stress actions of cortisol in effect, the body returns to normal after a few hours. Homeostasis has been achieved and a life-threatening situation avoided. Time to curl up by the fire and gnaw on one of those prehistoric spareribs!

Anti-Stress Hormone

Cortisol provides a very important secondary function here in controlling and reversing the fight-or-flight reaction. So important is this role that cortisol is often referred to as the 'anti-stress' hormone, potentially disrupting the stress-related disease processes. Stress-induced increases in cortisol protect, not against the source of stress itself, but rather against the body's normal reactions to stress, preventing those reactions from becoming excessive and damaging to the body. The lack of an adequate cortisol response to true stress in the chronically stressed individual poses an equally dangerous threat to health.

- **Skin:** Sweating, erection of hairs.

- **Brain:** Increased awareness and mental activity.

- **Eyes:** Pupils dilate.

- **Kidneys:** Retain fluid.

- **Metabolism:** Overall increased cellular metabolism.
  Carbohydrates: Increased breakdown of glycogen stores in liver and muscle to release glucose. Increases blood sugar. Increases glucagon levels. Reduces insulin secretion.
  Fat: Increases triglyceride breakdown to release free fatty acids. Increases the activity of hormone-sensitive lipase to further increase release of free fatty acids.

Chronic Stress

We have seen how the fight-or-flight mechanism works effectively to protect us when we're exposed to a threatening situation. However, where 'downtown man' differs from prehistoric man is in his perception of stress and his ability to resolve it. Downtown man's stress is predominantly cerebral — that is, it arises as a result of thought processes rather than a direct physical threat perceived through vision, hearing, or any other senses. Depending on the personality and lifestyle of the individual, stress may be limited to an occasional concern about work or it may extend to everything from personal and family relationships to personal health and world affairs.

Occasionally worrying about a situation or an event is commonplace — we have all had to sit for exams or attend an interview. The stress of this event is clearly not physical, yet our reaction is the same, the fight-or-flight response with all the associated hormonal upheaval and symptoms, such as anxiety, palpitations, poor sleep, and lower libido. Once the event is over, things should return to normal.

But the period of time that you remain stressed leading up to these events may be, depending on the individual, anywhere from a few hours to a few weeks. Even the coolest of downtown characters will remain stressed for far longer than his prehistoric ancestor unexpectedly encountering and fleeing from a ferocious animal. One study on the stress of surgery showed that ACTH and cortisol levels did not normalize for 24 hours after the procedure.

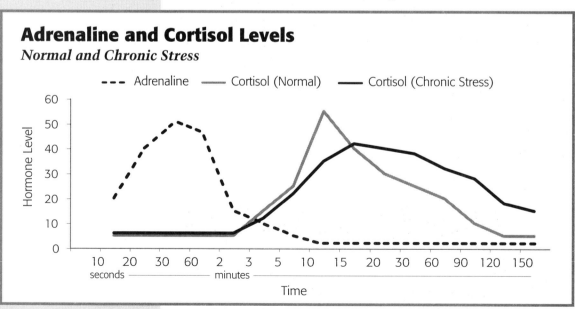

Adrenaline and Cortisol Levels
Normal and Chronic Stress

- - - Adrenaline   —— Cortisol (Normal)   —— Cortisol (Chronic Stress)

Now consider our friend downtown man who perceives many day-to-day events as stressful, including driving to work, meeting deadlines, maintaining performance, and trying to pay all the bills. He never actually switches off his fight-or-flight system. His hypothalamus remains active, releasing CRH and thus continually stimulating cortisol secretion. This is the basis of chronic stress — ongoing perceived stress and a persistent stress response without a healthy return to a normal, stable state.

Cortisol Levels

While it is generally agreed that the primary cause of the adverse metabolic and health-related conditions in chronic stress is due to overactivity or overproduction of cortisol, explanations as to how this develops are varied. Perceived stress (as opposed to physical stress) is certainly associated with increased cortisol release, although overall cortisol secretion in a 24-hour period may not be elevated even in a chronically stressed individual. Part of the difficulty in identifying a *raised* level of cortisol may be the large variation in normal values.

What is likely more relevant is the persistent secretion of cortisol and disruption of the daily cycle. The body appears to be able to cope with the regular daily rhythm and with occasional short-lived bursts of hormonal activity. After all, this reflects the original design and purpose of the stress response. However, chronic low-level secretion is disruptive to the hypothalamus-pituitary-adrenal (HPA) axis and damaging to many systems of the body.

Normal Cortisol Values

Plasma Cortisol	8:00 a.m.	5-23 micrograms/dL
	4:00 p.m.	3-16 micrograms/dL
	8:00 p.m.	< 50% of 8:00 a.m. value
Urine Cortisol	(24-hour collection)	20-90 micrograms/24 hrs.

Adrenal Fatigue

The reason behind the low-level secretion of cortisol relates to one of the major abnormalities in hormonal function seen in chronic stress, that of adrenal fatigue or exhaustion. The chronically stressed individual demonstrates an impaired adrenal response to stress and the release of CRH and ACTH. This is well recognized in athletic overtraining syndrome, a condition likened to the chronic stress syndrome.

Adrenal Exhaustion
Failure of adequate cortisol release impairs the body's ability to cope with true stress, such as infection or inflammation, while the persistent low-level secretion associated with chronic unresolved stress induces metabolic abnormality and tissue damage.

Faulty Feedback Controls

The most important disruption of the HPA axis in chronic stress may be the alteration in feedback control of the hypothalamus and pituitary by cortisol in the bloodstream. Tests on chronically stressed individuals (including those suffering from metabolic syndrome) reveal a reduced response to the dexamethasone suppression test. This test involves the injection of dexamethasone, a drug that mimics cortisol, in order to see how much it suppresses the hypothalamus, pituitary, and adrenal glands. In a normal test, dexamethasone will cause a significant reduction in CRH, ACTH, and cortisol. The fact that in stressed individuals this suppression is impaired indicates disruption of the normal control-feedback system.

The hypothalamus becomes insensitive to cortisol due to its chronic low-level secretion by the adrenal gland and altered daily cycle. This results in increased levels of CRH, produced by the hypothalamus in response to stress and no longer controlled by the feedback of cortisol.

Cortisol Resistance

Reduced response to cortisol or 'cortisol resistance' likely occurs through a down-regulation of cortisol receptors, a reduction in their numbers and sensitivity. This type of receptor abnormality is increasingly being recognized as central to HPA-axis disruption.

For example, in both depression and post-traumatic stress disorder (PTSD), CRH levels are increased. However, in depression, cortisol levels are generally raised, while in PTSD they are normal or low. In general anxiety disorder (GAD) and panic disorder (PD), there is reduced sensitivity to noradrenaline, and although CRH and cortisol levels are normal, feedback within the HPA axis is blunted.

These abnormalities are explained through variations in the responsiveness of the brain and HPA axis to the various hormones, mediated via alterations in receptor number and sensitivity. In depression, for example, there is effective cortisol resistance due to reduced cortisol receptor numbers, a similar scenario to that seen in chronic stress. In PTSD, there are increased receptors and receptor sensitivity, resulting in enhanced negative feedback. Therefore, despite chronic high CRH release, ACTH and cortisol stay low.

It seems paradoxical that despite reduced feedback and high CRH, cortisol levels remain within a relatively normal range. The answer likely lies not only in adrenal gland hypo-responsiveness, but also in a differential sensitivity of the hippocampus/hypothalamus and the pituitary gland. This is well demonstrated in post-traumatic stress disorder (PTSD), in which CRH levels are markedly elevated yet cortisol remains low or normal. In this condition, there is impaired negative feedback in the hypothalamus and enhanced feedback at the level of the pituitary. Thus, despite high CRH, the pituitary ACTH response is attenuated and the release of cortisol from the adrenal remains low.

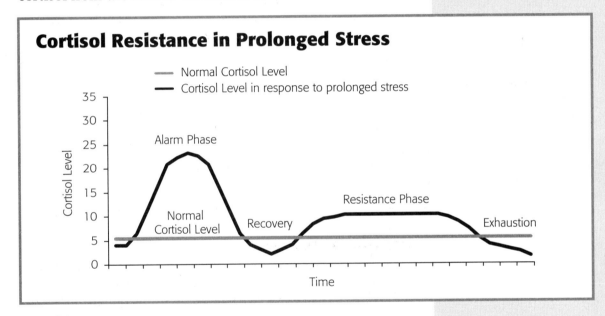

Central Stress Response

Studies on rats show that chronic stress increases CRH production in the amygdala and hypothalamus. The overall effect is to increase the responsiveness of the central stress pathways of the brain, leading to heightened anxiety and exaggerated reaction to minor stressors. CRH levels are increased with numerous central and peripheral effects, while the pituitary and adrenal glands remain relatively unresponsive. This results in a poorly executed peripheral stress reaction and inadequate feedback control.

Metabolic Syndrome

Cortisol is essential to the body for both the normal daily rhythm of waking and sleeping and to deal with stressful situations when they arise. Indeed, the cortisol reaction is vital for survival, particularly when considering physical stress such as injury or infection. Individuals suffering from Addison disease, a condition in which cortisol secretion is severely impaired, can die from something as minor as a chest infection. Patients on long-term steroid therapy for rheumatoid arthritis have a suppressed stress reaction with impaired cortisol production. They need to be given extra doses of cortisol in the event of surgery or infection to prevent a catastrophic system collapse and potentially death (addisonian crisis).

However, chronic stimulation of the adrenal gland, persistent cortisol secretion, and disruption of HPA feedback, which result from hyperactivity of the fight-or-flight stress reaction, have an extremely detrimental effect on the health and metabolism of our body.

Metabolic syndrome or syndrome-X is well recognized as the association of a number of health conditions in one individual. They include obesity (abdominal), high blood pressure, high insulin levels with insulin resistance, diabetes, high cholesterol, and increased risk of heart attack and stroke. Increased blood coaguability and gout are also associated with the syndrome. It affects a large proportion of the adult population of industrialized countries and likely represents the largest single threat to health in the upcoming decade.

Theories of Chronic Stress

Other medical research scientists have developed similar explanations of the mechanisms and effects of chronic stress, ranging from the pioneering work of Hans Selye to the recent work of Bruce McEwan.

Dr. Hans Selye and the General Adaptation Syndrome

We often refer to Hans Selye's general adaptation syndrome (GAS) when considering the adverse effects of chronic stress on the body. Selye's GAS was based on observations he made as a medical student in the 1920s. He noted that following physical or mental stress, humans and animals demonstrated a pattern of responses, which if untreated, resulted in illness and eventually death:

Stage 1   Alarm Reaction: the fight-or-flight response

Stage 2   Resistance: the cortisol reaction

Stage 3   Exhaustion: adrenal exhaustion, depleted energy reserves, failing immunity

The appearance of high blood pressure in metabolic syndrome has been likened to persistent stimulation of the "alarm reaction" in stage 1. However, the development of metabolic syndrome itself does not seem to fit clearly into either stage 2 or 3; rather, it has features consistent with both. The metabolic changes indicate a persistence of the resistance stage, whereas the impaired immunity fits more with the exhaustion phase. What is clear, however, is that the end point is the same, as the components of metabolic syndrome are not only debilitating — they are potentially lethal.

In Hans Selye's exhaustion phase, the adrenal glands fail to produce any further cortisol, resulting in a number of metabolic abnormalities, in particular low blood sugar. They also stop producing aldosterone, the hormone responsible for maintaining salt (sodium chloride) in the body. The combination of salt loss and inadequate glucose leads to cell damage and impaired ability to fight the ongoing stress to the body. Tissue death, organ collapse, and death ensue.

In chronic stress, the degree of adrenal fatigue is not as profound and, in general, the stressors on the body not so life-threatening — Selye's observations involved severe infection as the primary stressor. What we see is an inability of the adrenal glands to 'rise to the occasion'. Their ability to respond to a truly stressful event is weakened, resulting in fatigue, poor mental and physical performance, inadequate control over inflammation, and a reduced resilience of the body to disease. This component of chronic stress has been termed non-Addison hypoadrenia, subclinical hypoadrenia, and adrenal apathy, and constitutes one of the HPA axis abnormalities in this condition.

Metabolic Syndrome
Initial theories as to the development of this syndrome centered on diet, and while this is clearly an important factor, evidence is pointing to chronic stress, persistent stimulation of the HPA axis, and excess cortisol as being the primary cause.

Dr. Bruce McEwan and Allostatic Load

Another way to consider this exhaustion stage of chronic stress is as allostatic load, a concept recently introduced by Bruce McEwan. While the standard concept of the fight-or-flight response is as a homeostatic mechanism (from the Greek *homeo* meaning "the same" and *stasis* meaning "stable"), McEwan suggests that it is best seen as a series of allostatic mechanisms (from the Greek *allo* for "variable"), whereby the numerous systems of the stress response keep the body stable by being able to change on their own.

The abnormal situation of chronic stress is referred to as allostatic load, a dysfunctional state in which the neuroendocrine pathways and reactions of the stress response remain persistently activated, resulting in disease. McEwan concludes the underlying disruption of this unresolved stress load is an abnormal function of the normal HPA-axis feedback mechanism.

Summary

The fight-or-flight reaction is a protective cascade of hormonal events designed to protect us from threatening or stressful situations. It includes a rapid response mechanism (provided by the sympathetic system) and a sustained backup response (provided by the stress hormone cortisol).

Cortisol affects changes in many systems of the body, including metabolism, control of sugar and fat, blood pressure, immunity, sleep, and brain function. Under the conditions in which the stress response is supposed to work — brief exposure to a 'real' threatening stimulus, response, and resolution — these changes are beneficial to the body. However, the majority of our stressors are now 'perceived', that is, mental and not physical. Not only are they more frequent, they are not easily resolved. This results in persistent stimulation of the stress pathway and chronic low-level cortisol secretion.

In this state, cortisol is no longer beneficial, but becomes harmful to the body. The prolonged changes induced by cortisol, in association with lifestyle and likely genetic factors, produce a cluster of diseases, including obesity (abdominal), high blood pressure, high insulin levels with insulin resistance, diabetes, high cholesterol, and increased risk of heart attack and stroke. These have collectively been termed metabolic syndrome.

In addition, chronic stress leads to adrenal fatigue with impairment of the adrenal response to stress when needed for true emergencies, such as the control of inflammation. Chronic stress actually enhances the production of CRH in the brain, augmenting the central stress reaction. Impaired feedback of cortisol on the hypothalamus fails to control this overproduction of CRH, which itself has a number of detrimental effects on the function of the brain and body. Together, these disruptions of the stress response have adverse effects on numerous systems, including immunity, reproduction, the gut, the brain, bones, muscles, and joints.

If, in fact, chronic stress is caused by hormonal imbalance in the nervous and endocrine systems, then it makes sense that we should look for ways of restoring balance or homeostasis as a way of solving this problem. By adjusting and supplementing our diet, exercising, developing the ability to relax, and rethinking the way we perceive stressful situations, we can regain control of our stress pathways.

Look Ahead

In the next section of the book, we will consider numerous nutritional, physical, and mental treatments for chronic stress, providing the basis for a comprehensive management program. Then, in the final section we examine the link between chronic stress and disease, adding specific treatment strategies for disorders, including diabetes, heart disease, irritable bowel syndrome, chronic fatigue, migraine, and depression.

Stress Solutions

Anti-Stress Diet

Lowering Stress and Losing Weight

Mary, a 37-year-old patient, came to our office wanting to lose weight. She explained that despite eating well and exercising regularly, she had continued to gain weight, particularly around the mid-section. I went over her diet and exercise regime, tested her for thyroid and growth hormone insufficiencies, and found no specific problems. Her diet was balanced with protein at each meal, good quantities of vegetables, a small amount of fruit, and little to no high-glycemic foods. She maintained an exercise regime of 45 minutes to 1 hour of cardio 5 times a week, with 2 to 3 days of weight training. Despite her admirable attempts at positive lifestyle choices, she had continued to gain weight. Frustrated, she tried several over-the-counter diet supplements, with little to no success.

During our interview, we discovered that she never allowed herself any relaxation time, except when she was on holiday. And, whenever she was on holiday, she reported losing significant weight quickly, with a substantial decrease in bloating. This was despite a poorer diet, decreased exercise, and increased alcohol intake. When she returned home, she regained the weight rapidly.

The fact that she consistently lost weight while on holiday and gained weight at home, independent of diet and exercise, led me to think that stress was the main factor responsible for her unstable body weight. Mary is a lawyer who works long hours and raises two young children. She leaves little time for herself. She used exercise as her only stress management technique, but she usually rushed through it, her mind preoccupied with closing statements for an upcoming case.

We started Mary on a program of massage therapy, yoga, deep breathing, magnolia extract, and a vitamin B complex. Two weeks later, she had lost 3 pounds and overall felt much more relaxed. After one month, she had lost the 7 pounds that she had wanted to lose and has subsequently maintained this weight.

Mary now realizes the importance of keeping her stress levels down, and although her career does not always allow her as much free time as she would like, she makes a point of doing her deep breathing and yoga and taking cortisol reducing supplements like magnolia extract when life starts to get more hectic. She has now learned how to balance her lifestyle, allowing her body to function at a high capacity without causing damage.

"Stress" has become such an overworked word in our society that it is now considered normal to have stress. In fact, it is considered almost abnormal if we are not stressed. We may even feel guilty if we are relaxing or not being productive in some way. We have learned to equate productivity and success with being busy, and being busy with increased stress. In order to be successful, we must be stressed, this line of reasoning goes.

However, in association with this 'success', we live an unhealthy lifestyle, with a poor diet and a lack of exercise, the combination forming what is often termed overindulgence syndrome. The combination of chronic stress and raised cortisol causes metabolic disturbance that can lead to weight gain. In the long term, this abnormal state can lead to the complex of symptoms termed metabolic syndrome, including obesity, diabetes, high blood pressure, and cardiovascular disease.

Nutrition Basics

In order to understand how chronic stress can affect our weight unfavorably and how good nutrition can help reduce its effect, we need to review the basics of food metabolism, especially the relationship between two hormones, insulin and cortisol.

Food is traditionally divided into three main groups: fats, protein, and carbohydrates. Each food group affects the body differently.

Fats

Fat is also known as lipid. There are two main groups, saturated and unsaturated fats, differentiated by the number of hydrogen bonds between each link in a fat compound. Not all fats are bad — we do need some fat in the diet, especially unsaturated fats.

Saturated Fats

A saturated fat has all possible molecular bonds filled up or saturated with hydrogen and is considered solid in nature. It is found in animal fat. Because saturated fats contain completely filled bonds, they are quite stable, with no free bonds for other molecules to interact with. The role of saturated fats, or their breakdown unit, fatty acid, is extremely limited. They only serve as calories. Since they cannot interact with the body, they cannot aid in any bodily functions.

Unsaturated Fats and Essential Fatty Acids

Unsaturated fats are less stable because not all their bonds are filled with hydrogen. The empty bonds leave spaces that have the potential to react with other atoms or substances in the body. Unsaturated fats, especially *essential* fatty acids, play a vital role in the production of prostaglandins, cell membrane construction, hormone regulation, and many other body systems.

STRESS FACT CCK Hormone

Once ingested, fat molecules send a signal of satisfaction to the brain via the production of a hormone called cholecystokinin (CCK). Without this hormone, you would continue eating because your body would never receive a satiety signal. People on fat-free diets continually feel unsatisfied because they never receive the CCK hormonal message. They keep eating to try and achieve this feeling, even though they are not actually in need of food.

Brown Fat

Within the body there are two types of fat deposition. Brown fat, which is quite scarce and decreases in concentration as we age, exists only in certain areas of the body like the back of the neck and between the shoulder blades. We cannot produce more brown fat during our lifetime. Its main purpose is to generate heat through redundant metabolic cycling, a process by which calories are burned without producing any useable substances. This process occurs mainly in infancy and child-hood when it is vital for maintaining body temperature. It becomes less important with maturity.

White Fat

Most of the fat on the body is white fat, deposited subcutaneously (under the skin) in the abdomen or around the internal organs. This is the fat that changes in concentration throughout life — and this is the type of fat we talk about losing during a weight-loss program. The production of new fat cells only occurs during the first few years of life. Overfeeding in children can result in the production of excess fat cells, which then remain with us for life. By the time we reach puberty, the number of fat cells in our body is fixed. We can neither increase nor decrease their number (unless under the care of a surgeon!). However, the *amount* of fat each cell contains can vary tremendously, and this is the way in which we lose or put on fatty weight.

Protein

Protein is the basic building block of the body, the single most important nutrient. Protein is used for the growth of every cell in the body. Our brain cells, enzymes, many hormones, antibodies, muscles, and even blood cells are made of protein. Discounting water, over half the body weight of an average individual is protein. This protein is continually being broken down and replaced. Studies show that more than 90% of the body has completely turned over within one year. This process requires nutritional protein.

The addition of adequate protein to a diet helps control the release of sugar from carbohydrates into the bloodstream.

Thereby, the high peaks of glucose that stimulate insulin secretion are avoided. A more stable blood sugar translates into less sugar stored as fat and less stimulation of cortisol release, both of which aid weight loss.

 STRESS FACT Protein Deficiency

A deficiency of protein can result in serious malfunction in a number of systems. Poor immunity, muscle fatigue, slow tissue healing, and dry skin and hair are just a few symptoms of protein deficiency. Protein is also an important stimulus for weight loss. When the ratio of protein to carbohydrates in our diet favors carbohydrates, we tend to gain weight.

Amino Acids

When digested, protein is broken down into subunits called amino acids. There are 29 amino acids that form hundreds of different proteins in the body. The liver is capable of producing approximately 80% of the amino acids that we need. These amino acids are therefore considered nonessential to our diet. The other 20%, however, cannot be manufactured by the body and must be obtained from our diet.

Carbohydrates

Carbohydrates, unlike protein, vitamins, and minerals, are not considered building blocks for the body, but are short-term energy sources. Their breakdown product is sugar, also called glucose. To use them as fuel rather than store them as fat, we must ingest specific amounts at certain times and select particular types of carbohydrates.

Simple and Complex Carbohydrates

There are two main types of carbohydrates, simple and complex. Simple carbohydrates contain only sugars and starches. They are broken down very quickly because they have weak chemical bonds and thus raise blood sugar levels rapidly following ingestion.

Complex carbohydrates are a combination of fiber with or without sugar and starch. They provide the fiber that helps keep the digestive tract clean, promoting rapid transit through the bowel and binding to toxins that are subsequently expelled in the stools. Fiber cannot be broken down and thus cannot contribute to increased glucose levels in the blood. This is one explanation as to why complex carbohydrates that are high in fiber only contain one-third the amount of calories found in fat and simple carbohydrates. Not all complex carbohydrates are low in starch or sugar, even though they contain fiber.

Insulin and Glucagon

Sugar or glucose levels increase quickly after eating carbohydrates and slowly return to normal as the glucose is used by the body. However, blood glucose levels must remain at a fairly constant level for the body to function properly. Blood glucose balance is regulated by myriad hormones, most importantly, insulin and glucagon (not to be confused with glycogen, the storage form of glucose).

Insulin is produced in the beta cells of the pancreas. Sometimes referred to as the 'feasting' hormone or the 'storage' hormone, insulin is released when blood sugar levels rise and works by increasing the uptake of glucose from the blood and storing this sugar as glycogen and fat.

Glucagon is a hormone secreted from the alpha cells of the pancreas when blood sugar levels fall too low. It has the opposite effect of insulin. Glucagon functions in two major ways. First, it causes the breakdown of glycogen stored in the liver, a process known as glycogenolysis. Second, glucagon initiates gluconeogenesis in the liver, the formation of glucose from other molecules, such as amino acids, glycerol (from fats), lactate, and pyruvate. These two processes together promote the release of glucose into the blood to help raise sugar levels back to normal.

 STRESS FACT Carbohydrate Abuse

Insulin and glucagon work in tandem to help keep blood sugar levels within a narrow range. Large or continual swings in sugar levels from increased amounts of carbohydrate can produce an insensitivity reaction whereby more hormone is required to produce the same response, a response akin to drug addiction where higher concentrations of a drug may be needed to elicit the same reaction. This response takes many years of 'carbohydrate abuse' to develop, but when it does, we get into trouble not only with our weight but also with our health. We also become more susceptible to chronic stress.

The Hypoglycemia-Hyperglycemia Connection

*Hypo*glycemia is a condition in which blood glucose levels are abnormally low. This often occurs in reaction to *hyper*glycemia or high blood sugar levels following a high carbohydrate meal. After eating carbohydrates, the breakdown of food into sugar is quite rapid. This sugar is then delivered to the blood and glucose levels rise. The faster the breakdown of food into sugar, the faster the delivery of sugar, and the higher the blood sugar levels. Because the simple building blocks of carbohydrates are sugars and the bonds between them are weak relative to those of protein, a large amount of glucose is formed and delivered quickly to the blood after a meal rich in carbohydrates. Insulin is called upon to scoop up all this sugar and carry it out of the blood. Glycogen stores are full and blood sugar is therefore deposited as fat.

A few hours later, most of this meal has been stored as fat and our blood sugar levels are now too low, the result being hypoglycemia. Our body senses this and we feel very tired, dizzy, and possibly nauseated. Then our body begins to crave foods that will release sugar into the blood quickly, such as sweets or starches. It is a rare individual who craves a piece of chicken when they are hypoglycemic! Most of us indulge in carbohydrates, once again raising our blood sugar levels and starting the whole process anew.

Insulin Resistance

Most North Americans have grown up on a diet that is high in carbohydrates. Cereal or toast for breakfast, a sandwich for lunch, and pasta for dinner. Over the years our insulin-glucagon system has been overworked to the point of insensitivity. Our hormone responses have become exaggerated in order to achieve the same effect.

Approximately three out of four Americans have a slight to serious problem with their blood sugar level control mechanisms. This is known as insulin resistance, where there is a decreased reaction to insulin output, thereby stimulating extra insulin release. The extra insulin in our blood (hyperinsulinemia) acts as a barrier to using the body's existing fat by blocking access to it.

Carbohydrate Fatigue
If you're tired and hungry by 10:00 a.m. or 3:00 p.m. most days, take a look at your diet. Your breakfast or lunch was probably high in carbohydrates that create this problem and leave you vulnerable to stress.

 STRESS FACT Protein Catabolism

If we need glucose for energy and cannot access our fat, we must look to alternate sources. So, our body turns to our muscle and slowly eats away at our lean body tissue mass, a process called protein catabolism. Inside the muscle are mitochondria, fat burning units, which are subsequently lost, thereby decreasing our potential to lose weight.

For these reasons, if you eat a high-carbohydrate diet, it's almost impossible to lose weight while remaining in this biochemically undesirable state.

Diet and Stress

So where does stress fit into this picture? Whenever our brain (specifically the hypothalamus) perceives a stressful situation, it releases corticotropin releasing hormone (CRH). This hormone stimulates the pituitary gland to release another hormone called adrenocorticotropic hormone (ACTH) into the general circulation system. ACTH travels to the adrenal glands, our fight-or-flight stress glands. Here, ACTH directs the adrenal glands to release cortisol into the circulation, stimulating the physical stress response in the body. The initial sympathetic fight-or-flight response causes the same, albeit short-lived, response.

Cortisol acts to increase blood sugar levels in two ways: by releasing stores from the liver and muscle and by directing manufacture of new glucose in the liver from fatty acids mobilized from fat stores and from amino acids produced by breakdown of muscle. This helps prepare the body for the increased energy expenditure associated with resolving the fight-or-flight situation. This response is seen in both acute and chronically stressed individuals.

In one study, eight healthy volunteers were infused with cortisol, adrenaline, and glucagon over a 6-hour period to simulate a stressful situation. Their muscles were then biopsied at 6, 12, and 24 hours post infusion. They displayed characteristic changes to their muscle identical to muscle breakdown (protein catabolism). This process of muscular breakdown continued for 24 hours post infusion. Despite the fact that the stressor had stopped (the infusion was only for a few minutes), the reaction to the stress lasted the entire day.

Cortisol Activity

Releases muscle and liver stores of glucose.

+

Stimulates manufacture of glucose.

Results in increased blood sugar levels.

Increases release of fatty acids from fat stores into the blood.

Increases protein catabolism (muscle tissue breakdown)

Weight Gain

If stress and cortisol cause breakdown of fat stores, then why is stress related to weight gain? The answer lies with the effect of *chronic* stress. Under normal fight-or-flight circumstances, the stress response will lead to fat breakdown, although this is generally only short term, with the body switching rapidly back to storage mode once the danger is gone. However, as we have seen, chronic stress leads to persistent cortisol secretion, impaired feedback, and subsequent metabolic disruption.

Cortisol is extremely effective at raising blood sugar levels. While this may be beneficial when escaping from a marauding tiger, it's not needed when sitting in traffic or at a desk, times when our modern 'perceived' stress hits. Without exercise, the rise in blood sugar is profound. In response to this, the pancreas produces insulin. The effect of cortisol on the liver and muscle prevents storage as glycogen and storage is therefore predominantly as fat.

Although cortisol acts on fat cells to reduce storage and increase breakdown, this effect appears to be predominantly peripheral, that is, in the limbs. This may account for the tendency for excess fat to accumulate in the central abdominal region in high cortisol states, such as chronic stress, metabolic syndrome, and Cushing's syndrome (abnormally high cortisol secretion resulting from a tumor in the adrenal or pituitary glands). In addition, cortisol stimulation of the amygdala (part of the limbic system adjacent to the hippocampus) promotes excessive weight gain, particularly around the abdomen.

The insulin resistance associated with chronic stress and cortisol secretion further potentiates the problems associated with the ingestion of sugar and starch. People who are insulin resistant have a greater adverse reaction to the same glycemic intake of food. Thus, a bagel will result in higher blood sugar, more insulin, and greater fat storage in someone who is insulin resistant than someone who is not.

 STRESS FACT Metabolic Disruption

Insulin resistance develops as a result of chronically high blood glucose levels, excessive insulin secretion by the pancreas, and the effect of cortisol on peripheral tissues and fat stores. Insulin resistance is a state in which the body becomes less sensitive to insulin. A larger amount of insulin is needed to achieve the same effect. The combination of high cortisol and high insulin further propagates the metabolic disruption of the body, promoting fatty weight gain and muscle breakdown. In time, the pancreas becomes exhausted, leading to reduced insulin secretion and Type 2 diabetes.

Growth Hormone

Growth hormone (GH), produced by the anterior pituitary in response to hypothalamic release of growth hormone-releasing hormone (GHRH), has a number of important metabolic effects. One of these is its ability to force fat cells to release their stored fat into the blood as a source of fuel. In addition, it reduces their ability to store fat.

While acute stress appears to induce anterior pituitary activation, including an increase in circulating GH, this is only temporary. Chronic stress with HPA-axis disruption leads to a reduction in GH secretion (along with other anterior pituitary hormones, such as gonadotropin-releasing hormone (GnRH) and thyroid-stimulating hormone (TSH). This could potentially interfere with fat metabolism, swinging the balance in favor of storage.

Appetite

Stress and the subsequent production of cortisol also have an affect on appetite and feeding behavior. When released by the hypothalamus, CRH suppresses appetite. When cortisol is released, our body prepares to fight or flee, and as it does, our digestive system shuts down to better facilitate running away or fighting an attacker. Who needs to waste valuable energy on digesting food when a life is in danger?

As the stress response resolves, cortisol acts to inhibit CRH, thereby stimulating hunger. This aims to replenish energy reserves used up during the fight-or-flight episode.

Leptin

Leptin is a hormone produced by fat tissue to reduce appetite and increase energy expenditure, part of the body's control mechanism to maintain a steady weight. During starvation, reduced leptin levels allow conservation of energy by reducing metabolic rate, whereas in the well-fed state, its increased production by fat cells promotes calorie burning. Its daily cycle incorporates a peak at night, ensuring we continue to burn calories but don't feel hungry.

Leptin seems like the ideal hormone for controlling weight gain, but this is not the case. To start with, as a result of our evolutionary tendency to be faced with starvation more often than excess, the balance lies well in favor of weight gain. Reduced-calorie intake causes a rapid fall in leptin and subsequently a marked increase in appetite, despite the fact that our fat levels have not even begun to diminish. This is one reason why it is so hard to lose weight with calorie-deficient diets. Leptin levels increase with a high-fat diet (such as the Atkins diet). The health risks of such an elevated fat intake likely outweigh the benefits of weight loss.

Leptin's effect at reducing appetite is mediated by CRH, the hormone released by the hypothalamus as part of the stress response. CRH is a potent suppressor of hunger in acute stress and also increases anxiety and energy expenditure. Leptin stimulates the release of CRH from the hypothalamus.

Cortisol is a strong appetite enhancer, however, acting primarily through the inhibition of CRH secretion. We know that in obesity there is a degree of leptin resistance. The equilibrium between calorie intake and energy expenditure is maintained at an elevated 'set point'. Although the overall leptin level is increased (a direct effect of cortisol on fat cells), the daily cycle is blunted, resulting in a lower night-time peak, less energy expenditure, and the 'midnight munchies'. This correlates with an attenuated response of the hypothalamus-pituitary-adrenal (HPA) axis to stress.

An additional factor is the abnormal peak of cortisol levels between 2:00 and 4:00 a.m. seen in chronic stress. As levels begin to fall and the body switches to recovery mode, you will feel hungry, likely resulting in another surreptitious night-time trip to the fridge!

 STRESS FACT Leptin Resistance and Overnutrition

We know that in the chronically stressed state, the persistently high cortisol levels result in impaired feedback to the hypothalamus. It is likely that this also contributes to leptin resistance and the elevated set point with perceived starvation in the presence of excessive accumulation of lipid fats or adiposity. The combination of leptin resistance and overnutrition is thought to be partially responsible for diseases associated with obesity and metabolic syndrome in non-adipose tissues. These include diabetes and atherosclerosis (hardening of the arteries).

CRH

If the effect of CRH is to reduce appetite and increase energy expenditure, how is it that the chronically stressed individual with high CRH can put on weight? There is a degree of central CRH resistance within the brain, particularly in the areas of the hypothalamus controlling appetite, akin to the reduced sensitivity of the pituitary gland. In addition, in some individuals, cortisol may be a more potent inhibitor of CRH at this level, impairing the body's ability to burn calories. One further factor involves the amygdala (part of the limbic system adjacent to the hippocampus), which promotes excessive weight gain, particularly around the abdomen, following cortisol stimulation, independent of CRH.

Ghrelin

Ghrelin is a recently identified hormone produced primarily in the stomach. It has an effect on both the hypothalamus and the pituitary gland that appears to be the opposite of leptin. Ghrelin increases hunger and food intake, reduces fat utilization, and generally promotes metabolic efficiency. Rats given ghrelin show significant and rapid weight gain. Its levels are markedly reduced following gastroplasty (surgical stomach stapling) and may partially account for the success of this procedure in treating obese patients.

Ghrelin levels are increased during starvation and decrease following a meal or administration of glucose. This hormone primarily acts on the pituitary gland to increase release of growth hormone, but also influences hypothalamic hormone production. Studies showing ghrelin to stimulate production of CRH would appear contradictory, as this hormone is known to reduce hunger. Clearly, other factors are at play, and the rise in cortisol induced by ghrelin may account for part of its hunger-stimulating action.

Ghrelin does appear to be involved in the fight-or-flight response, its levels falling during acute stress and the subsequent catabolism (tissue breakdown) associated with energy production, and then rebounding during the recovery phase to rebuild stores. Ghrelin administration also induces anxiety in an animal model and increases cortisol. Production of ghrelin by the stomach increases significantly with physical or mental stress, as well as starvation (metabolic) stress. The stomach and ghrelin may play a pivotal role in the regulation of appetite and the response to stress.

✔ STRESS FACT Ghrelin Excess

Chronic stress may result in excessive ghrelin production that augments hunger and stimulation of the cortisol response. In addition, levels will be increased by the frequent low blood sugars associated with stress-related hyperinsulinemia. This pattern could feasibly contribute to both anxiety and weight gain.

Resistin

Resistin is a recently identified messenger molecule produced by fat cells — one of a new class of molecules called adipokines. Resistin, released specifically by abdominal fat cells, appears to induce insulin resistance and may be the link between central obesity and Type 2 diabetes. In addition, its effect on the cells of the blood vessel lining could also contribute to the increase in cardiovascular disease in these patients. Resistin levels are increased in patients with Cushing's syndrome (excess cortisol production) and they likely contribute significantly to the multiple diseases associated with metabolic syndrome.

Behavior

As we have seen, cortisol rapidly raises blood sugar levels, which are then normalized by the production of insulin. Persistently high cortisol levels induce insulin resistance, which means that higher levels of insulin are produced in response to the same sugar load. This inevitably leads to reactive hypoglycemia (abnormally low blood sugar). In order to correct this, our body will crave foods that will get sugar into the blood quickly. These are the highest glycemic index foods, sugars, and starches, such as chocolate and pastries. It is no coincidence that these are the foods that we crave when we are stressed.

Serotonin

Another reason that we may crave high sugar and starchy foods has to do with a chemical called serotonin, a neurotransmitter or chemical messenger within the brain. We like to call it our 'happy hormone' because its primary role is in the regulation of mood, sleep, and hunger. Serotonin activity is reduced in depression and accordingly is the hormone targeted by some antidepressant therapies. It is thought to induce feelings of well-being, calm, personal security, relaxation, confidence, and concentration. Serotonin is released whenever we consume high-glycemic carbohydrates, particularly chocolate, which is one of the reasons why we crave sweets and starches when we are sad.

When people first begin a diet or weight-loss program, there is an initial drop in serotonin as blood sugar levels stabilize. Even though these levels are only falling to normal — not below normal — the body still senses a change and reacts to this change. During this period, cravings for sweets and starches may exist in an attempt to increase both sugar levels and serotonin. Fortunately, once the body becomes more accustomed to the new blood sugar level, the cravings will dissipate.

Serotonin is made from the amino acid tryptophan. Insulin, released in response to a high blood sugar following ingestion of high-glycemic carbohydrates, removes glucose and some amino acids from the blood. However, it leaves tryptophan, resulting in relatively higher tryptophan levels in the blood and increased production in the brain. This is why we often feel relaxed and somewhat elated following a high-carbohydrate meal. Similarly, this is why we may crave sweets and starches or other foods that break down quickly into sugar when we are depressed or in other circumstances when serotonin is low, such as in women before their menstrual period.

Weight Gain
Another factor influencing weight gain in chronic stress is eating behavior. More often than not, people will gravitate toward high-sugar foods when they are stressed. The reason for this appears to be the insulin resistance associated with chronic stress.

Sugar Lows
In chronic stress, not only does altered carbohydrate metabolism increase the frequency and severity of 'sugar lows', thereby decreasing serotonin, cortisol also directly reduces serotonin production. Thus, our desire for sweets and starches is even higher.

✔ STRESS FACT So-Called Comfort Food

Cortisol is known to increase compulsive behavior, notably with respect to the use of drugs, alcohol, and food. Rats exposed to chronic stress increase their intake of comfort foods, those high in sugar or fat content. These foods appear to reduce levels of CRH in the amygdala and hypothalamus. Chronically stressed individuals may increase their comfort food intake as learned behavior to reduce central levels of anxiety-inducing CRH. In rats, such activity leads to increased abdominal fat stores and an intact feedback mechanism involving adipokine messengers acting to reduce HPA output. However, as we have seen, this mechanism is disrupted in humans with chronic stress, allowing unchecked accumulation of abdominal fat.

Certain foods are tryptophan-rich, such as turkey — thus the need for a snooze following the Thanksgiving meal. Unfortunately, a slice of turkey is not nearly as accessible as a chocolate bar when we need that serotonin!

Metabolic Syndrome

The metabolic consequences of weight gain and insulin resistance with hyperinsulinemia are sufficient to increase the risk of a number of diseases. Even with a low-fat diet, the vast majority of fat and cholesterol (more than 80%) comes from ingested carbohydrate and sugar under the influence of insulin. Associated conditions include high cholesterol, high blood pressure, cardiovascular disease, heart attack, and stroke, which, along with abdominal obesity, comprise the well-recognized metabolic syndrome or syndrome-X.

The role of a poor diet and chronic stress is central in the development of this metabolic condition. What is also of serious concern is that the other non-metabolic effects of stress on the cardiovascular system create additional damage, further increasing risk in these individuals.

Cortisol and Anorexia

An apparent paradox to our theories of cortisol and weight gain is anorexia, a condition in which individuals show high cortisol and low insulin levels with significant weight loss. As with chronic stress:

- Anorexics still show increased central-to-peripheral fat distribution.

- Depression and anxiety are common.

- Memory is impaired.

- HPA axis sensitivity is reduced.

The weight loss as opposed to weight gain may relate to an altered central conditioning that results in food avoidance rather than ingestion.

Summary

Not only are poor diet (high carbohydrate with insufficient protein) and cortisol (associated with chronic stress) responsible for the development of insulin resistance, the coexistence of all three propagate and accelerate metabolic disruption in the body. This leads to weight gain and, eventually, the development of obesity and metabolic syndrome, contributing to diabetes, high blood pressure, high cholesterol, and heart disease.

Can Stress Make You Fat?

The compounding factor of stress as a contributor in weight gain cannot be overemphasized. In our practice, we are continually faced with patients who say, "You know doctor, when I'm at work I eat well, I exercise regularly, yet I cannot lose any weight. Then I go on holiday, eat whatever I wish, drink alcohol, do very little exercise, and drop a few pounds within a week." We tell them the reason is simply because they relax. They lower their cortisol secretion, stabilize their insulin levels, and stop storing their food as fat. This is one of the major reasons why very stressed individuals can eat and exercise perfectly and not lose a pound, while others carelessly consume great quantities of food, often less-than-perfect foods, and still maintain their slim figure. So yes, stress can make you fat!

Similar findings in the research literature support this. In one study of middle-aged men, stress was found related to socioeconomic status and obesity. Low socioeconomic status and increased stress was associated with higher cortisol secretion and less inhibition of cortisol following dexamethasone administration — an indicator of chronic stress and altered cortisol feedback. These individuals had a higher incidence of abdominal obesity and diseases such as diabetes and high blood pressure.

This study shows us that the importance of controlling cortisol is not just about weight loss. It is also about disease control, its prevention, and treatment.

Dietary Prevention and Treatment of Stress

Is there a role for dietary change in the management of stress? Surely worrying about what to eat at every meal is only going to add to our daily anxieties! The answer, however, is "yes". And for a number of very good reasons:

1. *Rapid swings in blood sugar level actually act as a stressor on the body.* In fact, one of the tests that measure response of the HPA axis involves giving insulin to drop blood sugar. This stimulates release of cortisol. A diet that maintains a more constant blood sugar level will reduce stimulation of our stress response.

2. *A diet rich in high-glycemic carbohydrates (rapid breakdown to sugar) promotes the development of insulin resistance, a contributing factor to the adverse effects of chronic stress and metabolic syndrome.* Correcting your diet can reverse or prevent this.

3. *Correcting dietary imbalance and decreasing stress will reverse abnormalities in the fat hormone leptin.* Resistance to this hormone is thought to be responsible for increased weight gain.

4. *Controlling stress and weight may help reduce levels of resistin, an adipokine that induces insulin resistance.*

5. *A poor diet resulting in low blood sugar increases ghrelin release from the stomach.* This hormone acts on the hypothalamus and pituitary to increase appetite and impair the utilization of fat stores. It also induces anxiety. A good diet redresses this imbalance.

How Stress Can Lead to Weight Gain and Disease

Chronic stress leads to persistent cortisol secretion.

Cortisol raises blood sugar, causing release of insulin.

Insulin resistance develops from poor diet
and excessive cortisol.

High cortisol increases appetite and desire
for sugar and starch.

High cortisol impairs the fat control system.

⬇

High cortisol, insulin resistance, and increased appetite
lead to weight gain (central/abdominal).

⬇

High cortisol, insulin resistance, and weight gain
lead to metabolic syndrome, involving a variety
of common diseases.

Naturopathic Diet

We have developed a naturopathic diet as a healthy weight-loss and weight-maintenance program that does so by reversing abnormalities in metabolism and hormonal imbalances related to insulin resistance and hyperinsulinemia. As a weight-loss program, this diet helps to reduce weight by readjusting the balance of protein and carbohydrates in the diet. As a maintenance diet, it helps to prevent and treat diseases like obesity, diabetes (Type-2), high cholesterol, high blood pressure, atherosclerosis (hardening of the arteries), and heart disease. The ability of this diet to stabilize blood sugar levels and reduce insulin requirements prompted its use as a treatment for the chronic stress.

Diet Trends

Many different diets have been developed over time to try to slow down or stop our ever-growing weight problem and the diseases related to being overweight. Diet trends come and go, but despite varying degrees of initial success, the low-calorie, low-fat, and high-carbohydrate programs have *not* been shown to be consistently effective over time for weight loss or stress prevention and treatment. Even the latest high-protein diets have some serious shortcomings.

Low-Calorie Diets
Calorie-reduced diets flaunt their rapid weight loss, in some cases up to 5 pounds each week. This type of weight loss, however, causes other problems, which make maintenance of the reduced weight very difficult. Excessively rapid weight loss stimulates production of an enzyme known as lipoprotein lipase, forcing our bodies to store even more food as fat. These diets mimic starvation, a stressful state, and force the body to hold onto whatever food it is given as fat. Ultimately, this slows down our metabolic rate and therefore slows down weight loss. As well, the food groups chosen in these diets are unbalanced and disproportionately high in carbohydrates.

Low-Fat Diets
The popularity of low-fat diets waned with the realization that not only did they significantly increase hunger, they also significantly reduced HDL (good cholesterol) levels. Certain studies show that these low-fat diets may even increase the risk of heart disease by lowering HDL levels too far. Removing 'good' unsaturated fats from our diet is also dangerous for our health, for these fats are integral to the construction of cell membranes and the regulation of hormones, among other essential bodily functions.

High-Carbohydrate Diets
A diet high in carbohydrates seemed to be a logical solution to our weight-loss problem. Ingested carbohydrates are low in fat, low in cholesterol, and therefore lower in calories. So it made sense to eat primarily carbohydrates, such as pasta, rice, or potatoes, a regime promoted by *Fit for Life* and the Canada Food Guide, for example. Unfortunately, once the carbohydrates are ingested, this picture almost reverses due to the different hormonal secretions that occur in response to a high-carbohydrate meal.

There is, in fact, an increase in fat production and storage as well as a rise in blood triglyceride and cholesterol levels. These plain and simple carbohydrates become havoc-wreaking substrates that damage the body. Sadly, this diet had been advocated before any sound clinical data was collected. On paper, these foods look good, but in reality they have only increased our weight problem, accentuating the process of fat storage that we are now trying to reverse. A high-carbohydrate diet has also increased our risk of diet-related diseases.

High-Protein Diets

With the realization that carbohydrates were 'bad' came a revolution in dietary philosophy and the emergence of protein-based programs. Several high-protein diets have become popular, such as the Carbohydrate Addict's Diet advocated by Rachael and Richard Heller, Dr. Atkins' New Diet, and the Protein Power Plan diet developed by Michael and Mary Eades. These programs are biochemically well grounded. Their shared premise of reducing insulin secretion so that we do not store our food as fat is sound. Nevertheless, while they provide a foundation on which to build an effective protein-based diet, they lack many nutrients and are deficient in such valuable carbohydrates as fruits and vegetables. In addition, they can promote ketosis, the body's emergency response to lack of food. Its purpose is survival at the expense of health and therefore imposes added stress.

✔ **STRESS FACT** **Ketosis Dangers**

Ketosis results in symptoms such as nausea, dehydration, light-headedness, and bad breath. Toxic effects to the body include kidney damage. Ketosis may be fatal to diabetics and to the fetus in pregnancy. With respect to weight reduction, ketosis results in weight loss due to dehydration and loss of muscle tissue. Not only is this harmful to the body, but it can ultimately cause weight gain through the conversion of amino acids to fat. Studies have also shown that ketogenic diets alter fat cells to make them hungrier for fat storage.

Naturopathic Diet Principles

In order to achieve healthy and permanent weight loss, it is important not to deprive the body of any one food group — fat, protein, or carbohydrates. What we need is a relatively simple and convenient diet that enables immediate weight loss and long-term weight management without potential damage to our health. This involves retraining our bodies to use food as fuel rather than storing food as fat, restoring the biochemical balance needed to cope with everyday stress, and thus preventing chronic stress and the disease conditions associated with metabolic syndrome. The naturopathic diet is the basic treatment for chronic stress and the most effective preventive strategy.

The naturopathic diet we have developed in our medical practice achieves these goals by retraining our body to use food as fuel rather than storing it as fat, leading to permanent weight loss and increased energy levels without metabolic disruption. This is achieved with simple changes rather than with rigid dietary restrictions, in two stages.

The naturopathic diet is not a 'high-protein' diet but rather a balanced protein program with restrictions on high-glycemic carbohydrates. This diet is not a change in eating habits that we make temporarily until we lose weight and then return to the bad eating habits we had before. Any diet change that is not a lifestyle change only results in temporary weight loss. Just the same, there is no need to restrict ourselves completely from all the foods we love. By making a few additions to our diet (instead of restrictions), we will be able to eat almost anything we want after we have lost the weight. We can return to a large variety of different foods without any fear of regaining the weight. However, if we return to a diet of high carbohydrates and low protein, we run the risk of undoing all the metabolic changes that were brought about by the naturopathic diet.

Stage One: Weight Loss and Metabolic Retraining Stage

This stage of the naturopathic diet involves a limited period of time, for two reasons. The diet 'retrains' the body's metabolism in 2 to 8 weeks as a rule. During these weeks, blood sugar, and thus insulin levels, remain consistently low. The body learns the connection between protein and low glucose. The message it receives each time protein is ingested is that the blood sugar levels are low so it does not need to secrete insulin at a high rate. Once the body has practiced and consolidated this message for a period of time, we can then combine some higher-glycemic carbohydrates with our protein, and the insulin secretion will remain low.

Protein will always act as a cue, keeping the insulin release small and maintaining the weight loss.

The second reason for limiting the time period of this weight loss stage is that no one wants to be on a restricted diet forever! This is a very nutrient-rich diet that may be followed for long periods of time without adversely affecting your health. The foods recommended all contain high quantities of vitamins, minerals, and protein. These same foods are very low in 'empty calories' — calorie-dense foods that have little nutritional value. There is essentially no limit to the length of time we may stay in stage one. However, we most likely will stop losing weight once excess fat has been eradicated. Once stage one is complete, we can simply move into stage two, the maintenance stage. This is the balanced or homeostatic state where we will remain for the rest of our life.

Healthy Weight-Loss Guide

Most people will tend to lose weight in stage one of the naturopathic diet, on average 18 to 22 pounds over 8 weeks. However, not everyone with chronic stress wants to lose weight, and for this reason we will vary the amount of time in this stage depending on a number of factors:

1. If you are already at or close to your ideal weight, then it is unlikely that your metabolism has completely shifted to the abnormal hyperinsulinemic state. In this case, just 2 weeks in stage one is sufficient.

2. If you are slightly overweight (10 to 12 pounds), predominantly in the midsection of your body, you are likely in the early stages of stress-induced metabolic disruption. We would recommend 4 to 6 weeks in stage one, with adjustment depending on your starting weight and rate of loss.

3. If you are 15 pounds or more above your ideal weight, then you likely need a full 8 to 9 weeks in stage one.

For those individuals wishing to lose more weight at the end of the 8- to 9-week period, simply continue with stage one of the diet until you reach a desirable weight plateau.

Ideal Weight

There is much discussion as to what constitutes ideal body weight and how to calculate it. Unfortunately, as we all have different body types and different lifestyles, there is not an easy answer to this problem. The best-known technique to calculate the ideal body weight is by using the BMI or Body Mass Index.

Body Mass Index

The BMI scale was designed for a person of average height and build, between the ages of 20 and 65 years old, doing an average amount of activity. It was formulated to give people a general idea about how their weight and size puts them at a relative risk for certain weight-related diseases like diabetes and heart diseases.

This is a ratio of height versus weight. However, it does not take into account factors such as muscle mass, bone density and structure, or tissue hydration. In addition, it is not applicable to infants, teens, those over 65, body builders, pregnant or breast-feeding women, or endurance athletes.

Body-Mass Index Calculation

For the average woman, the ideal BMI is above 19.1 and below 25.8. For the average man, above 20.7 and below 26.4.

To calculate your BMI, take your weight in pounds and divide this by the square of your height in inches. (To change your measurements from pounds to kilograms, take the number of pounds and divide it by 2.2. To change your height from inches to meters, take the number in inches and multiply that by 0.0254.) For instance if a man was 5'10" or 70" tall and weighed 165 pounds, the calculation would be as follows:

Imperial Measure
$$165 \text{ pounds} / (70 \text{ inches})^2 = 23.9$$

Metric Measure
$$165/2.2 = 75 \text{ kilograms}$$

$$5'10" = 70 \text{ inches} = (70 \times 0.0254) = 1.77 \text{ meters}$$

$$75 / (1.77)^2 = 23.9$$

Thus for this individual the BMI would be 23.9

Body-Mass Index Chart

You can also calculate your Body Mass Index (BMI) using this chart.

BMI	19	20	21	22	23	24	25	26	27	28	29	30	35	40
Height (in.)	Weight (lb.)													
58	91	96	100	105	110	115	119	124	129	134	138	143	167	191
59	94	99	104	109	114	119	124	128	133	138	143	148	173	198
60	97	102	107	112	118	123	128	133	138	143	148	153	179	204
61	100	106	111	116	122	127	132	137	143	148	153	158	185	211
62	104	109	115	120	126	131	136	142	147	153	158	164	191	218
63	107	113	118	124	130	135	141	146	152	158	163	169	197	225
64	110	116	122	128	134	140	145	151	157	163	169	174	204	232
65	114	120	126	132	138	144	150	156	162	168	174	180	210	240
66	118	124	130	136	142	148	155	161	167	173	179	186	216	247
67	121	127	134	140	146	153	159	166	172	178	185	191	223	255
68	125	131	138	144	151	158	164	171	177	184	190	197	230	262
69	128	135	142	149	155	162	169	176	182	189	196	203	236	270
70	132	139	146	153	160	167	174	181	188	195	202	207	243	278
71	136	143	150	157	165	172	179	186	193	200	208	215	250	286
72	140	147	154	162	169	177	184	191	199	206	213	221	258	294
73	144	151	159	166	174	182	189	197	204	212	219	227	265	302
74	148	155	163	171	179	186	194	202	210	218	225	233	272	311
75	152	160	168	176	184	192	200	208	216	224	232	240	279	319
76	156	164	172	180	189	197	205	213	221	230	238	246	287	328

Body Fat Levels

The levels of acceptable body fat differ for men and women. For a female, the normal range is considered to be 15% to 22%, and for a male it is slightly lower at 15% to 18%. There are risks to being outside this range on either side. The risks associated with having too low a percentage of body fat are abnormal menstrual cycles, osteo-porosis, skin problems, thyroid problems, and sleep disturbances. The risks associated with being above this range are obesity, diabetes, heart disease, high cholesterol, and back pain. Body fat percentage can be measured using electronic sensors or calipers in what is known as the pinch test.

Protein

During both stage one and stage two of the naturopathic diet, you need to eat 15 to 25 grams of protein per meal, depending on your initial weight. This size is approximately equivalent to $3/4$ the size of your hand. You may exceed this amount slightly but not go under it. You require this much protein to instruct the body not to secrete insulin at a high rate.

Common protein sources are listed here. There must be one protein source from the list below at every single meal. Although there are other foods that contain protein, such as lentils or yogurt, they are not high enough in protein to be considered a protein source. Drink as much water as possible because the protein forces your body to pass more urine.

Common Protein Sources

- Fish
- Chicken/Turkey
- Red Meat
- Tofu (extra firm, low fat)
- Eggs (3 egg whites to 1 yolk)
- Protein Powders (use a whey protein powder, as it will also stimulate the immune system, with at least 15 grams of protein and only 3 or 4 grams of carbohydrate)
- Protein Bars (use bars that are high in protein but low in carbohydrates and fat; two-thirds of a bar is all that is needed for the protein portion of a meal and the rest may be snacked on later)
- Low-fat Cottage or Ricotta Cheese (approximately $1/2$ cup)

Legumes, such as lentils and chickpeas, are considered a carbohydrate because they are approximately 70% carbohydrate and 30% protein, so try to limit their use.

Carbohydrates and Glycemic Indices

You cannot just eat protein alone. Continual protein in high concentration by itself, without any carbohydrate, will stim-ulate ketosis, a starvation state in which the insulin and glucose levels are very low and glucagon levels rise. This is why you must add carbohydrates to your meals.

When considering carbohydrates, the glycemic index of the food becomes very important. Since all carbohydrates break down into sugar, select those that produce it in lower amounts and at a slower rate.

The glycemic index of food is a measure of the amount of sugar available in food to be delivered to the blood. The higher the glycemic index, the faster the sugar is transported into the blood, thereby raising blood sugar levels. Different foods have

Stress Solutions

different glycemic indices, and this is key to a weight loss or stress-reducing program. Pasta, bread, and potatoes, for example, have a very high glycemic index. Lettuce, mushrooms, and strawberries also contain carbohydrates, but have much lower glycemic indices and will subsequently not raise blood sugar levels excessively.

Now, a diet based strictly on very low-glycemic-index vegetables would be rather unpalatable, so this diet does allow a wider variety with increased flexibility even in stage one.

There are certain carbohydrates that are permitted in unlimited quantities — salads and most vegetables. Certain vegetables contain too much starch or sugar and will increase your blood sugar levels, although some of these (carrots, for example) are permitted in stage one because they contain many beneficial nutrients. By cutting out all the restricted carbohydrates from our diet, you will have lowered your blood sugars sufficiently to enjoy some of these high-sugar vegetables, safely.

Glycemic Index of Common Carbohydrates

The glycemic index (GI) is a ranking of carbohydrates based on their immediate effect on blood glucose (blood sugar) levels. Carbohydrates that break down quickly during digestion, causing a rapid rise in blood glucose, have the highest glycemic indices. Carbohydrates that break down slowly and release glucose gradually into the bloodstream have low-glycemic indices. This index compares the carbohydrates in various foods gram for gram. The benchmark is white bread, which is assigned a GI of 100.

- Benchmark: White Bread = 100
- Low GI = 55 or less
- Medium GI = 56 to 69
- High GI = 70 or more

GI of Common Foods

Food	GI	Food	GI
White Bread	100	Pizza	80
Instant Rice	124	Popcorn	79
Corn Flakes	119	Banana Muffin	70
Rice Krispies	117	Parboiled Rice	68
Jellybeans	114	Pasta	50-70
French Fries	107	Pumpernickel	66
Soda Crackers	106	All-Bran	60
Potato (boiled/mashed)	104	Banana	50
Melba Toast	100	Sweet Potato	54
Couscous	93	Skim Milk	46
Ice Cream	87	Lentils/Kidney/Baked Beans	40-69
Oatmeal (one-minute oats)	87	Orange Juice	46
Table Sugar (sucrose)	83	Apple	28

Restricted Carbohydrates

High-sugar carbohydrates need to be cut during stage one, including all breads or bread type products, such as bagels and muffins, all pasta, rice, bananas, potatoes, squash, corn, popcorn, yogurt, alcohol, and candy. This includes bread made with a grain flour other than wheat or rye, such as spelt and kamut flour, although a soy flour called Dr. Atkins' Bake Mix can be used as a substitute. This high-protein flour has no carbohydrate and makes very nice pancakes and muffins.

Limited Foods

Fruits need to be limited to a maximum of two pieces per day. Fruit is high in sugar and will force the body to secrete higher levels of insulin as well. One glass of juice is equal to one piece of fruit.

All dressings, mayonnaise, butter, nuts, and cheeses are allowed , but try not to use them excessively, for example, one slice of cheese and five nuts every other day. Do not replace the carbohydrates with fat.

You may have unlimited vegetables and salads, including carrots, beets, and peas, but those that are high in carbohydrate, such as potatoes and squash, remain restricted.

Naturopathic Diet Stage One Summary

This stage lasts 2 to 8 weeks, depending on your need to lose weight and your need to rebalance your blood sugar state.

1. Protein per meal: 15 to 25 grams.

2. Unlimited salads and most other vegetables.

3. Two pieces of fruit a day maximum, no bananas.

4. No grains, rice, pasta, or starches.

5. Very limited high-carbohydrate, low-protein foods, such as chickpeas and lentils.

6. Limited portions of dressings and condiments.

7. No alcohol.

8. Increased fluid levels by drinking more water.

Stage Two: Weight Maintenance and Metabolic Balance Stage

The maintenance stage of the naturopathic diet is a true lifestyle change that we can easily maintain for the rest of our life. Throughout this second stage, our energy levels will remain high, our weight stable, and our blood sugar will not show the large variations known to induce stress. Part of the maintenance diet is the addition of protein at each meal, but here the dietary choices expand, allowing us freedom to enjoy many different types of food. We can enjoy every food group and continue to protect ourselves against many food-related diseases at the same time. These benefits will last forever, as long as we balance our protein and newly introduced carbohydrates at each meal. The maintenance stage is thus not so much a stage as it is a permanent change.

Reintroduce Carbohydrates

During stage two, we begin to reintroduce some carbohydrates eliminated or markedly reduced in stage one. Now that your body has consolidated the protein/low glucose message, it is possible to add back carbohydrates at a higher concentration, along with the protein, without increasing insulin release. Blood sugar levels will not rise rapidly as they did before because the protein we are combining with the carbohydrates will slow the delivery of the sugar into the blood. This in itself will reduce the amount of insulin released. The reversal of insulin resistance and hyperinsulinemia achieved by stage one will further reduce the insulin response. Overall, less insulin will be secreted than before we started the diet. Slightly more insulin will be released during stage two than during stage one, and this will prevent further weight loss. However, it will not be sufficient to induce hyperinsulinemia.

The order in which you reintroduce the carbohydrates is very important. You must slowly integrate them back into the diet in a particular pattern. The sequence of reintroduction is determined by the glycemic index and type of sugar found in each carbohydrate. Fructose, the sugar found in fruit, is the first to be introduced. This is followed by glucose from whole grains and breads, then pasta, rice, potatoes and squash, and finally candy and alcohol. Adherence to this pattern minimizes large jumps in blood sugar levels and allows for easy adaptation of the body to carbohydrates.

The amount of carbohydrate reintroduced is also very important. Reintroduce a small amount of carbohydrate initially, approximately three parts protein to one part carbohydrate at each meal (for example, 21 grams protein with 7 grams carbohydrate). Remain at this 3:1 ratio of protein to carbohydrate intake for 4 to 5 days. A typical meal would be half a slice of bread, a piece of chicken, and unlimited salad or vegetable.

Stage Two Carbohydrate Reintroduction Order

1. Fruits
2. Whole Grains, Breads, Cereals
3. Pasta
4. Rice
5. Potatoes and Squash
6. Candy and Alcoholic Beverages

Weekly Weight and Anti-Stress Chart

To help you keep track of your weight, weigh yourself only once a week. It is important not to weigh yourself every day. Very few people lose weight consistently every day, since there will be minor fluctuations in your weight from water retention, salty food, hormones, and the natural weight-loss process.

Over the course of a week, weight will increase and decrease slightly, but by the end of the week, there should be, on average, a 2-pound loss. This chart will allow you to monitor the success of your weight-loss program while correlating it with your stress levels. You may find that weight loss slows or stops during periods of increased stress — a good way to test the effectiveness of your anti-stress diet program.

In the chart below, write down the date you begin stage one of the naturopathic diet and your stress-reduction program. Next, record your starting weight. During the initial 8 weeks of stage one, try to weigh yourself on the same scale and at approximately the same time of day each week. This will help to ensure a more accurate weight reading. Monitor your stress level daily using the 1 to 5 scale, with 1 being the lowest level and 5 the highest level of perceived stress (1 = calm, relaxed, stress-free; 5 = totally panic stricken and unable to cope).

Note: You can complete this program independent of a stress-management routine if you wish. However, if you find that your stress levels are staying high despite the diet, it is recommended that you incorporate a stress reduction program as part of your overall health plan.

Start Date:		Week 2 Date:	
Stress Level (1-5)	**Start Weight**	**Stress Level (1-5)**	**Week 2 Weight**
Day 1_____	_____	Day 1_____	_____
Day 2_____		Day 2_____	
Day 3_____		Day 3_____	
Day 4_____		Day 4_____	
Day 5_____		Day 5_____	
Day 6_____		Day 6_____	
Day 7_____		Day 7_____	

Hyperinsulinemia Signs

During this time period, watch for signs of hyperinsulinemia. Your body will become symptomatic when you ingest too many carbohydrates at once. You will feel tired shortly after the meal because your blood sugar levels may drop too low. Several hours later or perhaps the next day, you may feel bloated because your kidneys are not releasing enough salt. These signs will let you know that the ratio of carbohydrate to protein was too high and therefore insulin was secreted at a higher rate.

If none of these signs appear following the amount of reintroduced carbohydrate, then you can increase the amount consumed again. This time, consider a ratio of 2:1 protein to carbohydrate. Again, watch for signs and symptoms of hyperinsulinemia. If they do not appear, you a can continue to increase slowly the amount and type of carbohydrate until you have

Week 3 Date:		Week 6 Date:	
Stress Level (1-5)	**Week 3 Weight**	**Stress Level (1-5)**	**Week 6 Weight**
Day 1_____	_____	Day 1_____	_____
Day 2 _____		Day 2 _____	
Day 3 _____		Day 3 _____	
Day 4 _____		Day 4 _____	
Day 5 _____		Day 5 _____	
Day 6 _____		Day 6 _____	
Day 7 _____		Day 7 _____	

Week 4 Date:		Week 7 Date:	
Stress Level (1-5)	**Week 4 Weight**	**Stress Level (1-5)**	**Week 7 Weight**
Day 1_____	_____	Day 1_____	_____
Day 2 _____		Day 2 _____	
Day 3 _____		Day 3 _____	
Day 4 _____		Day 4 _____	
Day 5 _____		Day 5 _____	
Day 6 _____		Day 6 _____	
Day 7 _____		Day 7 _____	

Week 5 Date:		Week 8 Date:	
Stress Level (1-5)	**Week 5 Weight**	**Stress Level (1-5)**	**Week 8 Weight**
Day 1_____	_____	Day 1_____	_____
Day 2 _____		Day 2 _____	
Day 3 _____		Day 3 _____	
Day 4 _____		Day 4 _____	
Day 5 _____		Day 5 _____	
Day 6 _____		Day 6 _____	
Day 7 _____		Day 7 _____	

reached a 1:1 ratio. Should the symptoms of hyperinsulinemia appear earlier, limit your carbohydrate intake and return to the proportion previously used when you had no symptoms. While a final fixed ratio of protein to carbohydrate cannot be quoted because it differs from individual to individual, as a general rule, a ratio of one part protein to one part carbohydrate, excluding vegetables and salads, is a fairly good balance.

Dietary Balance
This is your state of dietary balance — the ratio of protein to carbohydrate that you can ingest to maintain a healthy metabolism without inducing hyperinsulinemia. At this balance between protein and carbohydrate, your blood sugar levels will remain steady, and, subsequently, so will your insulin secretion, weight, and cortisol.

Caffeine and Stress

The cup of coffee that most of us reach for in the morning to give us that 'wake-up' jolt may have more of a detrimental effect on our bodies than we think. At some point in our lives, most of us have consumed so much caffeine that we have experienced the jitters. We feel agitated, our limbs or extremities are shaky, our head feels fuzzy and drugged, and our stomach raw and nauseated. This situation represents an extreme example of the effect of caffeine. Smaller amounts, however, still impact the body in a similar, though less obvious manner.

Java Jolt

Even small amounts of caffeine can increase the body's stress response for up to 12 hours after consumption. Thus, even if your last cup of coffee is at 10:00 a.m., your body may still be reacting to it at 10:00 p.m. in the evening. This may augment the difficulty you already experience in falling asleep. There are numerous studies displaying the same ill effects of caffeine on the body, particularly when the body is under stress. All you have to do is take note of your own body next time you have coffee. Did your heart rate increase? Did you start to sweat a little more or feel a little more nervous or excited? Even though you may crave these reactions in the morning and feel you need them to get you going, remember that these physical changes are going to stay with you all day long, increasing your body's reaction to any stressors you face.

Reducing Caffeine Ingestion

The ideal solution for stress reduction is to cut out caffeine completely, at least in the short term. However, this needs to be done gradually. It is important that you do not cut out all caffeine at once. This is especially true if you are having 3 or more cups of coffee a day. If you do, you may go through withdrawal symptoms, such as headaches, irritability, short-temper, constipation, etc. To avoid this, cut down slowly.

1. Start by drinking the same number of cups of coffee each day, but changing each cup to half caffeinated and half decaffeinated for one week. Then change to one-quarter caffeinated and three-quarters decaffeinated.

2. Slowly drop the amount of caffeinated coffee until you are only consuming decaffeinated.

3. Colas, tea, and chocolate also contain caffeine so also be aware of your consumption of these substances.

Caffeine is a methylxanthine chemical that acts on many tissues in the body, and in particular stimulates the central nervous system. Pharmacological effects of caffeine include: stimulation of medullary respiratory centers, generalized enhancement of CNS cellular response to stimulation, increased heart rate, decreased peripheral vascular resistance, increased cerebral vascular resistance, smooth muscle relaxation, skeletal muscle stimulation, stimulation of gastrointestinal secretions, and diuresis. Caffeine may increase contraction of the diaphragm.

Caffeine is characterized as a central nervous system stimulant. It increases the response, function, and workload of our nervous system and therefore our fight-or-flight stress response. Caffeine also increases our metabolic rate. While this may seem like an ideal way to burn calories, when the stress response is chronically stimulated, metabolic changes actually result in weight gain.

Caffeine has several other detrimental effects on the body and the fight-or-flight stress response. Caffeine can significantly alter the production of our catecholamines (adrenaline and noradrenaline), alter blood pressure and heart rate, and change our sense of perceived stress.

One study conducted at Duke University Medical Center on 47 non-smoking coffee drinkers showed these changes. Caffeine significantly increased blood pressure and heart rate during the workday and into the evening, with a 32% increase in adrenaline excreted during the day. Caffeine was also shown to amplify the increases in blood pressure and heart rate associated with self-reported stress. These effects remained undiminished through the evening until bedtime. Similar studies show a dose-dependent response to caffeine. Stressful reaction to mental workload was exaggerated with prior coffee consumption when compared to caffeine-free individuals.

Alcohol and Stress

Many people look to alcohol to wind down after a hard day, promoting a relaxed feeling that 'helps' them forget about their stress. However, alcohol can have exactly the opposite effect. Alcohol intake can actually alter the activity of both the HPA axis and the opioid (endorphin) receptor system in a way that not only increases stress in the body, but can also influence further drinking behavior.

The way in which alcohol affects the body is complex and varies according to sex, age, and the amount of alcohol consumed. Studies indicate that ACTH and beta-endorphin levels are significantly reduced after drinking alcohol, more so in women than in men, and increasingly with age. CRH has a lesser effect on the pituitary and adrenal glands and the daily rhythm of cortisol release is disrupted. A decrease in endorphins exacerbates this effect by impairing relaxation. Independent of sex or age, the largest hormonal changes are seen after heavy drinking. Women seem to have a genetically greater response than men. An exaggerated response is correlated with the development of alcoholism.

Alcohol, like caffeine, dehydrates the body, which provides a physiological stress within the body. Its effects on the pituitary secretion of vasopressin or antidiuretic hormone (ADH) may also affect the HPA axis.

✔ STRESS FACT Alcohol Stressors

Alcohol acts as a stressor to the body, causing an increase in cortisol levels. With chronic use, this repetitive stimulation leads to a disruption of the HPA axis and reduced responsiveness of the stress response, a similar finding seen in chronic stress from other causes.

Anti-Stress Diet Diary

The role of the Diet Diary is to document the food you eat, its relationship to your emotions and stress level, and the effects that food has on the way you feel.

The Diet Diary will also allow you to link certain foods with certain side effects. You may discover that sugary foods increase your heart rate, that you begin to sweat after a cup of coffee, or that without protein at each meal, you have a crash in energy levels that leads to anxiety, irritability, or fatigue. For example, items containing red food dye may make you lightheaded and nervous. In these circumstances, you can easily pinpoint certain unpleasant emotions and physical symptoms that are associated with your diet. You can then make appropriate dietary changes to alter not only your immediate physical and emotional response to the foods, but also help alter the disruption in your overall stress response. In doing so, you will be making wise lifestyle changes that will help maintain a calmer, healthier, and happier you.

Using the chart, for each day of the diary try to note the following each time you eat. Even if you miss a meal or do not have a snack, complete the emotion and stress columns.

Caution: If any symptoms persist despite dietary changes, then it is important to go see your health-care practitioner. Together you can go through your food chart and identify links between your dietary problems to your symptoms. Without the chart, it becomes more difficult to see these links.

1. How you are feeling emotionally before you eat?

❑ Nervous ❑ Anxious ❑ Depressed ❑ Happy
❑ Content ❑ Angry ❑ Overwhelmed

2. How would you rate your stress level on a scale of 1 to 5?

1 = calm, relaxed, stress-free   5 = totally panic stricken and unable to cope

1   2   3   4   5

3. What did you eat?

Fats: _____   Protein: _____   Carbohydrates: _____
_____   _____   _____
_____   _____   _____

4. What physical or emotional effects occurred within 30 to 60 minutes after the meal?

Physical Effects

❑ Heart Palpitations   ❑ Fatigue/Loss of Energy
❑ Nausea   ❑ Gas/Bloating/Cramping
❑ Sweating   ❑ Diarrhea
❑ Stomachache   ❑ Headache

Emotional Effects

❑ Nervous   ❑ Content
❑ Anxious   ❑ Angry
❑ Depressed   ❑ Overwhelmed
❑ Happy

By reviewing your diary on a regular basis, you can begin to identify patterns in your eating behavior. Perhaps you always gravitate toward a sugary treat or salty snack when feeling anxious, or a large bowl of pasta when depressed. Recognizing such actions has two potential benefits:

1. You have found a way to identify your emotions and stress levels.

2. You can understand how your eating behavior relates more to emotions and stress than hunger.

Recognizing that eating certain food types is a reaction to your stress and not a cure, you can introduce stress-relieving alternatives instead of unhealthy products.

Anti-Stress Natural Supplements

Combating Overactive Adrenal Glands with Natural Supplements

James is a 41-year-old lawyer who has been trying to lose weight. He averages 80 hours of work a week, and, whenever possible, he rushes home and spends time with his children before they go to bed. He works out five times a week at 5:00 a.m. before heading to the office. He does 35 minutes of cardiovascular exercise and 30 minutes of weight training. He eats a very regimented diet consisting of organic lean protein sources like turkey, fish, and egg whites. This is complimented with nutritious low-glycemic carbohydrates, such as vegetables, salads, and fruits. Only rarely does he indulge in a glass of wine or a small dessert. Despite his compliance with diet and exercise, he has only lost 4 pounds in 3 months.

During our consultation, he told us that he feels very stressed, wakes consistently at 3:30 a.m. in the morning, and has a difficult time falling back asleep. He carries his weight only around his waist, despite his diligent abdominal workout routine.

After a physical and hormonal examination, it was discovered that his adrenal glands were overactive. The only form of treatment we added was a supplement combination to regulate the release of stress hormones and his physical and emotional response to stress. We used milk peptides, B vitamins, and theanine.

Within the first 10 days, he lost 3 pounds, and continued to drop 2 pounds every week thereafter until he reached his weight goal.

Improving our diet to restore hormonal balance in our bodies and thus to defend against chronic stress is certainly an effective treatment. However, the food we eat is not always adequate for the task, and we may benefit from dietary supplements of minerals, vitamins, and herbs.

Natural supplementation is the addition of vitamins, minerals, and herbs to the diet for preventive and therapeutic purposes. This philosophy of supplementation has gained greater acceptance over the past few years as we have become more aware of the deficiencies in our food. Not only are our fast-food choices lacking in vitamins and minerals, even our supposedly fresh vegetables and fruit are nutrient depleted. Our farm soils are exhausted, no longer enriched with natural minerals. Supposedly fresh foods have usually spent many days in storage or transport before making it to our plates. Food storage and processing generally destroys more than 50% of the vitamin/mineral content in that food, though variations exist between different nutrients within the food. Baking obliterates 100% of vitamin B-1, for example, while processing damages 80% of vitamin B-2. Given our overprocessed, stale, nutrient-scarce diets, it is easy to see why nutrient supplementation has grown in popularity.

Natural supplementation is just one weapon in a whole armory designed to help you beat stress. It should always be combined with other therapies discussed in this book, including diet, lifestyle changes, and physical modalities.

Not all supplements will work equally well for everyone. If you do not achieve adequate relief from one, you can try others from the following catalog of remedies. Just ensure you give them a chance to work, and do not change products too often. Natural supplementation for stress can begin to take effect within 2 to 4 days, but should be continued for at least 2 weeks before concluding it is ineffective.

Selecting and Combining Supplements

Taking every supplement indicated for a particular condition is never advisable. It is best just to choose a few different natural substances that work in different ways and then take the most effective dose of each supplement. Many people have the philosophy that more is better, and the greater the intake of supplements, the greater the benefit. However, what usually happens is that people sacrifice a sufficient dose of one supplement in order to take several others. Then the dose of each supplement ingested becomes too small to have a proper therapeutic effect. Also avoid taking multiple supplements if the routine becomes so cumbersome that you miss or forget doses. These are all good reasons why it is better to choose only a few specific products.

Not all supplements will work equally well for everyone. We have found certain natural remedies to be more successful than others. However, if you do not achieve adequate relief from certain supplements, try using others from the following catalog of remedies. Just ensure you give them a chance to work, and do not change products too often.

Supplement Safety
Supplements, although natural, can have side effects and interactions with other medications (both natural and pharmaceutical). Caution is advised with respect to self-prescription. Be sure to discuss any new medication or supplement with your medical or naturopathic doctor, particularly if you are taking a number of different therapies. Always let your treating doctors know every medication, natural or otherwise, you are taking. This is vital before invasive tests or surgeries.

Supplement Quality

Few of the nutritional companies that offer products to consumers have the financial resources and infrastructure to guarantee absolute purity of raw material supply. It is not uncommon to find heavy metals, pesticide residue, and toxic micro-contaminates in products. Our research has consistently led us to Jamieson Laboratories as one of only a few manufacturers that integrates clinical protocols to guarantee the pharmaceutical purity of their raw material supply. Other reliable suppliers include Sisu, Natura Pharm, Quest, Thorne, and Natural Factors. Many of these products are available at regular retail pharmacies, health food stores, and specialty natural supplement outlets. Remember, if the product you are looking for is not available, most pharmacies will special-order it for you.

Basic Terms

The term 'nutritional supplement' includes vitamins, minerals, enzymes and coenzymes, essential fatty acids, amino acids, and herbs.

Vitamins

Vitamins are defined as any constituents in the diet other than protein, fat, carbohydrate, and inorganic salts that are necessary for normal growth and activity of the body. They must be obtained from external sources, and a deficiency may result in specific diseases, depending on the vitamin.

Minerals

Minerals are essentially any inorganic substance found in the earth. Like vitamins, minerals must be taken in from an outside source and are necessary for proper bodily maintenance and growth. Minerals can be divided into two categories. 'Macrominerals' are those that the body needs in larger doses of milligrams or even grams. This includes such minerals as calcium, magnesium, phosphorus, and potassium. 'Trace' minerals are those that are required in much smaller amounts, in micrograms. This category includes iodine, selenium, and chromium, for example.

Enzymes and Coenzymes

Vitamins and minerals are essential components of enzymes and coenzymes. Enzymes are substances that stimulate different biochemical reactions in the body. Coenzymes aid the enzymes in this function. With proper nutritional supplementation, we can support certain enzymatic pathways to perform optimally, thereby speeding up certain reactions. If an enzyme is lacking a vitamin or mineral, it cannot function optimally and the process is slowed or halted. We must ensure adequate nutrient supplementation to accentuate certain bodily functions.

Essential Fatty Acids

Most people try to stay away from fatty foods, and for the most part, this is a wise decision. However, there are some fats that are actually beneficial — indeed, even essential to the body. Most people are approximately 70% to 80% deficient in essential fatty acids. The symptoms of a low dietary intake of essential fats are fatigue, dry skin and hair, constipation, depression, bloating, and arthritis.

Amino Acids

Amino acids are the component parts of protein molecules and are therefore needed for tissue repair, enzyme reactions, nerve and muscle function and recovery. Nonessential amino acids can be manufactured by the body, while essential ones need to be part of our diet.

Herbs

Herbal supplementation is the use of botanicals or natural plants as therapeutic agents. More than 70% of prescription drugs are based on plant formulas. It follows that by using the original plant we can achieve a similar result. Botanicals or herbs will often have the same physiologic effect as a drug. They will bind into the same receptors and produce similar outcome. The difference lies in strength. Generally, herbal medicine is much weaker, ranging from $1/100th$ to $1/1000th$ the strength of its pharmaceutical equivalent. Thus, the natural medications require more time to have an effect. However, the benefit is that their side effects are generally minimal. Once again, by combining both forms of therapy, we can achieve a maximum effect with minimal side effects. This is done by decreasing the dose of pharmaceuticals and enhancing the therapeutic effect with natural supplementation.

Vitamins

The family of B vitamins is used in many different areas of the body by the nerves, muscles, liver, skin, and brain. These vitamins are involved in many coenzyme reactions (helping an enzyme reaction take place) and thus are crucial to the function of the body. There are several different B vitamins, and although they are often supplemented together and do have similar actions, some of them have unique properties. For this reason, we have treated several B vitamins separately.

Vitamin B-1

Vitamin B-1 or thiamine is a water-soluble vitamin. It is a constituent of an enzyme called thiamin pyrophosphate and is required for oxidative decarboxylation of alpha-keto acids. Vitamin B-1 also has a specific role aiding nerve cell function by increasing the production of neurotransmitters or brain chemical messengers important for brain function and memory. B-1 has been shown to mimic the important neurotransmitter acetylcholine, thereby increasing the overall function of the brain.

Safety: No toxicity levels have been seen with B-1. Magnesium increases the efficacy of B-1 by helping to convert thiamin into its more active form. Alcohol, diuretics, and Dilantin have been shown to decrease the effect of thiamin on the body.

Dose: 50-100 mg per day

Vitamin B-2

Vitamin B-2 or riboflavin is also a water-soluble vitamin necessary for the production of energy and the burning of fat as it helps to increase mitochondrial output.

Mitochondria are the components in muscle that are responsible for breaking down fat and generating both heat and energy. Mitochondrial output also appears to affect stress-related migraine development. Clinical studies show significant benefit to migraine sufferers through B-2 supplementation.

Apart from these metabolic benefits, B-2 is also involved in recycling glutathione, the main free radical scavenger in the body. Free radicals mediate the cell damage caused by ingested and environmental toxins. Glutathione and other molecules mop up these free radicals and protect us from damaging pollutants. Low levels of riboflavin have been associated with certain cancers, especially esophageal cancer.

Safety: No toxicity has been seen with B-2. No interactions have been seen with riboflavin and other vitamins, minerals, or pharmaceutical drugs.

Dose: 50-100 mg per day

Stress Relief

Vitamin B-1
Vitamin B-1 aids the body by releasing energy from carbohydrates more quickly. Thus fewer carbohydrates are needed and consumed, and, as a result, a stable blood sugar level is maintained more easily.

Stress Relief

Vitamin B-2
Vitamin B-2 is important in weight regulation, assisting mitochondria in breaking down fat and affecting stress-related migraine.

Stress Relief

Vitamin B-3

Vitamin B-3 increases energy levels by maximizing glucose-burning capability. It also helps lower cholesterol.

Vitamin B-3

Vitamin B-3 or niacin is used in the maintenance of blood sugar levels, in detoxification, and in the production of energy. It functions as part of two enzymes, nicotinamide adenine dinucleotide NAD) and nicotinamide adenine dinucleotide phosphate (NADP). These enzymes are part of the glycogen cycle in which glucose and fatty acids are oxidized into energy. Thus B-3 or niacin is used in the production of energy from our food.

Niacin has also been used to help lower LDL, the bad cholesterol, and other lipoproteins in the blood. Its effects are also quite long lasting, and studies show that niacin actually can provide better overall results as compared to drugs like lovastatin.

Safety: Liver toxicity can be a side effect of taking too much B-3. This is only seen in doses ranging from 2 to 6 grams per day. The most common side effect is skin flushing or heat rashes and nausea. In order to decrease this side effect, a time-released B-vitamin complex is now available. Another version of niacin exists, known as niacinamide. This is a non-flushing version of niacin with no effects on the liver when used in appropriate doses.

Dose: 30-80 mg per day

Vitamin B-6

Vitamin B-6 or pyridoxine, like the other B vitamins, is water-soluble. B-6 goes into the production of serotonin and gamma-aminobutyric acid (GABA), neurotransmitters involved in preventing stress and depression while promoting relaxation. When there is a deficit of B-6 in the body, studies on rodents reveal an increase in sympathetic outflow, creating a high stress response and increased cortisol levels. An increase in blood pressure is also observed.

One way in which B-6 decreases the stress reaction is by altering the activity of the stress receptors themselves. B-6 or pyridoxal phosphate, its active form, has been shown to interact with the glucocorticoid receptors to decrease their sensitivity and activity. Thus supplementation with B-6 blunts the stress response.

In addition, B-6 helps relieve anxiety and depression in women with high estrogen or on the birth control pill. Vitamin B-6 also helps to regulate nerve conduction, reduce tissue damage seen in diabetes, and plays an integral role in the function of the immune system. A deficiency in B-6 results in decreased production of antibodies and immune cells, such as lymphocytes.

Stress Relief

Vitamin B-6

Vitamin B-6 is known as the anti-stress, anti-depression, and anti-anxiety vitamin. Supplementation of B-6 in both rodents and humans has been shown to decrease blood pressure and reaction to stress. B-6 also combats depression, as it is necessary for the production of serotonin, our body's happy hormone.

Stress Solutions

Vitamin B-6 is utilized in the production of hemoglobin, cellular turnover, and all new protein manufacture. For this reason, B-6 is very important in pregnancy, immune regulation, and skin and mucous membrane turnover.

Safety: Vitamin B-6 has been shown to express signs of toxicity when taken in large quantities and over long periods of time. Ironically, toxic symptoms include nerve damage and loss of muscle coordination. This is seen at levels higher than 2 grams per day

Dose: 50-100 mg per day

Vitamin B-12

Vitamin B-12, also known as cyanocobalamin, functions primarily as a coenzyme. Vital for production of new DNA, it is essential for the growth of all new cells, but particularly those involved with the blood, immune, and nervous systems. B-12 is therefore is an integral part of any therapeutic program involving these areas.

Deficiency of B-12 can lead to pernicious anemia and is associated with gastric upset and peripheral nerve dysfunction. Spinal cord involvement results in impaired sensation and movement disorder.

B-12 is also important for lowering homocysteine levels in the blood. Homocysteine is an independent risk factor in heart disease, and when elevated, greatly increases the risk of stroke.

Finally, B-12 is essential for brain function. B-12 acts as a methyl donor to many compounds in the body and is thus involved in neurotransmitter production.

Safety: No toxicity levels have been seen with vitamin B-12. B-12 is intimately linked to folic acid such that a deficiency in one will lead to a deficiency in the other. Treatment is usually combined.

Dose: 50-100 mcg per day

Vitamin C

Vitamin C or ascorbic acid is a water-soluble vitamin involved in the regulation of cortisol. In one double-blind, randomized study, performed on 60 healthy adults, subjects were given either 1000 mg of vitamin C 3 times per day or a placebo. They were placed under stressful situations, including public speaking and mental arithmetic under time constraints, and monitored for blood pressure, cortisol levels, and psychological responses. Results indicated that those participants taking

Vitamin B-12
Vitamin B-12 is essential for nervous system and immune function, as well as for promoting cardiovascular health. All of these systems are compromised by chronic stress.

Vitamin C

Studies have demonstrated the ability of vitamin C to lower stress-related cortisol secretion. Vitamin C reduces stress-related allergic responses, acts as the body's primary antioxidant, defends against viral infections, and promotes production of collagen and elastin, the structural protein in bones, tendons, cartilage, and other connective tissues.

vitamin C had lower blood pressure readings, significantly faster recovery from elevated cortisol, and reported less psychological distress.

Chronic stress is implicated in the potentiation of the allergic response, including dermatitis and asthma. Vitamin C reduces the production of histamine, the chemical responsible for allergic symptoms, such as rashes, itching, hives, and bronchial constriction. Vitamin C not only decreases the production and secretion of histamine from the white blood cells in an allergic reaction, it also helps break down or destroy existing histamine. The combination of these two effects helps minimize the symptoms associated with allergies and asthma.

Antioxidant Activity

Vitamin C is the most powerful antioxidant at work in the body. Antioxidants are substances that 'mop up' free radicals, the destructive molecules produced in the body as by-products of chemical reactions, exercise, inflammation, injury, metabolism of toxins, and stress. Free radicals damage cell membranes, structural tissues, and DNA. The body fights these free radicals with antioxidants, either produced endoge-

Antioxidants

Antioxidants are essential chemicals within the body that neutralize toxins, in particular free radicals, active molecules able to inflict damage on structural proteins and DNA within cells. The most effective and universal is glutathione, a molecule synthesized from the amino acids glycine, cysteine, and glutamine. Along with other antioxidants, such as vitamins A, C, E and the mineral selenium, glutathione counteracts oxidative damage from chemicals produced by metabolism within the body and those absorbed or ingested from the environment. It also controls the free radicals used by the immune system to kill foreign protein, such as viruses.

Oxidative chemicals and free radicals only serve to increase stress on the body. In addition, chronic stress reduces the availability of certain antioxidants, particularly glutathione. Adding an antioxidant supplement is a valuable part of a stress management program. It is important to take a combination as they have different effects and act on different types of free radicals. However, a lower dose of each can be used when taken in combination due to their synergistic effect.

Antioxidant Supplements

- Vitamin A   500 IU (international units) per day
- Vitamin C   500 mg per day
- Vitamin E   100 IU per day
- Selenium   50 mcg per day
- CoQ-10   15 mg per day
- Glutathione   15 mg per day
- Lipoic Acid   10 mg per day
- Pine Bark   100 mg per day
- Grape Seed Extract   50 mg per day

nously by the body (such as glutathione) or through antioxidant supplements (vitamin C, vitamin E, selenium, and coenzyme Q-10). Vitamin C not only possesses antioxidant properties itself, but also aids in recycling and potentiating the activity of other antioxidants. Vitamin C helps to regenerate oxidized vitamin E, for example, allowing vitamin E to continue its role in free radical scavenging. Vitamin C helps to potentiate the action of glutathione and superoxide dismutase, the endogenous free radical scavengers.

The antioxidant properties of vitamin C also play a role in heart disease, helping to decrease the oxidation-induced inflammation on the lining of the blood vessels and to neutralize oxidized cholesterol in the blood, decreasing platelet aggregation. Oxidized cholesterol is much 'stickier' than non-oxidized cholesterol and therefore has a greater affinity to bind to the walls of the blood vessels and increase atherosclerosis.

Antiviral Activity
Vitamin C possesses antiviral properties. It has the ability to inhibit viral replication and, in addition, maintains the strength and integrity of the tissues that first come in contact with a virus, such as the mouth, nose, and throat. If these mucous membranes remain strong and free of inflammation, they are better able to neutralize at this level an incoming virus, such as a cold of flu virus, without allowing it to pass farther along into the body.

Vitamin C is essential for the manufacture of collagen and elastin, working with iron molecules to activate enzymes that hydroxylate the amino acids proline and lysine to complete the protein. Without strong collagen and elastin, our skin would deteriorate, gums would bleed, and wound healing would become less efficient. These are some of the many signs of scurvy, a disease of vitamin C deficiency.

Safety: In doses up to 3 grams per day, vitamin C is well tolerated with no side effects. As it is water-soluble, any excess is simply excreted in the urine and stools. However, in very high doses, for example, 10 grams per day, there are concerns with the formation of kidney stones and the development of acidosis (too much acid in the body). The evidence for these side effects is, however, inconclusive. An excess of vitamin C can lead to loose bowel movements or diarrhea. This is a sign that you need to decrease your dose. The dose at which this arises is different for each person, but usually does not occur at doses at or below 3 grams per day.

Dose: 1-3 g per day. Can be increased temporarily during infections (including colds and flu) or periods of vigorous exercise to

5 grams per day (or bowel tolerance). The daily dose has been the subject of much debate. Ingested fruits and vegetables often contain inadequate doses of vitamin C, although these amounts are reduced by other factors, such as coffee intake and exercise. Megadoses of vitamin C are recommended by some authorities (up to 10 grams per day), but evidence about the effectiveness of this regime is limited.

Minerals

Magnesium

Magnesium is the second most abundant mineral in the body. Approximately 60% of it resides in the bone, 26% in the muscle, and the remaining is distributed in the soft tissues and fluids of the body. Magnesium functions in more than 300 different enzyme reactions in the body involved in energy production, muscle contraction, and regulation of electrolytes, among many others.

Magnesium is required to control the balance of blood sugar levels and the sympathetic fight-or-flight hormones. In one study, supplementation of 400 mg per day of magnesium in non-obese, elderly individuals significantly improved glucose tolerance and insulin response to sugar.

When studied in the laboratory, cells from the adrenal medulla released more catecholamines and cortisol when they were suspended in magnesium deficient solutions. In athletes, magnesium supplementation reduces exercise-induced stress hormone release, indicating a protective and stress-modifying role for this mineral in acute stress.

Magnesium is partly responsible for any reaction in the body requiring energy. Magnesium is used to produce ATP, the body's stored and available energy source. Without sufficient magnesium, the production and use of ATP decreases greatly. ATP is required to fuel or energize almost every reaction in the body, from muscle contraction to hormone production. A lowered ATP production has significant ramifications for the body. In the case of stress, it greatly increases the adrenal response and subsequent release of catecholamines and cortisol.

Magnesium plays a large role in cardiac control and regulation. It is often referred to as nature's calcium channel blocker because of its ability to decrease vascular resistance, effectively opening up blood vessels and lowering blood pressure. However, in the presence of magnesium deficiency, stress increases risk of cardiovascular damage. This includes hypertension, coronary artery spasm, abnormal heart rhythm, and sudden cardiac death. A low magnesium-calcium ratio increases vessel constriction and promotes formation of blood clots. Low magnesium also increases constriction of the airways in the lungs in asthma.

Safety: Due to the powerful effects that magnesium can have on the heart and blood vessels, check with your health-care practitioner for the correct dose. This becomes even more important if you are on calcium channel blockers or other cardiac medications. Outside of these restrictions, magnesium is considered very safe and well tolerated by most. In very high doses relative to calcium, magnesium can soften stools.

Dose: Supplementation of magnesium is often based on weight. On average, a safe and effective dose of magnesium is 5-10 mg of magnesium per kilogram (2.2 pounds) of body weight. In a very active individual, exercising regularly and utilizing magnesium stores for muscle contraction and repair, a higher dose (10 mg/kg of body weight) is recommended.
It is recommended that a combined magnesium-calcium supplement be used as the two minerals complement each other with regards to function. For calcium, the recommended dose is 1000-1500 mg per day.

Calcium

Calcium is the most abundant mineral in the body, constituting up to 2% of our entire body weight. While the majority of calcium lies within the bones, this mineral is essential for many reactions in the body that take place outside of the bones.

Calcium's best-known function is the role it plays in the prevention and treatment of osteoporosis, the thinning of the bones that leads to an increase risk of fractures. Since 15% to 20% of hip fractures result in fatal complications, the maintenance of bone density becomes very important. The main mineral lost from bone in osteoporosis is calcium. Without it, bone loses density and strength. Insufficient intake of calcium in the diet impairs bone formation in younger individuals and increases loss in older people.

Calcium also plays an integral role in the regulation of blood pressure. Studies have shown a direct correlation between low blood calcium levels and high blood pressure. The mechanism behind this is two-fold. First, calcium works with magnesium and potassium to regulate fluid levels within the blood vessels themselves. Second, calcium aids in the muscular control of small blood vessels. By allowing relaxation of the wall muscles, size is increased, thereby lowering blood pressure. In pregnancy, calcium is used in higher doses not only to provide building material for the bones of the fetus, but to prevent preeclampsia (very high blood pressure during pregnancy).

Calcium is also used to enhance muscle control and repair. Calcium works in tandem with magnesium to improve contractility and therefore muscle strength. Calcium and magnesium are also responsible for muscle relaxation. Together, these two minerals play a vital role in prevention of muscle cramping, injury, and pain.

Safety: Calcium is generally a very safe mineral. When taken in very high doses for a long period of time (2 to 3 grams) there is a risk of developing kidney stones and calcium deposits in the muscle or soft tissues. Because the parathyroid controls the movement and use of calcium in the body, individuals with a parathyroid disorder should consult a health-care practitioner before supplementing with calcium. Calcium absorption is decreased by caffeine, soda pop or other carbonated drinks, stress, high levels of protein and sugar, and increased exercise.

Dose: 1000-1500 mg per day

Herbs

Magnolia Bark

Magnolia bark (*Magnolia officinalis*) is a traditional Chinese medicine herb used since 100 AD for treating what the Chinese refer to as blocked or stagnated qi or chi (pronounced "chee"). Qi in Chinese medicine is the energy and life force of the body. When qi is blocked, it causes symptoms such as low energy, emotional distress or anxiety, digestive complaints, dizziness, and alterations in the sleep cycle. In Western medicine, this would equal chronic stress and fatigue.

Magnolia bark contains many different therapeutic compounds, the two most often used and studied being the biphenols called magnolol and honokiol. However, other ingredients such as beta-Eudesmol and bornyl acetate have also proven to have great therapeutic potential. These ingredients possess anxiolytic or anxiety-reducing properties.

The use of magnolia for stress reduction has been clinically evaluated in several different studies. One study examined a crude extract from magnolia bark containing all four ingredients. The study was performed in a lab setting on cells extracted from bovine adrenal gland. Stressors were placed on the adrenal cells through the application of high-dose potassium. Potassium in this setting depolarizes the cell membrane, mimicking stress. The production of catecholamines (our fight-or-flight sympathetic hormones) was then monitored. Following this, each of the four magnolia ingredients was added to the cells and once again the levels of the stress catecholamines measured. All four ingredients had an inhibitory effect on catecholamine production, with honokiol and bornyl acetate producing the greatest reduction in stress hormones. The results of this study indicate that the inhibitory effect of magnolia bark may be associated with its pharmacological effects on the nervous system.

Another study performed on mice also displayed the therapeutic benefits of magnolia in conjunction with other natural herbs. A combined formula of magnolia, ginger (*Zingiber officinalis*), *Perila frutescens*, and *Poria cocos* was given to stressed mice. The antidepressant and anti-stress effects of this complex of herbs was shown to produce near identical relief of symptoms to that of administered Prozac.

Magnolia has also been found to possess potent antiallergy properties. Administration of magnolia bark extract to rats significantly reduced IgE (allergy-mediating immunoglobulin) and histamine production during an induced allergic reaction. In addition, there was also a decrease in antitumor necrosis factor production (tumor necrosis factor being the major antiviral and antitumor immune cell). This reaction was seen both *in vitro* (isolated rat cells in the lab) and *in vivo* (in the live rat).

Safety: No side effects have been seen with magnolia bark extract. In some people who are used to the stress 'high', fatigue may ensue for the first couple of days. It is important to note that this is not sedation, but rather a return to normal energy levels, not the falsely elevated energy levels we often refer to as an adrenaline high.

Dose: For the average 140-150 pound adult, 125-200 mg of extract three times per day on an empty stomach

Passionflower

Passionflower (*Passiflora incarnata*) has been used medicinally for centuries, as a sedative by the Aztecs and as an antispasmotic and anxiolytic stress reliever by Europeans. Some of the first clinical studies were performed in Italy, where passionflower was observed to decrease brain excitation and prolong sleeping hours with no adverse side effects. In France, a multicenter study of anxious patients was carried out to evaluate a plant extract containing botanicals, including passionflower. The group taking the plant extract had significantly greater improvement in symptoms than the group taking a placebo.

Stress Relief

Magnolia Bark
In both traditional Chinese and Western medical traditions, magnolia bark is used as a general anti-stress and antianxiety herb. The anxiolytic or stress-relieving effects of magnolia have often been equated with the effects of benzodiazepines such as Valium, a pharmaceutical antianxiety drug. However, benzodiazepines can cause sedation that makes daytime activities quite difficult.

Magnolia bark extracts do not have any of the sedating or sleepy qualities. Although most people do sleep more soundly when taking them, it is an indirect effect through cortisol reduction rather than direct sedation. In this way, magnolia becomes a very important agent in the treatment of panic disorders, anxiety, and stress.

A further double-blind, randomized, controlled study in 2001 compared passionflower directly to a pharmaceutical antianxiety drug, Oxazepam, in 36 patients with anxiety disorder. There was no significant difference between groups with respect to anxiety reduction, but the passionflower group demonstrated far less sedation and impairment of daily function.

Safety: While drowsiness or sedation is rare, it can occur in some individuals in higher doses (over 750 mg per day). If you are affected, caution is recommended when driving or operating machinery. There is one case report of heart arrhythmia in self-medicating patient taking a high dose.

Dose: 250-1000 mg of dried herb per day. Passionflower is most frequently prescribed in combination with other herbs.

Hops

Hops (*Humulus lupulus*) has been an essential part of the brewing industry for decades, making it by far the most commonly used herb ever. Much of the sedating and relaxing effect of beer is due to hops.

Safety: Hops is an allergenic herb and has resulted in acute respiratory distress and skin rashes in those sensitive to it. It should not be given to people with depression due to its hypnotic effects. Hops has also been shown to have a slight estrogenic effect and therefore can disrupt menstrual cycles. It should not be used in pregnant women or those with estrogen sensitive cancers.

Dose: 250-500 mg before bed

Valerian

Valerian (*Valeriana officinalis*) has been historically used as a sedative, anticonvulsant, and muscle relaxant. Research has shown its effect to be mediated in part by interaction with the gamma-aminobutryic acid (GABA) and serotonin neurotransmitter pathways in the brain. Valerian also appears to inhibit the breakdown of GABA, increasing availability of this relaxing chemical. It may react with the GABA-A receptor, the site of action of benzodiazepines such as diazepam (Valium).

Safety: Valerian is contraindicated in children under 3 years of age and should not be used in pregnant women. Valerian should not be used in combination with other pharmaceuticals affecting GABA, such as the benzodiazepine family or other central nervous system depressants. Always advise your doctor, surgeon or anesthetist if you are taking this supplement.

Dose: 500-800 mg before bed

St. John's Wort

St. John's wort (*Hypericum perforatum*) has a long history of use starting with Hippocrates and Galen, who originally used it for wound healing and pain. Today, St. John's wort is used extensively for its effects on mood and emotion.

St. John's wort has several different properties, but the two main actions are as an antidepressant and as an antiviral. There are two main active ingredients responsible for these effects, hypericin and isohypericin.

Antidepressant

St. John's wort has a clear pharmacological effect on a number of neurotransmitters in the brain. It prevents re-uptake of serotonin, GABA, dopamine, and noradrenaline, potentiating the effects of these chemical messengers. GABA is the main inhibitory neurotransmitter of the brain and central nervous system. St. John's wort, by increasing GABA activity, decreases nervous stimulation, induces relaxation, and provides some sedative effect. Serotonin activity is reduced in depression. By effectively slowing the re-uptake of this neuro-transmitter, St. John's wort prolongs its activity. The role of serotonin in anxiety remains unclear, but relates to the relative activity of a specific receptor (the 5-HTP 1A receptor).

Clinical studies reveal that St. John's wort is useful in the treatment of mild to moderate depression. Of importance, is that this occurs without the alterations in sleep and EEG (electroencephalography) patterns that normally accompany pharmaceutical tricyclic antidepressants. In several studies, St. John's wort was very well tolerated and patients reported no side effects. In patients taking St. John's wort, there was a 60% reduction in depressive agitation and anxiety, with a 43% reduction in sleep disorders. In a comparison group receiving the antidepressant fluoxetine, only a 40% reduction in these symptoms was observed. St. John's wort was much better tolerated than the pharmaceutical fluoxetine.

Studies performed on rats evaluated how the animals performed in a maze and how much time was spent in different sections of the maze, a test used to determine the levels of stress felt by each rat. This was then compared to other stress symptoms, such as gastric ulceration, adrenal gland weight, and spleen weight. As stress increases, so does the weight of the adrenal gland, as it is the stress organ and

St. John's Wort
St. John's wort is effective not only in control of mild depression, but also in the treatment of anxiety. This is achieved without the common side effects experienced with many psychotropic drugs. There are, however, significant interactions with a number of pharmaceutical drugs and anesthetics.

must increase production of hormone and function when under stress. The spleen is an immune organ and should therefore decrease in weight under stress, as the stress hormones secreted inhibit the production of various immune factors. Following a 14-day study, several factors were noted. The first was an increase in adrenal gland weight and a decrease in spleen weight, indicating the activation of the stress response and inhibition of the immune system. Increased gastric ulceration was also seen. In addition, a significant reduction in learning was seen, accompanied by both anxious and depressive behavior, both inside and outside of the maze and a decrease in sexual activity. The rats that received St. John's wort before entering the maze demonstrated a significant reduction in all anxiety symptoms and quantitatively less increase in adrenal weight or reduction in spleen size.

Side Effects: Although there are very few incidences of reported side effects with St. John's wort, a few symptoms have been seen. These often occur after prolonged use at high doses (over 6 months with 500 to 600 mg, 4 times per day). These symptoms include photosensitivity, constipation, dry mouth, and gastric irritation.

St. John's Wort should not be used in conjunction with other pharmaceutical drugs as it may alter their action or efficacy. These drugs include the MAOIs, SSRIs, dibenzazepine derivatives like amitriptyline, the sympathomimetics like amphetamines and ephedrine, and foods high in tyramine. St. John's wort has only been studied on mild and moderate anxiety and depression and not severe or suicidal depression.

Dose: 250-400 mg, 3 times per day when the extract is standardized to 0.3% hypericin. It is best to take St. John's wort on an empty stomach since food will decrease the rate and amount of active ingredient delivered to the body.

Kava Kava

Kava kava (*Piper methysticum*) has been used in the treatment of anxiety and stress since the 18th century when the British explorer James Cook first discovered its benefits in the South Pacific.

The main active ingredients in kava are the kavalactones. They have shown to have a particular attraction toward the GABA and benzodiazepine receptors (the relaxing and, more importantly, sedating receptors), although this is still under debate. Kava kava has also been shown to induce EEG changes that resemble the effect of diazepams (antianxiety drugs). In addition, Kava has displayed anticonvulsant activity by

Kava Kava

Kava kava has very significant anti-stress and antianxiety effects that may be employed with caution in a stress-reduction program.

blocking the sodium ion channels that create the increased voltage in the brain. This, in turn, brings about feelings of calmness and relaxation.

Recent studies have revealed the anti-stress qualities of kava kava. One study performed on rats showed that kava had a similar anxiolytic behavior to that of diazepam. Several other studies investigating the efficacy of kava kava in the treatment of anxiety displayed its positive anxiolytic properties. The reviews concluded that kava kava extract is superior to the placebo in the treatment of anxiety and is a very safe option to consider.

Side Effects: Following excessive consumption (5 to 6 times the recommended dose), some skin irritation and scaling has been seen. Slight dizziness and grogginess have also been reported. This herb has been banned in several countries, including Canada, due to concerns with respect to liver toxicity. For those with liver damage or a family history of liver damage, discussion with your health-care professional is recommended before use.

Dose: 50-100 mg of kava extract standardized to 70% kavalactones, 2-3 times per day on an empty stomach.

Lavender

Lavender (*Lavendula angustifolia)* is one of the most versatile herbs used in an oil form. Traditionally, it was used for its impressive healing qualities that stems from the natural antibiotic and antiseptic (cleaning) qualities of lavender. Recently, lavender has been shown to improve and promote sleep, decrease the activity of the nervous system, reduce anxiety and depression, and improve moods.

Although there is little scientific data to support the benefits of lavender, there is a great deal of subjective evidence. One study examined 17 patients with cancer living in a hospice. These patients were treated with the essential oil of lavender infused in a humidifier on 3 different days before treatments. They were assessed for levels of pain, anxiety, depression, and sense of well-being, as well as physical changes, such as blood pressure and pulse. The results demonstrated a positive, although small, change in blood pressure and pulse, but a large change in anxiety, depression, well-being, and pain as compared to the days where only water was administered in the humidifier.

A similar study examined the EEG activity, alertness, and mood of 40 healthy adults following the use of lavender oil extracts. Participants were given mathematical equations to perform before and after a 3-minute treatment with lavender.

As a control, one group received a 3-minute placebo treatment. The group receiving lavender displayed increased beta-wave activity on the EEG, indicating increased sedation and relaxation. This was confirmed by their verbal reports of feeling less depressed, more relaxed, and generally better overall. In addition, their math scores were better. Not only did they complete the mathematical equations faster, but they were also more accurate with their computations.

Side Effects: Although side effects are rarely seen with lavender oil, some people may experience an allergic reaction on the skin to the oil. This usually only occurs if the dose is too strong or the oil is applied directly to the skin without blending it with a neutral massage oil. In very rare cases, nausea, headaches, and chills have been reported. It is not clear whether lavender is safe during breastfeeding or pregnancy, so it should be avoided during these times, for fear of uterine stimulation. Because lavender can affect the central nervous system, people taking medications that also affect the same area, such as diazepam and lorazepam, should consult their health-care practitioner before extensive use of lavender oil.

Dose: Lavender is most often used topically in an essential oil: 1-4 drops are used, massaged gently into the skin. When used as an inhalant, 2-4 drops may be added to 3 cups of boiling water and infused in a vaporizer. As a tincture (liquid oral form), 20-40 drops up to 3 times per day in warm water to be sipped.

Amino Acids

Theanine (Green Tea)
Theanine or L-theanine is an amino acid commonly found in the leaves of green tea.

Traditionally, theanine was used as a flavoring agent, but after discovering its ability to counteract the stimulatory effects of caffeine, its use as a therapeutic substance was investigated. In one study, rats were given caffeine regularly and their brain waves monitored using EEG. Following administration of caffeine, the brain-wave pattern of the EEG indicated significant excitation at minimal doses. The subsequent administration of theanine reversed the stimulatory effects of caffeine, returning the EEG to normal.

The relaxing effect of theanine is due to an increase in alpha waves, one of the four main types of brain-wave activity. Alpha waves represent a 'relaxed alertness'. There is no sedating effect, only relaxation, with theanine. This, too, has been clinically demonstrated. The higher the administered dose of theanine, the greater the alpha-wave response. Q waves (related to sedation and doziness) in both groups remained unchanged at all doses.

L-theanine also stimulates production of gamma-aminobutyric acid (GABA), a neurotransmitter that inhibits the release of dopamine and serotonin and promotes relaxation.

In addition to relaxation, L-theanine is observed to lower blood pressure in hypertensive rats.

Theanine has other beneficial properties, including action as an antioxidant with chemotherapeutic effects. Free radicals have the potential to bind to the DNA of any cell, causing cell damage, cell death, or potentially cancerous mutation. Theanine has the interesting property of increasing the delivery of chemotherapeutic drugs to tumors. Early studies show that by combining theanine with doxorubicin (a chemo drug), tumor weight could be halved due to the effects of the drug alone. This result was not seen when the theanine was not given simultaneously. Theanine appears to selectively carry the drug to the tumor cells, leaving the healthy cells alone.

Safety: No side effects or toxic levels of theanine have been reported. Studies on the effects of theanine indicate that its effect is blunted by simultaneous ingestion of caffeine. Therefore, a decaffeinated green tea product is recommended.

Dose: 100-300 mg, 3 times per day, depending on stress levels

Milk Peptide Hydrolysate

Milk contains a high concentration of peptides or chains of amino acids. An infant's enzyme system is very immature and has only a trace amount of pepsin, the enzyme that breaks down many of these peptides. Because they do not break down, larger peptide chains result. The trypsin hydrolysate decapeptide is one particular sequence of amino acids that is 10 units or amino acids long found in milk and has been shown to possess strong anxiolytic properties. This may account for the soothing effect mother's milk has on the child, beyond satisfying the stressful situation of being hungry.

In adults with high levels of pepsin, the small amount of this peptide found in normal milk is rapidly broken down. However, by increasing the ingested concentration above pepsin capacity, adults will also absorb some of the anxiolytic decapeptide.

Therapeutic Activity

Clinical research has revealed how this milk breakdown product exerts its therapeutic activity. One study looked at 24 healthy volunteers (12 men and 12 women). They were evaluated according to the Cattell Anxiety Scale under stressful circumstances with and without the consumption of this protein peptide. A comparative, randomized, double-blind, controlled study was employed. Subjects had to complete mental tasks, rapidity tests, and anxiety questionnaires while being monitored for blood pressure, heart rate, cortisol, and ACTH levels, in addition to their test performance. The study revealed that when the subjects performed the tests following ingestion of the protein peptide, their scores improved greatly. In addition, they noticed that the cortisol levels did not rise as high, and that their ACTH levels did not change. When they took the tests without the peptide, their cortisol levels rose, as did their ACTH. Blood pressure remained lower following use of the peptide, while heart rate remained unchanged.

Other studies revealed that the protein peptide exhibited diazepam-like effects on stress responsiveness of the HPA axis. It has been speculated that decapeptide binding into the GABA receptor is not complete — that is, it does not act equally at all receptor sites. The sites that are not filled are those responsible for sedation. This may be why benzodiazepines, such as diazepam, which fill all receptors, have a strong sedative effect, while the protein peptide does not.

Safety: To date, there are no side effects known with protein decapeptides.

Dose: 150-200 mg, 2 times per day

5-HTP

5-HTP or 5-hydroxytryptophan is the molecule converted in the brain to serotonin, one of our most important neurotransmitters. Serotonin pathways are responsible for control of mood, hunger, sleep, and aggression. Abnormalities in functioning of this system are found in depression, anxiety, and other psychological conditions.

The work of many scientists over the past two decades has shown that serotonin is a daytime neurotransmitter responsible for mood (anxiety and depression), impulse control, pain control, and obsessive behaviors. Serotonin is also the precursor to the production of our sleeping hormone, melatonin, in the pineal gland. Human clinical studies have revealed that not only does a decrease in serotonin induce a poor sleep, but that sleep patterns are greatly improved following supplementation with 5-HTP.

Normally, 5-HTP is synthesized from tryptophan, an amino acid or breakdown product of protein, with the help of vitamin B-3. A further step under the influence of vitamin B-6 then completes the conversion to 5-HTP. Tryptophan is readily

Stress Relief

5-HTP

5-HTP helps to induce relaxation by increasing the production of serotonin and dopamine, and by suppressing noradrenaline activity. 5-HTP is very useful in promoting proper sleep and relieving both anxiety and depression.

broken down by the liver or used as a protein building block for hormones, muscles, and other tissues in the body. Only what is left over is then converted into 5-HTP. If there is deficiency in tryptophan, there is a subsequent deficit in 5-HTP and serotonin. A high carbohydrate meal increases available tryptophan in the blood by raising insulin and promoting rapid transfer of glucose and other amino acids into the tissues. This leaves a relative excess of tryptophan, which can then be converted to 5-HTP and serotonin. This is thought to be the basis of the reassuring euphoria associated with candy or ice cream! A similar, though more soporific, effect is gained from eating foods high in tryptophan, such as turkey.

Side Effects: Despite the fact that 5-HTP already naturally exists in the body, occasional upset stomach or increased abnormal euphoria can be seen at high doses (200 mg, 2 times per day). 5-HTP can interfere with MAO inhibitors, tricyclic antidepressants, and SSRIs, such as Prozac, Paxil, and Zoloft. 5-HTP supplementation should be avoided when on these medications.

Dose: 50-100 mg twice per day. Taking tryptophan as a supplement, rather than 5-HTP, does not seem to work that well, as it is only partially converted to 5-HTP and other by-products may be harmful. In addition, it does not pass easily into the brain. By taking 5-HTP orally, the conversion is bypassed and this molecule transfers easily through the blood-brain barrier, a filter around the brain that acts as a protective barrier, allowing only certain substances through. In addition, as opposed to tryptophan, 5-HTP is not used to make any other proteins in the body, so there is no competition for it outside the brain.

Other Anti-Stress Supplements

Essential Fatty Acids
The fats that are actually good for us are known as essential fatty acids (EFAs). EFAs come in a variety of different shapes and sizes, and they perform a multitude of different functions in the body. For instance, fats surround each cell in the body and act as a barrier, protecting the cell from metabolic toxins and allowing hormones and enzymes to bind to it. Fats are also an energy source for the body.

The relative ratio of the various kinds of EFAs in the body is crucial in the production of prostaglandins. Prostaglandins are hormone-like substances that are important in the regulation of many bodily functions, such as blood pressure, pain, inflammation, swelling, allergic reactions, blood clotting, and more.

Essential fatty acids are also of vital importance in the maintenance and integrity of the myelin sheath that covers most nerves. EFAs are natural anti-inflammatories that also have stool-softening effects to help regulate the bowel movements without the stimulation of laxatives.

Types of Essential Fatty Acids

There are four main types of essential fatty acids: omega-3, omega-6, omega-7, and omega-9. These are unsaturated fats, meaning they have one or more double bonds connecting their chemical structure. It is this double-bond property that allows them to interact with other substances in the body.

Omega-3 Essential Fatty Acids: Omega-3 fats are broken down into three different groups. The first are alpha-linoleic acids, found in flaxseeds, hemp seeds, canola, soy, walnuts, and dark green leaves. The second group are stearidonic acids found in black currants. The final group, eicosapentaenoic acids, are found in cold-water fish like salmon, mackerel, sardines, and trout.

Omega-6 Essential Fatty Acids: Omega-6 fats are also broken down into three different groups. The first group is the linoleic acids (LAs), found in safflower, sunflower, hemp, soybean, pumpkin, and sesame. The second group, gamma-linolenic acids (GLAs), are found in borage oils, evening primrose oil, and black currant seed oil. The final group of omega-6 fatty acids are the arachidonic acids found in meats and other animal byproducts.

Omega-7/9 Essential Fatty Acids: Omega-7 is found in coconut and palm oils. These fatty acids do not play a crucial role in the treatment of inflammation, back pain, and arthritis. Omega-9 fats are also called oleic acids and are widely abundant in olives, almonds, avocados, peanuts, cashews, and macadamia oils.

EFA Balance

The main goal of essential fatty acid supplementation is to decrease the production of arachidonic acid and increase the production of eicosapentaenoic (EPA) and dihomo-gamma-linoleic acids (DHGLA). These latter two are the final products of omega-3 fatty acids and omega-6 fatty acids, respectively. The important issue, then, becomes achieving the correct balance of different fats in the body in order to decrease inflammation. The most favorable ratio of omega-6 to omega-3 essential fatty acids is approximately 4:1. However, it is important to note that most dressings and oils in the grocery store contain omega-6 oils. Thus, many people are already consuming it in high quantities. In fact, many people are consuming a ratio of 15:1 of omega-6 to omega-3 fatty acids. The most viable solution is to increase the omega-3 fatty acids. This is easily achieved by consuming more flaxseed oil, which has a relative ratio of 1:3 of omega-6 to omega-3 fatty acids.

Safety: Essential fatty acids are very safe. There is no real toxicity level associated with them. However, they can cause some gastrointestinal changes, such as belching, after consumption and loose stools when the dose is too high. If you already have loose stools, it is advisable to drop the dose in half.

Many essential fats come from cold-water fish, so it important to ensure that you are not allergic to these sources. Fish oil supplementation can have an effect on blood clotting. In high doses, it can slightly thin the blood and should therefore be used with caution if you are taking blood-thinning medication, such as warfarin, heparin or high-dose aspirin. If you are predisposed to easy bleeding and are on high doses of other vitamins that can contribute to thinning of the blood, such as vitamin E and C, then you should consult a health-care practitioner to determine the correct dose for you before starting essential fatty acid supplementation.

Dose: In order to determine which fatty acid supplementation is best for you, it is important to consider all the different fats already in your diet. If you generally follow a very low-fat diet, then you should consider a mixed essential fatty acid supplement that contains both omega-6 and 3, with a slightly higher concentration of omega-3 to counteract the hidden omega-6 fatty acids that will undoubtedly exist in your diet.

Stress-Related Bowel Disorder Supplements

These supplements can be used for stress-related peptic ulcer disease, irritable bowel syndrome, and inflammatory bowel disease.

Slippery Elm, Marshmallow, and Cabbage

These demulcent herbs help soothe irritated and inflamed mucous membranes such as the bowel.

Dose: 250 mg of each, 2 times per day

Acidophilus (Probiotic)

Acidophilus is a natural 'good' bacteria that normally inhabits the gut, regulating pH levels and controlling the growth of 'bad' bacteria.

Dose: 2 capsules (10 billion bacteria per cap) per day on an empty stomach

Digestive Enzymes

Digestive enzymes can be taken as a supplement. Capsules contain a full spectrum of enzymes normally produced by the stomach, pancreas, and liver to aid in the digestive breakdown of proteins, carbohydrates, and fats.

Dose: 1-3 capsules per meal

Immune System Supplements

These supplements can be used for stress-related immune compromise and viral infections, low CG syndrome, allergies, and skin conditions.

Oregano Oil

Oregano oil is a natural antimicrobial herb that helps fight viruses, bacteria, yeast, fungus, and parasites in the body.

Dose: 30 drops, 2 to 3 times per day

Olive Leaf Extract

Olive leaf extract is a natural antiviral that helps to decrease the replication of viruses and increases production of the antibodies that fight viruses. This can be used on a long-term basis without overstimulating or fatiguing the immune system.

Dose: 500 mg, 1-3 times per day

Activated Whey Protein (HMS-90 or ImmunePro)

Activated whey protein is a milk peptide containing cysteine that increases the production of glutathione, an amino acid vital to effective functioning of the immune system.

Dose: 5 grams per day

Zinc

Zinc is a mineral that promotes wound healing throughout the body and supports the integrity of mucous membranes in the throat, nose, and gut. It also has antiviral properties.

Dose: 25 mg per day

Quercitin

Quercitin is a bioflavonoid extracted from citrus fruits. It acts to stabilize mast cells to decrease histamine release and control the allergic reaction.

Dose: 500 mg, 2 times per day

Weight-Management Supplements

Garcinia Cambogia

Garcinia cambogia is a herb that has been shown to inhibit the formation of fat from food (lipogenesis).

Dose: 350 mg, 30 minutes before a meal

Citrus Aurantium

Citrus aurantium is a herb that helps mobilize fat to be burned more easily without any stimulation.

Dose: 150 mg, 30 minutes before a meal

Conjugated Linoleic Acid

Conjugated linoleic acid is a fatty acid that prevents the breakdown of muscle during dieting and stress and only allows the body to utilize fat as a fuel source.

Dose: 2000 mg per day

Sleep Supplements

Melatonin

Melatonin is the 'sleeping' hormone of the body produced in the pineal gland. It regulates our sleep-wake cycle.

Dose: 4 mg before bed

Pain Supplements

Capsicum

Most forms of capsicum are administered through a cream and applied topically over the affected painful area. The skin is supplied with many small nerve branches that then lead back to the main 'trunks' of the nerve. When capsicum is applied to a nerve branch, substance-P, released from nerve fibers in response to pain, is depleted simultaneously in all connecting branches.

Side Effects: The main side effect experienced with capsicum is a redness, irritation, and initial burning of the skin. This generally only lasts for a few minutes after application, and will subside with each following application until it is no longer experienced.

Caution: Do not use on damaged, inflamed, or broken skin.

Dose: Creams generally range from 0.025% up to 0.075% of capsicum. It is wise to start with a lower concentration cream and slowly build up as needed.

Anti-Stress Exercise Therapies

The Stress-Relieving Power of Exercise

At 45 years of age, Gordon was found to have high blood pressure, high cholesterol, and borderline diabetes at his yearly physical. He had already started the naturopathic diet, but had never been involved with any form of regular exercise. He also reported feeling stressed both at work and at home. He was having trouble sleeping through the night.

The first problem we encountered was trying to fit an exercise routine into his hectic life, but he agreed that his health was important enough to make some serious priority decisions. He agreed to commit to 30 minutes of exercise, three times per week. This could include activities like Tai chi that incorporated a relaxation component. In addition, he would do 30 more minutes of relaxation work, 2 days a week. He used walking meditation, yoga, and deep breathing for his relaxation program.

We started him on our Exercise Program for Beginners but he was able to progress to the Intermediate Program after only 6 weeks. He bought some simple weights and a fitness ball for use at home, thus adding a component of strength training and core conditioning (which incidentally greatly improved his grumbling back discomfort!).

Gordon currently has normal blood pressure and blood sugar. His cholesterol is almost back to a level where it poses no risk to his health. He reports feeling fitter, more energetic, less stressed, and sleeps soundly most nights.

Exercise is beneficial not only for weight reduction and cardiovascular health, but also for stress management. The runner's 'high' that entices individuals to head out in the early hours of a mid-winter morning can have a very therapeutic effect on the body. Fortunately, you do not need to run 5 miles at 6:00 a.m. in temperatures well below freezing to achieve this wonderful sensation. The chemical alterations that occur can happen at any hour of the day, but do require at least 30 minutes of exercise to achieve them. Not all people experience it, and the time required for hormonal alterations to occur can vary between individuals.

Exercise Basics

Before starting any exercise program, you should consult your health-care practitioner. It is also very important that you

Stress Solutions

perform each exercise properly. If you exercise with an incorrect technique, you may do yourself more harm than good. And do start slowly. If you have exercised in the past, but have been inactive for the past few years, do not expect your body to be capable of returning to the exercises you were doing before at the same intensity. This, too, increases your risk of harm or injury, from both cardiovascular and musculoskeletal perspectives. Start slowly, and build from there. Don't get discouraged! You should anticipate a 6-month program to reach the state of fitness you desire and to help restore balance or homeostasis to your stress response system.

Program Components

Whatever type of exercise program you choose, it should involve three main components: stretching, strength training, and cardiovascular exercise. Ideally, you should perform stretching exercises daily and alternate strength training with cardiovascular exercise from day to day.

When you perform the same exercise over and over again, the muscles become very efficient. Thus, you will reach a point where you are actually burning fewer calories and gaining less strength, despite performing the same actions at the same rate of intensity. By alternating the type of exercise you perform and the level of intensity, you can increase the amount of work performed during the same amount of time. Second, it is important to alternate the muscle groups that you use. By exercising the same muscles over and over again, you can inflame, irritate, and weaken them, leaving them more susceptible to injury or harm. A muscle group needs 48 hours of rest. You can still exercise every day, just alternate muscle groups. For example, upper body one day, lower body the next.

You will get a better work out by varying the type of cardio and weight program, alternating running, cycling, and swimming, as well as changing exercises for certain muscle groups. If you really love one type of cardiovascular work, then you can vary the intensity of that workout. For instance, if you love to run, then instead of simply running 30 to 40 minutes at the same pace each time you go running, change your program around, running hills one day, small sprints with interval rests the next.

By alternating the type of exercises you do and the muscle groups you use, you will strengthen a wider variety of muscles, while giving each muscle group time to recover and rest. There is great truth to the adage "It is the rest that makes you strong." Easy-to-follow exercise programs are described here and can be expanded with the help of a personal trainer.

Exercise-Induced Hormonal Changes

During exercise, several highly beneficial changes take place in the endocrine system that counteract the dangerous effects of the chronic stress response.

1. Growth Hormone (GH): Within the first 2 to 5 minutes of exercise, there is an increase in GH, the body's anti-aging hormone. Growth hormone helps to burn fat and release energy, build more muscle and improve sleep.

2. Endorphins: After 25 to 30 minutes of exercise, other changes occur in the group of hormones called endorphins, chiefly dopamine and serotonin. Dopamine induces feelings of relaxation, and serotonin — our 'happy' hormone — increases a sense of overall well-being and happiness. In addition to these hormones, a sub-unit of endorphins known as enkephalins is released. Enkephalins are similar to morphine and produce a euphoric state or 'high'. As enkephalins are not identical to morphine, they do not have the adverse side effects of constipation and lack of mental control and awareness.

3. Alpha Waves: An increase in alpha-wave brain activity is seen after exercise. Alpha waves bring about relaxation. This is the brain-wave activity present before sleep or felt during various forms of relaxation therapy.

Exercise Options

When doing any exercise program, it is important to choose exercises that you like. If you hate every step on the treadmill, get off and ride the bike. If you don't like exercising indoors, then head outside. If you don't like exercising alone, then grab a friend and join a class or set a date to work out regularly together. Whatever your style of exercise, it is important that you enjoy it. This does not mean that you will look forward to it each and every day, especially at the beginning. However, as you progress through the workout schedule and start to see and feel the positive effects, you will start to enjoy the workouts most of the time, and even miss performing them if circumstances arise.

Your body may be sore after a workout. This is normal. There are inflammatory waste products that can build up in muscles after a workout. This sensation will decrease as your body gets used to working out regularly. Stretching, drinking more water, and increasing your circulation with gentle walking the day after will help to lessen this buildup. If at any time you feel a sudden, sharp or unusual pain during movement, stop exercising. If the pain is severe or persistent, see your doctor to ensure that you have not sustained a significant injury.

Stretching Exercises

Make sure you warm up before you stretch! Trying to lengthen a cold muscle is difficult, painful, and may cause injury. A short period of aerobic activity may suffice, or try a hot shower, sauna, or hot tub.

No matter what area of the body you are stretching, in order to increase flexibility and elasticity of the muscles, ligaments and tendons, you need to push a stretch to the furthest possible range of motion. There should be no pain involved with the stretching process. Take the stretch just to the point before it hurts and hold it for 60 seconds. Ease into it slowly and don't bounce while stretching, just hold. There may be some discomfort (not pain) involved in this at first, and it may take weeks to months before you can take a stretch to its full range. However, if you keep working at it, each time you stretch, you will take the stretch a little bit further.

In order to determine how much discomfort you should endure before causing injury, use correct posture and motion through the stretch as your guide. For example, if you have to bend a nearby joint, like the knee, in order to move that hamstring stretch a little further, then you are compromising the stretch and risking injury. Go as far as you can in the correct position without having to compensate in another area of the body when you push further.

Stretching is one area where 'no pain, no gain' is a bad slogan to follow. While a good stretch should induce some bearable discomfort, pain is an indicator that you are not sufficiently warmed up and are beyond your current ability range.

Stretching is often relegated to the last few minutes of a workout. This is probably the biggest mistake you can make. An adequate stretch program should comprise at least 15 to 20 minutes.

Benefits of Stretching

1. Reduces risk of injury during exercise or other activity.

2. Improves muscle function.

3. Prevents muscle 'tightness' with associated postural compromise.

4. Increases muscle blood flow and clears metabolic waste products.

5. Valuable exercise for relaxation and stress relief.

Exercise Pace

With any exercise program, start at your own pace. As long as your heart and breathing rate are elevated, the speed or intensity does not matter. As your fitness improves week by week, your strength will build and your pace will naturally increase. You can also increase the intensity of many of the workouts simply by exercising on an incline (up hill) or increasing the resistance of the machine (gears on bike).

Note: It is recommended that you have a full physical examination by your doctor before starting a new exercise program.

Stretches Most Useful for Stress Reduction

There are seven main types of stretching: static stretching, active stretching, dynamic stretching, passive stretching, isometric stretching, proprioceptive neuromuscular facilitation, and ballistic stretching. They vary in their intensity and complexity, some requiring a second individual to assist.

In order to determine which type of stretch is best suited for you, seek out advice from a trainer or health-care worker. If you have exercised and stretched in the past, start slowly on your own. Begin with the easier stretches, such as the static, active, and dynamic stretches. These are the ones most appropriate for relaxation and stress relief.

Static Stretching

Static stretching is the simplest type of stretch. The muscle or joint is taken through a slow and controlled range of movement until the limitations in the muscle or joint are reached. The stretch is held for a minimum of 15 seconds and for up to 30 seconds, if possible. In order to achieve this, the muscle group or joint is not pushed quite as far as it is in active stretching.

The stretch is performed slowly, in a controlled manner, with enough support to ensure that no sudden movement occurs.

Active Stretching

Active stretching is probably the most popular and best-known form of stretching. It involves stretching the muscle to the limits of motion and then holding that position for a short period of time, around 10 to 15 seconds. The stretch is held 'actively' by the individual whose muscles are being stretched, rather than having another person hold the limb in position. This active contraction in the opposing muscle groups actually helps relax the muscles being stretched. It is a more aggressive stretch than the static stretch and is used to increase flexibility and to strengthen opposing muscles.

This type of stretch is best used after exercise as a warm-down.

Dynamic Stretching

Dynamic stretching, as the name implies, involves moving the body gradually through a movement. This is done with increasing speed as the stretch progresses. As opposed to ballistic stretching, where there is bouncing and small, fast movements, dynamic stretching employs long, controlled movements that gently take the muscle or joint to the limits of the range of motion and not beyond.

This type of stretching is very beneficial for increasing flexibility and warming up muscles before an aerobic activity, but can also be used after exercise.

Other Stretching Exercises

Passive Stretching

Passive stretching is also called relaxed stretching because most of the work involved here is not performed by the person whose muscles are being stretched. The muscle group being stretched is usually held in place by another individual or occasionally by another body part. This type of stretching is particularly useful for muscles that are extremely tight or in spasm. It also helps to clear metabolic waste products in muscle after a workout and is therefore often used as a cool-down stretch.

Isometric Stretching

Isometric stretching helps to increase the strength and integrity of the muscle being stretched while increasing flexibility. It involves moving the muscle or joint to its full range of motion, and rather than simply holding it there, applying a resistant force in the opposite direction. The force is applied for 10 to 15 seconds and then relaxed for 20 seconds before repeating. Best used after a workout, it is not an ideal stretch for beginners or when there is damaged tissue.

Proprioceptive Neuromuscular Facilitation (PNF) Stretching

PNF stretching is a very useful and popular type of stretching among athletes. A combination of isometric and passive stretching, it involves resistance placed upon the muscles while in tension. The muscles are put through the fullest range of motion that the muscle bed or joint will allow. However, rather than one continuous movement, the motion is stopped frequently and an opposing resistance force is applied. The resistance is applied for at least 20 seconds before moving the muscle through further range and applying resistance again. Between each force application in a new position there should be at least a 20-second rest to allow the muscle to recuperate and recover before firing once again.

This type of stretch, is not suitable for injured areas of the body and is best used with a knowledgeable trainer or health-care worker who can assist you.

Ballistic Stretching

Ballistic stretching uses the momentum of a body part to create a force that will allow the body to move beyond the normal range for that joint or muscle. This is a type of stretch that helps to increase circulation quickly and warm up the muscles and joints. It is a bouncing type of motion, where the muscles are used like springs, bouncing in and out of a stretched position. This type of stretching needs to be performed very carefully in a warmed muscle to prevent injury.

Stretching Exercises for Stress Reduction

Low Back Stretch
Lying on your back, pull both your knees to your chest until a comfortable stretch is felt in the low back.

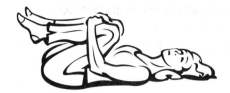

Lumbar Rotation Stretch
While lying on your back, draw one knee toward your chest, then slowly bring your bent leg across your body until a stretch is felt in the low back and hips. Repeat with opposite leg.

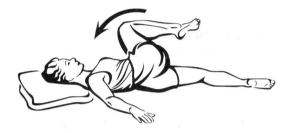

Press Up
Lying on your stomach, press your upper body upwards with your arms. Exhale and sag your stomach toward the ground. Keep your hips on the floor and relax.

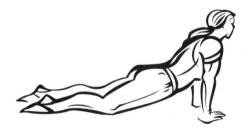

Groin Stretch
Sitting down, place your heels together and pull your feet toward your groin until a stretch is felt in the groin and inner thigh.

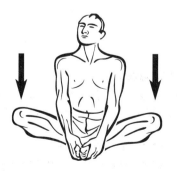

Shin and Quadriceps Stretch

Lying on your side, grasp your toes and pull your heel toward your buttocks until a stretch is felt in the front of the shin and thigh. Repeat for opposite leg.

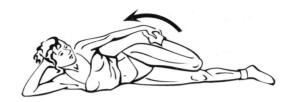

Seated Hamstring Stretch

Sitting upright, tuck your right foot near your groin with your left leg straight. Keep your back straight and head up. Lean forward until a stretch is felt in back of your thigh. Repeat for opposite leg.

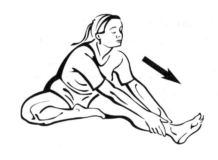

Calf Stretch

Standing upright with your hands against a wall, step forward keeping your back leg straight and on the floor with your feet pointed straight ahead. Move your hips forward until a stretch is felt in the calf. Repeat for the opposite leg.

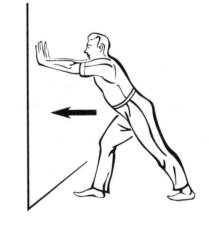

Achilles Stretch

Standing upright with your hands against a wall, slightly bend both knees with one foot back. Move hips forward until a stretch is felt in your lower calf and Achilles tendon. Repeat for opposite leg.

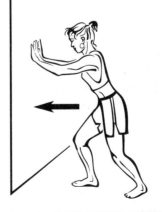

ITB Stretch

Standing upright, cross your left leg behind your right. Lean to the right until a stretch is felt over your left hip. Repeat for the opposite leg.

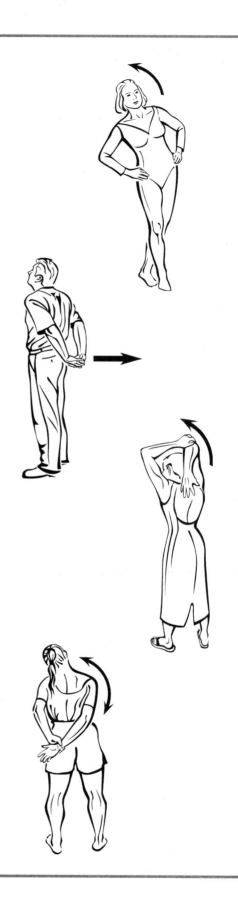

Chest and Biceps Stretch

Standing upright, lace your fingers behind your back and squeeze your shoulder blades together. Slowly raise and straighten your arms.

Triceps Stretch

Standing upright with your hands above your head, gently pull on your left elbow with your right hand until a stretch is felt along the back of the left upper arm. Repeat for the opposite arm.

Neck Stretch

Standing upright with your hands behind your back, grasp your left arm above the wrist and pull downward and across your body. Tilt your head to the right. Repeat with opposite arm.

Strength-Training Exercises

The second component of exercise involves strength training — muscle force and muscle endurance. Muscle force is the ability to contract against resistance — basically how much you can lift. Muscle endurance is the ability to contract repeatedly — how long can you lift for.

Strength training does not mean using heavy weights. Start with a weight that actually feels too easy. Get used to the exercise and get your muscles used to resistance training. Only then can you gradually and carefully increase resistance.

For strength-training and weight-lifting programs, the same philosophy applies. Do not push yourself too quickly, and alternate your program. It is important that you alternate muscle groups, not working the same muscles each time.

For individual programs, it is best if you consult with a personal trainer to ensure that you are using proper technique and form to prevent injuries. They can also help you determine how much weight you should be using for each set.

In general, if you are looking to tone up and lose weight, you should lift lighter weights and perform more repetitions (15 to 18 reps). If you are looking to build muscle mass and gain muscle bulk, then you should lift heavier weights and perform fewer repetitions (8 to 12 reps).

Strengthening Exercise Basics

1. Muscle force is increased by exercising against high resistance with few repetitions.
2. Endurance is increased by exercising against lower resistance with a higher number of repetitions.

Good Pain vs. Bad Pain

Strengthening exercises should not be painful. However, it is not uncommon to experience discomfort afterward. This may be after a few hours or even the next day. Individuals who are accustomed to exercise will recognize this as the 'healthy' muscle ache indicative of a hard workout.

Learning to distinguish 'good' from 'bad' pain is essential for making progress. You may need to consult a therapist or other practitioner to learn the difference. Adequate warm-up, controlled exercise with slow resistance increments, and sufficient stretching along with modalities such as heat and ice will minimize discomfort from your workout.

Strength-Training Terminology

Resistance: the force against which you work during an exercise. This may be just body weight against gravity or it may involve external weights, elastic bands or pulleys.

Rep (short for repetition): one complete movement of an exercise, for example, one leg-lift, one biceps curl, one sit-up.

Set: any number of reps comprise a set. Strengthening involves sets with a low number of reps (8 to 10), while endurance is built with low resistance and a higher number of reps (15 to 20).

Bad Pain Indications

The following are indicators that you are doing more harm than good with your exercises:

- Sudden sharp pain that occurs during exercise.
- Pain that radiates or spreads beyond the exercised area.
- Pain that fails to subside after resting the muscle for at least 2 to 3 days.
- Pain that persists and prevents you from progressing with your program.

Strength-Training Exercises

Below is a basic guideline that you can use for each muscle group.

Chest Exercises

Chest Press

Preparation: Lie on your back on a bench. Dismount barbell from rack over the upper chest using a wide oblique overhand grip. Be sure to have a spotter assist you.

Execution: Lower weight to upper chest. Press bar until arms are extended. Repeat.

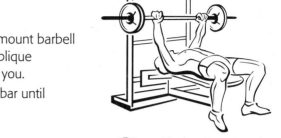

Incline Chest Press

Preparation: Lie on your back on an incline bench. Dismount barbell from rack over the upper chest using a wide oblique overhand grip. Be sure to have a spotter assist you.

Execution: Lower weight to upper chest. Press bar until arms are extended. Repeat.

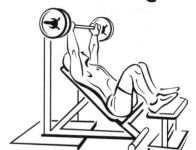

Back Exercises

Wide-Grip Pulldowns

Preparation: On a trapezius pulldown machine at the gym, place your hands slightly further than shoulder width apart on the grip bar.

Execution: Pull down while keeping the back straight. Pull the bar down in front of your face rather than behind your back and do not lock your elbows on the return motion. You can add weight to the machine as you improve.

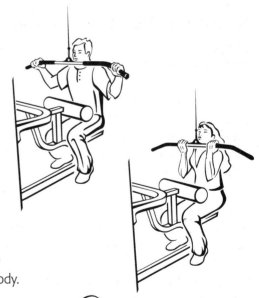

Close-Grip Pulldowns

Like wide-grip pulldowns but hands closer together (about shoulder width) and palms facing toward body.

Seated Row

Preparation: On a rowing machine, sit with your back straight and elbows bent at 90 degrees.

Execution: Pull the grip bar past your body, bringing your elbows past your back. Concentrate on trying to get your shoulder blades to touch.

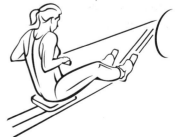

Arm Exercises

Bicep Curl

Preparation: Sit back on a 45- to 60-degree incline bench. With arms hanging down straight, position two dumbbells with palms facing in.

*Execution:*With elbows bent and back to sides, raise one dumbbell and rotate forearm until forearm is vertical and palm faces shoulder. Lower to original position and repeat with opposite arm. Continue to alternate between sides.

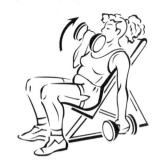

Tricep Extensions

Preparation: Kneel over bench with arm supporting body. Grasp dumbbell. Position upper arm parallel to floor.
Execution: Extend arm until it is straight. Return and repeat. Continue with opposite arm.

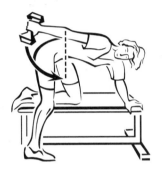

Hamstrings/Quadriceps and Bottom

Lunge

Preparation: Stand straight, with or without support of a chair.

Execution: Step forward with one leg, and bend until your knee has formed a 90-degree angle, then return back to standing. Always keep your knee and foot aligned. Do not let your knee go beyond your ankle.

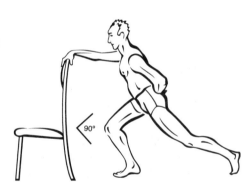

Leg Press

Preparation: On a leg press machine, place your feet shoulder width apart, with your knees bent to a 90-degree angle.

Execution: Slowly straighten your legs out, but do not lock them. Start with the lowest weight, and slowly build up.

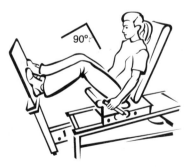

Squat

Preparation: Stand against a wall with your legs slightly wider than shoulder width.
Execution: Tilt your pelvis back, straightening your abdomen, then bend your knees, and lower your body down, keeping your back straight at all times. Make sure your knees stay over your ankles. Looking down, you should be able to see your toes at all times (although ideally you should be looking ahead during the exercise). Do not let your buttocks drop below the level of your knees.

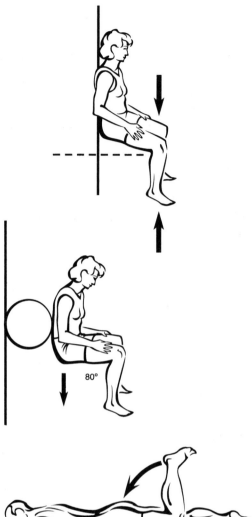

Ball Squat

Preparation: Face away from a wall and place an exercise ball between you and the wall
Execution: Squat, allowing the ball to roll down as you move. Hold the squat with the knees at about 80 to 90 degrees for 5 seconds or longer as your strength improves.

Hamstring Curl

Preparation: Lie prone, face down.
Execution: Keeping your thigh to the floor, lift your heel up toward your buttocks. This can be done at home or on a machine with weights.

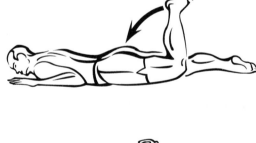

Leg Extensions

Preparation: Sit in a chair with your hands braced under the seat.
Execution: Extend your leg out straight, slowly lower it again by 20 to 30 degrees, and then raise it again. Do not let your knee fall all the way back to 90 degrees. A weight can be added around your ankle to increase resistance and the extension can range to 45 degrees.

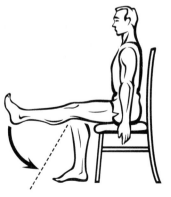

Abdominal Exercises

Pelvic Tilt

Preparation: Lie on your back, knees bent and feet on the floor.

Execution: Contract you abdominal muscles and tilt your pelvis so as to flatten your low back to the floor. Hold for 15 to 20 seconds. Repeat.

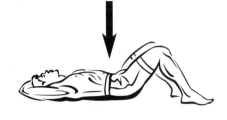

Full Sit-up

Preparation: Lie on your back, knees up, feet on the floor, and hands beside your ears.

Execution: Lift your body until your elbows touch your knees. Count to three and release. Repeat. You may tuck your feet under something to increase stability.

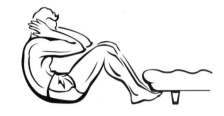

Oblique Sit-up

Preparation: Lie in the full sit-up position.

Execution: Take your elbow up to touch the opposite knee. Repeat on the other side. Crossing one leg over the other makes this exercise even easier.

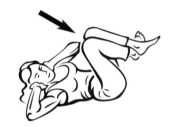

Bridging

Preparation: Lie on your back, knees up, and feet on the floor.

Execution: Lift your buttocks and pelvis off the floor until your back is straight. Hold for 20 seconds. Repeat.

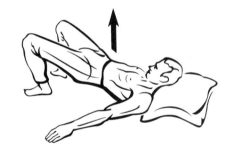

All-Fours Extension

Preparation: Rest on all fours — hands and knees.

Execution: Keeping the body straight, extend the opposite arm and leg and hold for 10 to 15 seconds. Repeat on the other side.

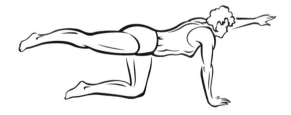

Plank Hold

Preparation: Lie prone, face down.

Execution: Lift your body up onto your elbows and toes. Make sure your back is straight. Hold for 30 seconds. Repeat.

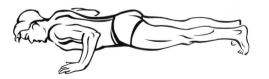

Cardiovascular Exercise

Cardiovascular exercise is the third crucial component of any exercise program and plays a key role in stress management. By cardiovascular exercise, we mean walking, running, swimming, biking, elliptical training or playing an active sport at a pace that increases your heart rate. It is most important that you enjoy your exercise. Try to pick something that appeals to you or makes you feel good. This might involve a group fitness class at your local gym, a dance class, or even gardening.

Warm-Up and Cool-Down

Make sure you warm-up for 5 to 10 minutes by performing your planned activity at low intensity. Then stretch the principal muscles used in the activity for a further 5 to 10 minutes. This will prepare your body and muscles both physiologically and psychologically for exercise and help prevent injury.

As important as the warm-up, the cool-down should be performed at 50% to 60% maximum heart rate for about 5 to 10 minutes. This is followed by stretching for 15 to 20 minutes to complete your workout.

Cardiovascular Exercise Components

- **Frequency:** To improve fitness and maintain optimum body fat, you should perform cardiovascular exercise at least 3 times a week.
- **Duration:** Cardiovascular exercise should be performed for at least 20 minutes at a time.
- **Intensity:** Percentage of maximum heart rate should be monitored during the workout.

Frequency, Duration, Intensity

Frequency, duration, and intensity are the three important components of any cardiovascular program.

Frequency

To gain cardiovascular benefit, it is recommended that you exercise at least 3 times a week and ideally 3 to 5 times. If you are just starting to train, then you will need a good 24 to 36 hours between sessions to allow adequate recovery and to reduce injury and exhaustion risk. This can be gradually increased as you become fitter.

Duration

Exercise duration should be at least 20 minutes and is best when varied between 20 and 60 minutes. However, beginners should take things very cautiously and start at low intensity for 5 to 10 minutes, gradually increasing duration over a few weeks. Always increase duration before you increase intensity; walk for longer before you start to walk faster.

Intensity

The easiest way to monitor the intensity of your workout is to measure your heart rate. This should be done at rest, during, and on completion of your session. Some fitness machines have built-in heart rate monitors and may even have cardiovascular programs you can follow. You can buy a separate heart rate monitor to wear (chest devices are most accurate) if you are exercising outside or on other types of equipment. Or you can take your pulse, preferably at your wrist. Count the number of beats in 10 seconds and multiply by 6 or count for 15 seconds and multiply by 4 to get a value of beats-per-minute (bpm).

When considering how hard you are pushing your cardiovascular system, you can monitor your heart rate during exercise. To calculate your target heart rate so that you may work out at the appropriate range for your level of fitness, follow the simple calculation below.

If you feel tired during a workout, slow your pace down rather than stopping. If you feel light-headed or dizzy, stop the exercise, sit down, and rest. Always remember to see your doctor before starting an exercise program if you have never exercised before or have a health condition that exercise may aggravate when performed improperly. If you are concerned about your program, team up with a personal trainer. A trainer can help keep you motivated, ensure that you perform each exercise correctly, and alter your program as you improve.

Measuring Your Heart Rate

1. Find your pulse at your wrist or on the front of the elbow.
2. Count beats per minute (bpm) at rest, during exercise, and before the cool-down.
3. Measure your heart rate (bpm):
   Number of beats in 10 seconds multiplied by 6
   or
   Number of beats in 15 seconds multiplied by 4
4. Calculate your 'maximum' heart rate = 220 minus your age = xx
   maximum beats per minute (bpm).

Heart Zone Training

Using your heart rate to determine intensity is called heart zone training. It uses percentages of your age-adjusted maximum heart rate. This is most simply determined by subtracting your age from 220. So, if you are 45, your age-adjusted maximum is 175 bpm. A more accurate assessment is a Max Heart Rate fitness test but this needs to be performed by a professional.

Healthy Heart Zone (Pace 1): This is exercise performed at 50% to 60% maximum. This is the lowest level at which benefit is achieved and is generally a good starting point for beginners. It has been shown to reduce blood pressure, cholesterol, and body fat, but not to greatly improve fitness.

Fitness Zone (Pace 2): This involves exercise at 60% to 70% max and adds cardiovascular fitness and greater fat-burning potential. You should aim to reach at least this level within a few weeks of starting to train. The advantage of this level is that it generally involves less stress on the musculoskeletal system and spine.

Aerobic Zone (Pace 3): This is where you really begin to increase your cardiovascular endurance and efficiency. Performed at 70% to 80% max, it greatly improves heart and lung function. It also burns far more calories and is therefore more effective for weight loss.

More advanced training includes anaerobic and interval training, which will not be discussed here. Further information is easily obtained from books, the Internet, or a personal trainer.

Healthy Cardiovascular Exercise Stages

1. Warm-up: 5 to 10 minutes

2. Stretching: 5 to 10 minutes

3. Exercises: Healthy Heart Zone = 50% to 60% of maximum, 20 to 60 minutes

    Fitness Zone = 60% to 70% of maximum, 20 to 60 minutes

    Aerobic Zone = 70% to 80% of maximum, 20 to 60 minutes

4. Cool-Down: 50% to 60% of maximum, 5 to 10 minutes.

5. Stretching: 15 to 20 minutes
    Some people find the concept of 'perceived exertion' easier to follow. Ask the question, 'on a scale of 1 to 10, how hard am I working?' 1 is rest, 10 is flat-out.

    • Healthy Heart Zone = 5 to 6
    • Fitness Zone = 6 to 7
    • Aerobic Zone = 7 to 8
    • Above 8 = working too hard, slow down!

Cardiovascular Exercise Program for Beginners

Cardiovascular exercise should be done 3 times a week. It is important to build up slowly. The exercise should be done for 30 minutes at a time; however, you should never just attempt 30 minutes of high intensity cardiovascular exercise if you do not exercise regularly. Start slowly and gradually build up your stamina. You may choose any form of exercise you prefer, whether it is cycling, running, walking, swimming, or playing active sports. Check off each stage once completed.

Pace 1 = 55% (Healthy Heart Zone)
Pace 2 = 65% (Fitness Zone)
Pace 3 = 75% (Aerobic Zone)

Day 1: 30 minutes
- 5 minutes slow comfortable exercise at Pace 1, where you can easily maintain a conversation.
- 5 minutes at Pace 2, where it is easy to maintain conversation but you could not chat the entire time.
- 5 minutes at Pace 1.
- 5 minutes at high intensity Pace 3, where you are breathing heavily and cannot talk.
- 5 minutes at Pace 2.
- 5 minutes at Pace 1.

Day 2: 30 minutes
- 30 minutes of any type of cardiovascular exercise at a medium Pace 2. You should feel tired after the 30 minutes, but able to complete it without needing to stop.

Day 3: 30 minutes
- 10 minutes at Pace 2.
- 5 minutes at Pace 3.
- 5 minutes at Pace 1.
- 10 minutes at Pace 2.

By alternating the type of exercise you do, and the intensity at which it is performed, you will maximize your workouts in the shortest period of time.

Cardiovascular Exercise Program for Intermediates

This program is for those people who have exercised in the past, but have never pushed themselves, tried a different form of exercise, or stuck to the program week after week. For these people, you will be able push for longer periods of time and at higher intensity. An 80% maximal heart rate for this group will be more of a workout than it was for the beginner group.

Pace 1 = 55% (Healthy Heart Zone)
Pace 2 = 65% (Fitness Zone)
Pace 3 = 75% (Aerobic Zone)

Day 1: 40 minutes
- 5 minutes slow comfortable Pace 1, where you could easily maintain a conversation.
- 10 minutes at a medium Pace 2, where it is easy to maintain, but you could not chat the entire time.
- 10 minutes at high-intensity Pace 3, where you are breathing heavily and could not talk.
- 10 minutes at Pace 2.
- 5 minutes at Pace 1.

Day 2: 45 minutes
- 45 minutes of any type of cardiovascular exercise at a medium Pace 2. You should feel tired after the 45 minutes, but able to complete it without needing to stop.

Day 3: 40 minutes
- 10 minutes at Pace 2.
- 20 minutes at Pace 3.
- 10 minutes at Pace 2.

Any of these workouts can be easily varied by running at a slower pace or uphill.

Anti-Stress Physical Therapies (Bodywork)

CASE STUDY

Bodywork for the Mind

Marian is a 38-year-old patient who had just started a new job when we first saw her in our office. She was very excited about her position and the opportunities it offered. She was delighted with the people she worked with and enjoyed the work itself. Although it entailed longer hours than she was used to, she felt she was handling it quite well.

Three months into the new job, Marian started suffering from frequent headaches. She had rarely experienced headaches in the past, but remembered them occurring, in particular, when she was very stressed, during final exams at school and when her parents separated. She reported that the headaches rarely occurred on weekends, but would build during the work week. She would feel the muscles in her shoulders get progressively tighter, and no amount of stretching or aspirin would relieve the pain. Despite the positive nature of her new job, it was still triggering her stress response.

We felt Marian was suffering from tension headache, a diagnosis also suspected by her family doctor after a number of investigations. We advised her to try some relaxation therapy and bodywork. She began massage therapy once a week and received a short course of acupuncture. Even after her first treatment, she reported that her neck tension and 'fuzzy' head had resolved for the first time in months. She persisted with the massage work along with stretching, meditation, and deep breathing. We gradually reduced and eliminated her acupuncture treatments.

With this program, Marian found that the frequency of her headaches diminished and eventually resolved. She was then able to stretch the appointments to every 2 weeks. By 6 months, she was performing regular at-home relaxation exercises and seeing her massage therapist once a month.

Physical therapies for stress incorporate 'bodywork' techniques that involve the individual alone or the hands of a practitioner. Although the mental and physical aspects of relaxation therapy are intimately intertwined and often overlap, physical therapies generally relate to touch and movement. Bodywork with a practitioner includes massage therapy, reflexology, and acupuncture. Self-directed or instructional bodywork includes yoga, tai chi, and shiatsu.

Finding a Bodywork Practitioner

There are several characteristics to look for when searching for the appropriate practitioner to help you reach your therapeutic goals.

Licensing

No matter what type of therapist or practitioner you are looking for, the most important credential is licensing. You need to ensure that you are with someone who has been fully trained, and that they are accountable for their actions to a board or governing body. This should help to make sure that each practitioner has your best interest at heart and will treat you in a professional manner.

Because licensing boards and regulations vary among provinces, states, and countries, it is important to thoroughly investigate the guidelines set out for your area. Most provinces or states have specific licensing protocols for each profession. These will be clearly stated in that profession's licensing body association. Information on credible associations and licensed practitioners can be easily found on the Internet in most cases.

There are fine distinctions to be made in some cases. When looking for a massage therapist, for example, search for a registered massage therapist, and not simply a masseuse. A masseuse needs only to take a short training course in massage, which does not teach or test the therapist in anatomy, physiology, or other relevant medical and therapeutic courses. A registered massage therapist is completely trained and experienced in massage as a therapy, not just a back rub, and is well versed in contraindications.

Graduating Schools

Within most professions, whether it be law, traditional medicine, or complimentary medicine, the curriculum between schools can differ. If you have heard positive remarks from one school and not another, or prefer to go see a practitioner who has graduated from a specific school, you may research this too. You can do this in a variety of ways. The licensing board of each profession will have a record of the school each practitioner graduated from.

Alternatively, if there is a specific practitioner you would like to see, but wish to know this information first, call the practitioner's office.

Specialties

Although the training of each practitioner is similar, some health-care workers have gone on to do more research on their own in one particular area of interest. The majority of their work may be in this one field, yet they continue to treat other health issues as well. If there is one specific health issue that you wish to address, you may choose to find a practitioner who has a little more experience in the field. Again, as they have received similar training, any licensed health-care worker should be able to treat you, but the choice is yours.

To search out this information, the best way is to look up the type of treatment you are looking for — for example, weight loss — and the type of practitioner — for example, naturopathic doctor. If a practitioner specializes in one such area, this information should be readily available. However, if this information is not posted on the Internet, you may simply search or call the appropriate association for a list of the practitioners and their specialties.

Location
While it is important to have your practitioner accessible, it may often be worth traveling a little farther if you find one you have good rapport with or one who specializes in a certain field. Minimizing the stress associated with travel and parking is a consideration. Try to choose appropriate appointment times.

Number of Years in Practice vs. Current Knowledge
Most licensed professionals are required to take continuing education courses so the quality of care and level of current knowledge should be identical. Most types of therapy get better with experience, but that does not mean that a new graduate is not qualified to help you. It is more important that you trust your health-care professional.

Male or Female
For any type of therapy, the sex of the practitioner should be irrelevant. All health-care workers should treat you professionally and kindly, to the best of their ability. In saying that, the most important feature between a patient and practitioner is trust. If you are not comfortable relaxing with your massage therapist or describing personal symptoms to your doctor, then you will not receive the best possible treatment. You may feel less vulnerable or simply more comfortable with a certain gender of health-care worker. If you do, it is important that you acknowledge that preference and seek out a practitioner accordingly.

Word of Mouth
Information provided by other patients is very useful. There is nothing more valuable than praise about a practitioner given by someone you trust. This will give you an idea about their practice, their personality type, their specialties, and whether or not that style suits you. Do not forgo the above criteria just to meet this one, but word of mouth, whether it is positive or negative, is most likely your most valuable tool in selecting a practitioner to help you reach your therapeutic and health goals.

Massage

The relaxation benefits of massage therapy are not just subjective – massage has been shown to decrease both noradrenaline and cortisol levels in the blood, urine, and saliva. That wonderful feeling you get at the end of a massage is not just from lying down quietly for a period of time. There is a significant therapeutic effect from receiving regular massage therapy, which clearly goes far beyond simple musculoskeletal pain relief.

Massage Therapy

Defined as the treatment of disease or injury through the manual manipulation of body tissues, massage is thought to decrease stress levels by relieving pain. Massage breaks down scarring and adhesions, increases circulation and metabolism, and promotes resorption and metabolism of toxins and residua of inflammation.

Pain Relief

Massage affects our experience of pain in two ways. First, pain is felt when sensors in the skin, muscles, joints, and other tissues are stimulated. These sensors send messages through nerve fibers to the brain where the sensation is interpreted. Massage gently stimulates adjacent fibers, sending another set of messages to the brain. This acts like an overload on the system so that not all of the messages get to the brain. As the massage sensation is 'new' or 'different' from any chronic or constant pain, it lessens the sensation of the true pain, even though the massage is not actually painful.

Second, massage has also been shown to stimulate the release of enkephalins and endorphins, the body's natural painkillers. These hormones act on the same receptors as powerful drugs, such as morphine, reducing the awareness and intensity of pain and inducing a feeling of calm and relaxation.

Stress Hormones

Massage also decreases levels of the stress hormones cortisol and noradrenaline. In one study, 30-minute daily massages were performed for 5 days in a row on 52 patients hospitalized for anxiety and depression. When compared to similar hospitalized patients that did not receive massage therapy, the treated group had lower stress hormone levels in the blood, urine and saliva, and greater subjective reduction in anxiety. This finding was supported by medical staff observation of behavior, with treated patients much less anxious and more cooperative.

Other studies have been performed on adults measuring salivary cortisol levels and EEG patterns with and without massage. While both groups reported decreased depression levels at the end of the 5 weeks, only the massage group reported decreased stress levels at work. A similar study in hospitalized bulimic patients found an immediate reduction in anxiety and depression in those patients receiving massage therapy noted by self-reports from the patients and observed reports by their doctors. In addition, those undergoing the massage therapy had significantly lower cortisol levels and increased dopamine levels (relaxing hormone), and showed improvements on several other psychological and behavioral measures.

Other studies on patients undergoing surgery have offered insight into how massage benefits the body. Patients who received a massage before surgery displayed decreased anxiety symptoms according to medical staff reporting. This was supported by significantly lower blood pressure readings, pulse rates, and norepinepherine/epinephrine levels after the massage and after surgery in the massage group. The control group showed increased levels of all the stress hormones. This study helps to illustrate, both from a subjective and objective point of view, the positive impact that massage can have on stress and anxiety, not just from an emotional point of view, but from a physiological one as well.

Immune System and Allergies

Massage therapy offers other beneficial effects associated with relaxation, one of which is an increase in immune system function. Further studies show how massage therapy can reduce cortisol levels in children with asthma. This has a significant effect on their disease. Massage also helps to increase local circulation, improving the flow of nutrients to an area, thereby increasing the amount of available material for healing. An increase in circulation will also help to remove the inflammatory chemicals, which not only contribute to further inflammation, but can act as free radical stimulators that hinder healing. Massage promotes the resorption and metabolism of toxins and the residua of inflammation.

Inflammation

Massage helps to increase local circulation, improving the flow of nutrients to an area, thereby increasing the amount of available material for healing. An increase in circulation will also help to remove the inflammatory chemicals, which not only contribute to further inflammation, but can act as free radical stimulators that hinder healing and add biological stress to the body.

Safety

Contraindications are few. Following acute injury or a severe flare-up of an existing injury, or in the presence of an open wound, local massage would not be advisable in that area. However, distant massage or massage therapy performed on other parts of the body is advisable to help increase the effects of the immune system and decrease inflammatory mediators, and cortisol levels. In order to receive these benefits, massage can be performed anywhere on the body. It is avoided in certain cancers to avoid spread of the disease.

Massage Therapy at Home

Simple massage techniques can also be practiced at home to help relieve stress.

1. Use a massaging showerhead, which augments the benefits of superficial heat from the water.

2. Move a simple wooden roller-type massager back and forth across the neck, back or feet.

3. Use commercial electric massagers with or without heat.

4. Have a partner apply slow, gentle, finger, thumb or hand pressure.

Types of Massage Therapy

There are several different types or techniques that fall under the umbrella of massage therapy.

Swedish Massage

Probably the best-known technique, Swedish massage involves long strokes along the superficial layers of muscle fiber. This massage uses strokes such as effleurage, which are smooth gliding motions across the soft tissue applied with both hands.

Effleurage

Effleurage is used to gently relax the muscle fibers. Swedish is often combined with active and passive movements of the joint to help stretch the muscle, ligaments and tendons.

Deep Tissue Massage

Deep tissue massage is another popular form of therapy used to release chronic patterns of tension in the body with slow, deep finger pressure and strokes on contracted muscles. Unlike Swedish massage, this type of massage focuses on deeper layers of the muscle. Deep tissue massage can be sore or tender during the treatment, but subsides rapidly following the treatment session.

Friction Massage

Friction massage involves a type of stroke that is very effective for pain and inflammation. It includes deep circular movements applied to soft tissues or muscles, often at right angles to their orientation, causing a degree of friction. The result here is to increase the blood flow to the area and help break down adhesions and 'muscle knots'.

Petrissage

Petrissage or kneading massage involves squeezing, rolling, and kneading the muscle bed. This is used in most types of massage with varying degrees of depth and strength. It usually follows effleurage as a way to loosen the muscle fibers and prepare the area for deep tissue or trigger point work.

Trigger Point Therapy

Trigger point therapy, also known as myotherapy or neuromuscular therapy, is the application of concentrated finger pressure to irritated and painful areas in the muscle, otherwise known as 'trigger points'. This type of therapy is used to help relieve spasms and localized pain within the muscle.

Tapotement

Tapotement is a technique used where the therapist places the sides of the hand on the patient's tissues and applies short vigorous taps in a repetitive and rhythmic motion.

Massage Holding Patterns

by Amanda Webber, Registered Massage Therapist

In my career as a registered massage therapist, I have spent substantial time and effort performing deep tissue massage, 'fighting' my way into muscles that refused to 'let go'. However, I have come to realize not only how unnecessary such an approach is, but also that it is entirely ineffective. Even those few clients who seem to relax, appear, upon careful examination, appear simply to have displaced the muscle tension to another part of their body.

I believe the underlying cause of muscle tension or spasm is a 'holding pattern'. For example, when we are feeling angry or frightened or when we are suffering from depression or guilt, the way we hold our body reveals this emotion to others. This likely represents a phylogenetically primitive form of communicative body language, akin to a cat arching its back or a dog snarling. What we often do not consider, however, is that when exposed to prolonged periods of distress, the body begins to adopt these emotional postures as its 'normal' state. Eventually, despite the fact that the emotional event has passed, the body remains locked in position. We have all heard the saying; "If you're not careful, your face is going to stay that way!" While this is admittedly a little extreme, it does contain an element of truth.

In this way, stress is translated into the body's musculature and fascia as contracture, or holding patterns. Unfortunately this is not something we easily surrender.

Relaxation, the foundation of massage, has somehow been forgotten. People have come to see the wide range of healing benefits massage offers and expect 'results' ranging from increases in restricted ranges of motion and decreases in pain levels, to the reduction of swelling.

However, I have found that many of the problems encountered in my practice are a direct result of the stress in my client's lives. Most of them hold onto their stress, resulting in damage to all systems of the body, including the muscles and fascia, producing holding patterns. Any attempt at healing without addressing the underlying problem is like administering aid to a soldier who remains lying on the battlefield; while one wound may be treated, other wounds are being sustained.

The body's natural state is health. Any deviation from this is an 'active' response by the body. In the case of muscle tension, the active process is the clenching that produces holding patterns. Unfortunately, these patterns become so ingrained that we are not even aware of them. A massage that brings awareness to the body, revealing to it that the muscles are not only tight, but are in fact actively contracting, is the key to relieving both muscle pain and the stress that causes it. It is a gentle awareness that demands nothing be done, nothing be achieved — just the opposite. By inducing a calm and balanced state, the active process is halted, allowing true relaxation and release.

The body has within it a vast inner potential for healing, exceeding anything a practitioner can pass on. The greatest healing that I can bestow upon a client is to return them to a place of stillness, where they themselves can access their own inherent resources.

Aromatherapy

Aromatic healing oils can be used during a therapeutic massage. These essential oils are absorbed both through inhalation and through the skin during a treatment. Throughout the massage, lymphatic drainage, muscle releases, and spinal pressures are applied to target the nervous system, and affect every organ and muscle of the body. Each oil has a different effect, ranging from detoxifying and relaxing effects to increasing energy levels.

Aromatherapy Essential Oils for Relaxation and Stress Relief

- Amber
- Bergamot
- Camphor
- Cedarwood
- Lavender
- Poppy
- Ylang-Ylang

Ways to Use Essential Oils

- Diffuser (a small metal bowl heated by a candle)
- Bath (a few drops in a warm bath)
- Massage Oil (mixed with other oils)
- Facecloth (a few drops in a facecloth or sponge in the bath or shower)
- Perfume

Reflexology

Reflexology originated in the Far East and Egypt as a form of therapeutic touch. Clinically, it dates back to 1913, developed by Dr. William Fitzgerald, an ear, nose, and throat specialist. He was one of the first in the medical community to notice the anesthetic effects on the body resulting from pressing on specific 'pressure points'.

Reflexology is said to help clear toxins and help remove waste materials from the body, increase the energy pathways, and restore balance back to the body. This is achieved by stimulating one or several of the 7000 sensory nerve endings on the feet. In doing so, a specific message is sent to the brain and spinal cord, where this information is deciphered and the appropriate response is sent to the target area of the body, such as the liver. Reflexology practitioners have identified specific pressure points on the feet that relate or have a 'reflexive' relationship to every part of the body.

Stress Relief

Reflexology
Although there is no clinical data to support the therapeutic effects of reflexology, there are many anecdotal and subjective reports of stress and anxiety reduction, increased well-being and relaxation. As this is a noninvasive, non-dangerous form of relaxation, its physiologic benefits may yet be clinically proven.

Treatment Procedure

A reflexology treatment lasts approximately 1 hour. The patient is fully clothed during the treatment and usually lies flat on the floor or on a massage table. Sometimes, a patient may be treated while sitting up, particularly if this assists in the treatment, such as with clearance of secretions from the lungs.

The reflexologist applies pressure to the specific points on the feet while gently massaging the entire foot. As this occurs and stimulates other areas on the body, the patient may experience symptoms like a runny nose, increased urination, and perspiration. These are all said to be detoxifying effects from the reflexology treatment.

Reflexology Pressure Points

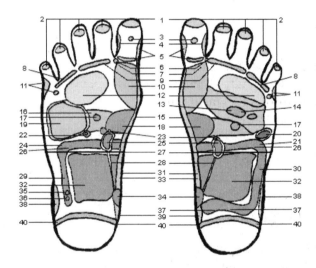

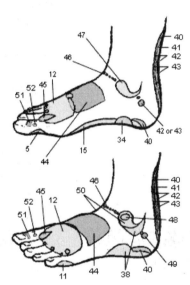

1. Top of Head
2. Sinuses
3. Pituitary Gland
4. Temporal Area
5. Neck, Cervical
6. Upper Lymph Area
7. Parathyroid Gland
8. Ears
9. Eyes
10. Thyroid Glands
11. Shoulder
12. Lungs and Bronchi
13. Heart Area
14. Heart
15. Spine, Vertebra
16. Pancreas
17. Solar Plexus
18. Stomach & Duodenum
19. Liver
20. Spleen
21. Spleenic Fixture
22. Gall Bladder
23. Adrenal Glands
24. Hepatic Flexure
25. Kidneys
26. Transverse Colon
27. Waist
28. Ureters
29. Ascending Colon
30. Descending Colon
31. Lumbar
32. Small Intestines
33. Sacral
34. Bladder
35. Ileo-Caecal Valve
36. Appendix
37. Sigmoid Flexure
38. Hip and Lower Back
39. Coccyx
40. Sciatic Area
41. Rectum
42. Uterus
43. Prostate
44. Breast
45. Lymph Drainage
46. Fallopian Tubes
47. Lymph Nodes (Arm Pit)
48. Sacroiliac Joint
49. Ovary or Testicle
50. Lymph Nodes (Groin)
51. Maxilla/Submaxilla (Jaw)
52. Tonsils

Acupuncture

According to Chinese medicine, most stressed individuals have an excess of energy, but the flow of this energy is blocked, resulting in fatigue and ill health. Acupuncture in stress management aims to remove the blockage, allowing the energy to flow and dissipate, thereby reducing the overall stress response and adverse effects. Many people may not think of the insertion of acupuncture needles as a relaxing or calming treatment for anxiety and stress, but the effects can be just as powerful as any other type of bodywork. Bodywork aims to access information and energy in the body and channel it into a more free-flowing form.

Acupuncture

Acupuncture is a therapeutic method for promoting natural healing of the body through the insertion of needles. Although acupuncture is relatively new to the Western world, it has been used therapeutically in Asia for more than 2000 years. Western medical studies have shown that endogenous opioids or endorphins can be released upon insertion of a needle, thus affecting pain and anxiety.

Qi (Energy)

Energy in traditional Chinese medicine is called Qi or Chi (pronounced "chee"). Qi circulates through the meridians and heals the body. The body continually generates small but detectable charges of energy. The flow of this energy influences growth, maturation, relaxation, and muscle tone, as well as the production of hormones and enzymes — in fact, the functioning of the entire body.

Traditional Chinese medicine teaches that there are a series of 12 energy channels that run through the body, known as meridians. These meridians are somewhat like blood vessels and nerves, serving as the routes through which energy is dispersed and nutrients are delivered. Much like a defect in an artery or nerve causes pain, inflammation, swelling, and other pathology, so does an obstruction in a meridian.

There are hundreds of specific points along these meridians, each point acting like a reservoir of potential energy for that meridian. If there is a block or problem in the meridian, the energy can be released and flow restored by stimulating a certain acupuncture point or points. This helps to heal the meridian and to re-establish a beneficial flow of energy through the body. The kidneys and heart are the two main organ systems in Chinese medicine that will require rebalancing during times of stress.

Nerve Stimulation

In Western medicine, acupuncture is described as a stimulation of the nervous system by inserting a needle into the body. This stimulation causes a release of specific chemical substances that influence the muscles, spine, and brain. These various chemicals then bring about the relief of pain, a decrease in inflammation, relaxation, and a calming or stimulative effect in order to bring balance back to the body.

Acupuncture can be used in two different ways: to increase energy in an area where it may be deficient by stimulating the Qi; and to decrease excess energy in an area that is considered overstimulated by relaxing, dispersing, and calming the Qi. The difference lies in the insertion of the needle and whether or not the needle is manipulated further during the treatment.

If we are trying to increase energy, we insert the needle while twisting it in both directions as it enters the skin. In addition, we periodically twist the needle in both directions throughout the treatment (or use electrical stimulation), and spin the needle in both directions when taking it out at the end. This is said to excite the Qi in that area and increase energy levels.

Relaxation

In order to calm an area or relax a stressed individual, not only are the points the practitioner chooses important, so is the way the needle is moved. To calm an area, the needle is inserted gently while twisting only in one direction, clockwise. We do not spin the needle during the treatment and we do not use electrodes. At the end of the treatment, we spin the needle counter-clockwise as it is removed. We do not at any time spin the needle in both directions if we are trying to relax the Qi in that particular area.

Kidneys and Heart

The main areas of focus in acupuncture for stress treatment are the kidneys and heart. Kidneys in Chinese medicine are akin to the adrenal glands in Western medicine. Anatomically, the adrenal glands sit on the top of the kidneys. If the adrenals are overworked or exhausted, they can cause an alteration in kidney Qi energy. The heart in Chinese medicine controls emotions and sleep. When one has been going through an emotional or stressful period, an alteration in heart energy or Qi can be seen.

As many people present with different symptoms from stress, such as bowel problems or headaches, other organ systems can be added in to complement the treatment. For instance, if a bowel problem is present, then stomach and spleen channels would be treated in addition to kidneys and heart. If headaches are a problem, then liver points may be used. However, much like Western treatment, if the problem arises initially from stress and HPA-axis dysfunction, then this must be treated first.

Acupuncture Meridians

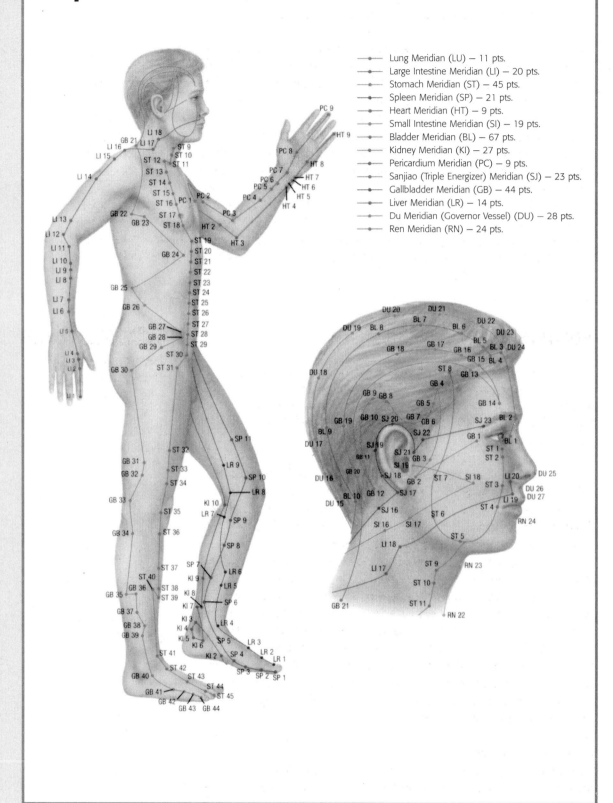

Lung Meridian (LU) — 11 pts.
Large Intestine Meridian (LI) — 20 pts.
Stomach Meridian (ST) — 45 pts.
Spleen Meridian (SP) — 21 pts.
Heart Meridian (HT) — 9 pts.
Small Intestine Meridian (SI) — 19 pts.
Bladder Meridian (BL) — 67 pts.
Kidney Meridian (KI) — 27 pts.
Pericardium Meridian (PC) — 9 pts.
Sanjiao (Triple Energizer) Meridian (SJ) — 23 pts.
Gallbladder Meridian (GB) — 44 pts.
Liver Meridian (LR) — 14 pts.
Du Meridian (Governor Vessel) (DU) — 28 pts.
Ren Meridian (RN) — 24 pts.

Rei-Ki

by Shula Starkey, Advanced Level 2 Usui Rei-Ki Practitioner

Rei-Ki is a therapy that aims to renew life-force energy, creating inner calm and well-being, thus combatting stress. This energy flows as hands are placed on the client, slowing the brain-wave pattern to a meditation level of 8 to 10 hertz. The energy enters via the crown of the head, following the energy pathways that parallel the nervous system.

Rei-Ki energy is used by the body where it is needed most. Practitioners believe that most ailments are a manifestation of a past action, perception of a situation, or bad habit that has not been confronted and resolved. Life-force energy disperses this negativity, sometimes releasing a healing crisis. By releasing us from the memory of past negative experiences and bad habits, it enables us to move forward, minimizing the impact of future stressors.

Rei-Ki can also target a specific area, such as the adrenal glands. Exhausted adrenal glands resulting from continuous stress can be addressed by placing the practitioner's hands directly over the area of these glands, giving them a healing energy boost. While Rei-Ki does not, in itself, profess to 'cure' in the medical sense of the word, it enhances life force to promote the innate healing ability of the individual.

Shiatsu

Shiatsu is another form of therapeutic body treatment, an ancient healing practice that literally means finger pressure in Japanese. The art of shiatsu is based on a combination of the knowledge of traditional Chinese medicine and Western physiology and anatomy.

Similar to reflexology, shiatsu employs the application of pressure to specific points. The difference here is that the points are very specific acupuncture points along various energy meridians in the body. These energy meridians or channels are located all over the body, so shiatsu treatments involve physically treating the entire body, not just the foot.

One study evaluating the effectiveness of shiatsu on stress clearly demonstrated this point: 25 volunteers had a 10-minute shiatsu treatment, or a similar treatment where the pressure was applied to other areas of the body, not on the acupuncture points. Before and after the treatment, patients were asked to record their stress levels, in addition to using the bispectral index (BIS). Pressure applied to the acupuncture points significantly reduced the BIS values and verbal stress scores when compared to the control group receiving pressure on non-acupuncture points.

Treatment Procedure

Like reflexology, these treatments also take place with the patient fully clothed, most often lying flat on the ground, as the therapist combines stretches and joint movements or limb

Stress Relief

Shiatsu
Since clinical research still remains limited, shiatsu should not be the only form of treatment used in any therapeutic plan. However, there is extensive credible research on acupuncture. Since the principles of shiatsu are similar to acupuncture with similar 'points' being treated but without needle insertion, the therapeutic benefit of shiatsu has great potential.

rotation while pressing on the acupuncture points. Shiatsu is said to affect all levels of the body, the physical, the emotional, and the spiritual. Shiatsu treatments usually last one hour and are not usually associated with any adverse effects. Like any form of body treatment, muscle stiffness, fatigue, headaches or other mild symptoms may occur.

Craniosacral Therapy

Craniosacral therapy is a type of physical treatment that works through the mobilization of the cerebral spinal fluid surrounding the brain and spinal cord.

The sacral rhythm of cerebral spinal fluid is said to be an indicator of mobility of the connective tissue, body symmetry, and vitality. This sacral rhythm occurs at 6 to12 cycles per minute and correlates with the pressure of the cerebral spinal fluid and with breathing rhythms. Craniosacral practitioners feel this pattern as a widening and narrowing pulse-like sensation that is reflected throughout the body. The pulse varies in symmetry, amplitude, and quality, depending on the individual. The role of the therapist is to follow the pulse through the tissue, rather than forcing it to change direction.

Treatment Procedure

During craniosacral treatments, the patient lies down flat on a table and the therapist begins by placing his or her hands at the base of the neck or occiput to sense the craniosacral rhythm. Once it is found, the practitioner then follows this rhythm and unblocks any restrictions. This may take the practitioner over the head, down the back, or over the body. Patients undergoing this treatment may sense that fluid is moving in the body or in the head — or they simply feel a release of a tight muscle or tissue. The treatments can induce both physical and emotional symptoms, such as headaches or tears as various restrictions are released. Each patient's reaction is unique, depending on the type of restriction and where it is located.

Yoga

Yoga is a type of exercise program that aims to bring a sense of balance to the body and the mind. It is best known as a physical practice utilizing gentle stretching, breathing, and relaxation techniques. Each of these techniques follows a specific pattern or sequence that helps to relax the mind and energize the body.

Craniosacral Therapy

Craniosacral therapy aims to release stress-related restrictions in the flow and rhythm of the cerebrospinal fluid that leads to pain, inflammation, emotional disturbances, and other disruptions of bodily function. While clinical research associated with craniosacral treatment is very limited, there do not appear to be any adverse reactions with this treatment, nor contraindications. Craniosacral therapy may be a beneficial form of noninvasive stress management.

Practice

Yoga practice begins with concentration on breathing to quiet the mind. When the mind is quiet, the release of cortisol, our stress hormone, decreases. Next follows a series of gentle movements and poses that help to strengthen and lengthen the muscles. This also helps to increase the circulation through the body, which in turn provides new nutrients to damaged or inflamed areas of the body, helping to sweep away metabolic by-products.

Effectiveness

Studies have been performed monitoring stress and its response to yoga. In one study, seven yoga instructors were examined for brain-wave activity and cortisol levels while they were performing yoga exercises. A significant change was seen. All participants displayed a marked increase in alpha-brain-wave activity, indicating increased alertness with enhanced relaxation. Reduction in cortisol levels directly correlated with these changes in brain-wave activity.

Similar studies have demonstrated the physiological and psychological effects of Hatha yoga. In one study, healthy women were divided into two groups. The first study group performed daily yoga exercises and the control group sat in a comfortable position and read books during the same time period. All participants were measured for heart rate, blood pressure, cortisol, growth hormone, and a variety of psychological parameters, such as anxiety, aggressiveness, life satisfaction, and coping mechanisms. At the end of the study, no significant differences were seen in blood hormone levels, but those performing the yoga exercises displayed much lower blood pressure readings and reported significant differences in all psychological factors, such as decreased excitability, decreased aggressiveness and anger, increased life and job satisfaction, better coping skill to stress, elevated overall mood, and decreased somatic complaints.

Safety

There are essentially no contraindications for yoga. Some people may need to limit the range of motion through some of the exercises. Such caution is advised for those with a total hip replacement (due to decreased stability in the joint); practicing yoga should be discussed with your surgeon. Some individuals may need to begin more slowly with the exercises and build up their strength and flexibility. It is important not to push the body too far. Pain on a movement is indicative that you should move through the exercise with care.

Yoga Breathing and Stretching Exercises

Child's Pose

Preparation: Sit on your heels, bend forward, and rest your arms and head on the floor.

Execution Sequence:

As you exhale, let your hips drop toward your heels. At the same time, let your head, arms, and shoulders also drop. See if you can feel the ripple through your back as your spine releases.

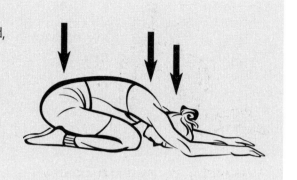

Sun Salutation

Preparation: Start standing with your hands in a prayer position.

Execution Sequence:

1. While exhaling, drop your weight on to your heels.

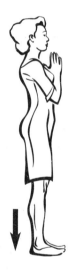

2. While inhaling, drop your arms and bring them up over your head in a circular motion, making a long gentle arch with your back.

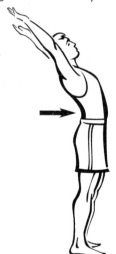

3. While exhaling, bend forward, dropping your head below your knees and stretching your hands to the floor, palms down.

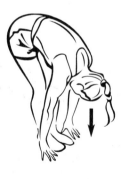

4. While inhaling, step forward with your right leg into the lunge position.

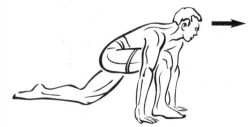

5. While holding your breath, step your other leg back into the 'plank pose'.

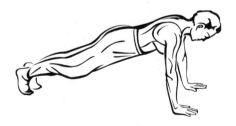

6. While inhaling, round your back and lower your head in the 'cat pose.'

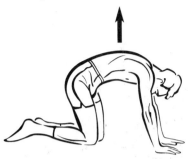

7. While exhaling, dip you chin and chest to the floor

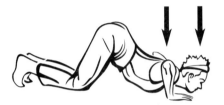

8. While inhaling, lower your pelvis to the floor and raise your head with your arms into the head-up 'dog pose.'

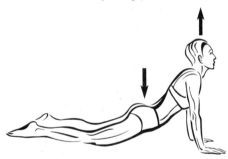

9. While exhaling, press down with your wrists and raise your pelvis into the head-down 'dog pose.'

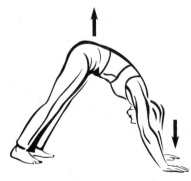

10. While inhaling, step forward with your left leg into the lunge position.

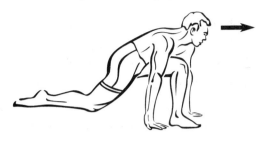

11. While exhaling, bend forward, dropping your head below your knees and stretching your hands to the floor, palms down.

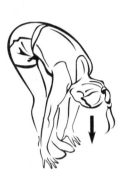

12. While inhaling, drop your arms and bring them up over your head in a circular motion, making a long gentle arch with your back.

13. While exhaling, come back to standing straight and bring your hands together into a prayer position.

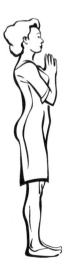

Tai Chi

Tai chi is often referred to as a moving form of yoga combined with meditation. There are many different forms of Tai chi, otherwise known as 'sets', each consisting of a different sequence of coordinated movements. These movements mimic the natural movements seen in animals and birds, but unlike the staccato movements of these animals, Tai chi is performed in a slow, continuous, even motion. Many of the movements stem from various martial arts practices, such as QiGong. Tai chi has been used therapeutically with the elderly and injured for decades and has spread to all ages as a form of warm-up, cross-training, and body awareness exercise. Practicing Tai chi 3 times a day meets the American Health Association standards for exercise.

Yin-Yang

Tai chi is based on the principle of 'yin' and 'yang' forces, which can be likened to opposite sides of a coin or opposing characteristics of the same detail. For example, female-male, hot-cold, dark-light are all yin-yang characteristics. The goal of Tai chi is to bring about a balance between the two sides. This is achieved by fostering the flow of Qi, the life force or life energy in the body that runs along a series of meridians. This restores the natural harmony or balance within the system and ultimately relieves the pain or heals the injury.

Breath Control

Breathing is a very important component of Tai chi. In Tai chi, you are taught to breathe fully from the abdomen to relax the mind, as in meditation, but to do so with awareness, not to make the mind 'blank'. Each breath should be processed by the mind in a graceful and active manner.

The movements of Tai chi are timed with the breath. As one extends out or forward, the breath is exhaled. The breath is inhaled as the movement returns to the center of the body, or a neutral position. In doing so, you are able to bring together both the mind and the body in a simultaneous awareness that allows for better musculoskeletal functioning.

The basic movements in Tai chi are pushing movements with the hand that works to move all the joints through their full range of motion. The muscles 'learn' which fibers should contract first, in a coordinated sequence of stimulation to increase strength, range of motion in a joint, and decrease injury. The gentle movements of Tai chi also help to smoothly rotate all the joints and stretch them, freeing up the blocked Qi that can create pain.

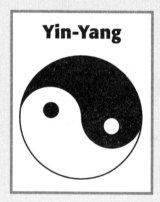

Yin-Yang

Anti-Stress Mental Therapies

CASE STUDY

Saying 'No' and Breathing Deeply

Simon is a 28-year-old business man who, having become aware of the impact his stressful lifestyle was having on his health, wanted to incorporate mental relaxation therapy into his daily routine. However, he was convinced it would be too time-consuming and was uncertain whether he had the right personality to see it through.

We informed him that to gain benefit he did not have to disappear to the top of a mountain for 10 hours of yogi-like transcendental meditation 3 times a week. Rather, by combining simple lifestyle changes with some brief self-guided relaxation exercises, he could quickly see significant improvements in his overall stress level.

Simon began by starting a stress journal so that he could identify and avoid situations he knew would be stressful. He began to say 'no' rather than always taking on more tasks than he could ever hope to complete. He listened to relaxing music in the car and rented comedy films rather than horror or tragedy. For more formal relaxation, he practiced deep breathing during the day and completed a simple 3-minute mediation at least 5 days a week.

Simon now finds he is more relaxed and productive, his stress level markedly reduced. He has time for some of the longer meditation exercises and has noted improvements in his interpersonal relationships and enjoyment of life.

Much of the stress in our lives relates to our perception of the world around us and our place in the world. Many people are able to simply 'let stress roll off of them'. These people seem to be able to filter out what is important to them, and what they need to worry about, placing importance only on those things they want to change and can change. Other individuals in the same situation may find different things important, or overemphasize other things, leading to a feeling of loss of control, stress, and anxiety. Because we each perceive and react differently to situations, it is easy to see the truth in the saying, "One man's stress is another man's pleasure."

Fortunately, there is a host of therapies designed to overcome 'perceived' stress and help restore balance to our stress response before we develop related illnesses.

Relaxation Techniques

There are several different techniques used to improve relaxation as part of a stress management program. Anything that makes you feel better is stress management. That could be renting a funny movie, having tea with a friend, listening to music, or just breathing.

Controlled Breathing

This process is used to relax the body and free it of tension. Although it is used to quiet the mind and decrease sensory input, deep breathing is very different from sleeping. In fact, during this exercise, you become more aware of your surroundings. Deep breathing requires conscious effort to do it correctly. Breathing uses both the voluntary and involuntary parts of the nervous system.

Simple-Breathing Exercise

1. To begin, simply start by being aware of your breathing. Sit quietly and watch your breath as it moves in and out of the abdomen. Breath deeply so that your diaphragm and abdominal muscles, not just your lungs and chest, are rising and falling. Do this for 15 minutes a day. You should notice your body becoming quiet and a decrease in heart rate and blood pressure.

2. From here you can then move into progressive relaxation. Lie down and take several deep breaths. Feel for tension in the body in the form of muscle tightness or inability to let that muscle 'go'. Then concentrate on the feet. While you do so, take a big breath in, hold it for 5 to 10 seconds (or as long as you can without feeling light-headed or uncomfortable), and tense the muscles in your feet. As you slowly exhale, slowly release or relax the muscles in the feet.

3. Next, do the same for the calf muscles. Continue this exercise upward in different areas until you get to the head. Here, rather than trying to tense the muscles of the head, lift it slightly off the floor or pillow. Hold it up while you hold your breath. Once again, as you exhale, release the muscle contraction in the neck and allow the head to sink into the pillow or floor.

This process can be repeated as frequently as needed. It helps the body to let go of tension and muscle tightness.

Deep-Breathing Exercise

Deep breathing is a simple, yet highly effective technique for relaxation and stress reduction. It requires no special equipment, no particular location, and very little training. It can be used in an instant to calm the mind for a few seconds or as part of a longer relaxation program. With experience it becomes an essential first step toward the deeper state of meditation.

State of Calm

The aim here is to become aware of the relaxed state deep breathing can achieve. By practicing the technique, you can then use it more quickly in situations you find stressful — once familiar with the sensation of calm associated with this breathing pattern, it will only take one or two breaths to return to that state in a stress emergency.

Daily Routine and Stress Emergencies

Deep breathing can become part of your daily routine. You may wish to deep breathe for 5 minutes in the morning before you leave for work, when you get home or just before bed. In addition, the technique can be used during the day to alleviate stress and control anxiety-inducing situations. In this latter situation you will have to modify the exercise. For example, closing your eyes may not be practical (or safe!). You may not be in a comfortable spot and only have time for a few breaths. However, once you are familiar with the relaxation that deep breathing brings, you can use it to defuse your stress at any time, whether in traffic, a supermarket line, or a board meeting.

Steps

1. Find a quiet, comfortable place to sit. Turn off distractions such as radio, television, or telephone. Rest your hands on your knees or clasp them lightly in your lap.
2. Close your eyes and let your mind be aware that it is time to relax. Repeating a word such as 'calm' or 'peace' a few times may help at this point.
3. Become aware of your breathing. Rather than it be an automatic activity occurring in the background, concentrate on each breath. Feel the air entering and leaving your lungs over four or five breaths.
4. Breathe in through your nose and out through your mouth to start with and then, as your breathing deepens and you start to relax, in and out through your nose.
5. Try to breathe more deeply, using your diaphragm and abdomen rather than just your lungs.
6. As your breaths get deeper, pause very briefly between inhaling and exhaling, being aware at that point of the oxygen and energy filling your body.
7. Pause slightly between exhaling and inhaling, allowing your body to completely relax at that very moment.
8. Try counting during inhalation and exhalation. Start with a count of three on breathing in and five on breathing out. If this feels comfortable increase the exhalation count a little at first and then the inhalation count.
9. As you breathe, feel yourself relaxing and sinking deeper into the chair.
10. Continue as long as you wish.
11. Once you have completed the exercise, open your eyes, return your breathing toward normal, and stretch. Bring your arms out straight, then raise them slowly above your head, allowing them to touch before bringing them back to your side. Do this three times.
12. Get up slowly rather than standing up right away to allow your body time to adapt.

Note: During the exercise, do not hyperventilate. If you begin to feel dizzy or sick, open your eyes and stop the exercise. Concentrate on something else until your breathing returns to normal and any untoward sensations have passed.

Visualization

This is another technique used to help both the mind and body relax by providing it with positive thoughts and temporarily steering the thoughts away from the 'worries' of your world. It is believed that your thoughts influence how you feel and act. If you continually dwell on the negative thoughts and processes, then you are more likely to be an unhappy and unsatisfied person. However, if you change those thoughts into happy and positive ones, then your mood and behavior will most likely follow that change. Visualization is a therapy used to help elevate your mood and direct your thoughts to positive ones.

Visualization Exercise

1. Start by sitting quietly and thinking of a place or an object that is pleasing to you, for instance a waterfall. Then begin to visualize all of the surroundings. Imagine the water rushing down and falling into the pool below. Then look up to see the mountains surrounding the pool and follow the pool of water down a stream, visualizing the flowers and the trees along the banks.

2. Next, introduce your other senses. Imagine how the air smells, the sounds you may hear, and how the soft grass feels beneath your feet as you walked alongside the river.

3. As you move along, you can hear yourself saying, "I feel calm," or "I'm letting go of my tension" and see it float away down the river.

4. Once your body learns to associate this place with feeling relaxed and happy, you can go to this place anytime you feel nervous, anxious, or depressed and replace those negative feelings with calm ones.

Meditation

Meditation comprises a number of practices that aim to calm and quiet the active mind. By concentrating on one particular element, such as a sound, an image, a word, or one's breathing, intrusive thoughts that induce stress are excluded. Most people fill their mind with constant thoughts of past memories or future plans. Both have a tremendous ability to induce stress and disturb calm. The desired end result of meditation is to focus the mind on the present, allowing the body to feel, breathe, and exist in the 'here and now', rather than in the past or future.

During meditation, we are not trying to remove all external stimulation. However, while experiencing and appreciating sounds, smells, and images, they are allowed to drift through the mind without being dwelt upon.

Proven Effectiveness

There is ample evidence to demonstrate that meditation induces significant physiologic changes in the brain and body. The practice generates a profound alteration in the way our mind and body interact. Evolved as we are, the reactions of our body remain quite primitive, still under the influence of the older, less developed areas of our brain. The fight-or-flight response, for example, is mediated by the 'primitive' hypothalamus and brainstem with little influence from the developed 'thinking area' of our brain, the cerebral cortex. Studies on individuals experienced in meditation, such as yogis or Zen practitioners, found them to achieve a state of restful alertness, relaxed yet receptive. In addition, they were able to slow their heart rate and breathing rate, reduce their metabolism, increase their skin resistance, and induce a calm alpha rhythm on brain-wave recording.

How to Meditate

While there are many different meditation disciplines (Transcendental Meditation (TM), Zen Buddhism, Kundalini and Hatha Yoga, etc.), they all share a few essential principles and practices.

Quietness and Isolation: You need to be in a place where you will not be disturbed by other people, or devices such as telephones, pagers, radio, or television.

Comfort: You need to be comfortable in your posture, clothing, and environment.

Time: You need to set aside a certain amount of time that you are comfortable with. Whether you choose 3 minutes or 30 minutes, you need to complete the entire time period.

Attitude: You need to be open to the process of meditation and its desired goals. Peace and happiness are an ideal starting point.

Breathing: A key component to all meditation exercises is calm and controlled breathing. Practice this first.

Do not be disheartened if your first attempts at meditation seem to be a battle of wills between you and the thought processes of your active mind. This is very normal and will subside as you get more experienced. Recognize the intrusive thoughts for what they are and let them drift by like clouds in a blue summer sky without dwelling upon them.

Physiologic Changes During Meditation

- Lower metabolic rate
- Reduced oxygen consumption
- Reduced heart rate and blood pressure
- Slower breathing
- Increased parasympathetic nervous system activity
- Reduced sympathetic (fight-or-flight) nervous system activity
- Reduced skin electrical resistance (a measure of 'anxiety')
- Reduced lactate (produced by muscle metabolism)
- Increased alpha-rhythm activity (calmness) in brain EEG recording
- Reduced activity in the reticular formation (brainstem area responsible for stimulation)

Meditation Exercise #1

3-Minute Seated Meditation

Once practiced, this meditation can be used almost anywhere, allowing you the ability to calm your mind and body throughout the day. You should first learn this technique at home in a comfortable quiet place, but later on it may be used at work or on a train, for example.

1. Find a room where you can sit comfortably. You may choose to sit in a chair to support your back, or you may prefer to sit cross-legged on the floor.

2. Wear loose comfortable clothing, but ensure you are not too warm or too cold.

3. Turn off the television, radio, or other devices, and unplug the telephone.

4. You may play some music with natural sounds, such as ocean waves or bird songs.

5. Close your eyes.

6. Take 5 deep breaths. On your first inhalation, slowly count to 3. Then start to exhale on a count of 3. On the next breath, again inhale to 3, and exhale to 5. On the third and subsequent breaths, inhale to a count of 3, and exhale to 7. Increase the counts on either inhalation or exhalation if you feel that you can comfortably.

7. While continuing to breath, now concentrate on relaxing muscle groups throughout your body. Start with your forehead and face. As you exhale, feel the muscles in this area calm and relax. Release all tension from them. This may take a few breaths to complete. Then move on to your shoulders and repeat the same exercise. Gradually work your way down through your trunk, along your legs, and finally into your toes.

8. Once you are completely relaxed, continue to breathe and focus on your breath as it moves freely through the relaxed muscles. Remember to breathe deeply, using your diaphragm.

9. On completion of the exercise, open your eyes, slightly increase your breathing, and begin to slowly move your limbs before standing. Do not stand up immediately; rather, do it in stages to allow your body to adapt.

Meditation Exercise #2

10- to 15-Minute Quiet Place Meditation

This exercise can be performed daily or two to three times per week, depending on your available time and level of stress. Generally this will be done at home. It is an ideal exercise for relaxing at the end of the day.

1. You may wish to set aside a room or area that can be used as your meditation sanctuary. You can light some candles and incense for added ambiance. You may want to turn off or dim the lights, and as with all relaxation exercises, turn off distractions. Tell other members of your household that you do not want to be disturbed for 10 to 15 minutes.

2. Wear loose comfortable clothing but ensure you are not too warm or too cold.

3. You may play some music with natural sounds, such as ocean waves or bird songs.

4. Close your eyes.

5. Take 5 deep breaths. On your first inhalation, slowly count to 3. Then start to exhale on a count of 3. On the next breath, again inhale to 3, and exhale to 5. On the third and subsequent breaths, inhale to a count of 3, and exhale to 7. Increase the counts on either inhalation or exhalation if you feel that you can comfortably.

6. While continuing to breath, concentrate on relaxing muscle groups throughout your body. Start with your forehead and face. As you exhale, feel the muscles in this area calm and relax. Release all tension from them. This may take a few breaths to complete. Then move on to your shoulders and repeat the same exercise. Gradually work your way down through your trunk, along your legs, and finally into your toes.

7. Once you are completely relaxed, continue to breathe and focus on your breath as it moves freely through the relaxed muscles. Remember to breathe deeply, using your diaphragm.

8. Allow yourself to relax, sinking into the floor or bed. Imagine you are sinking slowly through a cloud, floating gently downward.

9. You can focus on your breathing or on a mantra, a pleasant thought on which you can concentrate as part of your relaxation exercise. It may be a particular word or sound such as "Om" (pronounced "ohm"), "peace" or "calm;" an image such as an ocean, a rainbow, or a forest glen; or an object like a statue or simple picture. If your mind begins to drift into a chain of thought or stress awareness, remain calm, recognize the intrusion, but refocus on your breathing or mantra.

10. Once you have completed this exercise, open your eyes, take 3 deep breaths, and gradually begin to move. Stand up slowly.

Meditation Exercise #3
10- to 20-Minute Walking Meditation

Walking meditation provides both a source of relaxation and exercise. It can be performed anywhere, although ideally it should be somewhere quiet with few distractions. An early morning walk in the summer is an excellent idea since it is light enough to be out before the morning bustle begins.

1. Make sure you are in comfortable walking attire.

2. At the start of your walk, relax with a breathing exercise. Take 5 deep breaths. On your first inhalation, slowly count to 3. Then start to exhale on a count of 3. On the next breath, again inhale to 3, and exhale to 5. On the third and subsequent breaths, inhale to a count of 3, and exhale to 7. Increase the counts on either inhalation or exhalation if you feel that you can comfortably.

3. Begin to walk, breathing slowly in over 3 to 4 steps and out over 4 to 5. Walk at a comfortable pace but not too slowly. Allow your arms to swing freely with shoulders relaxed.

4. Appreciate beauty in the images you pass — the blue sky, the flowers, the birds singing. Use these as your mantra. If your mind slips into thoughts of work, for example, refocus your mind on a particular tree, the warmth of the sun's rays, or the sound of a cricket.

5. At the end of the walk, complete the exercise with some deep breaths and simple stretches.

Music

Under normal everyday stressors, the excitatory parts of the brain are continually firing. This creates an imbalance in brain functioning, and furthers the fight-or-flight response. Music has been shown to balance this and reinforce the relaxation response. Music has a real potential to decrease the physiological and psychological aspects of anxiety and stress. This makes for a very pleasant and affordable tool for stress management.

Music Therapy

Many of us put on music to relax after a hard day at work or to dance to before going out for a night on the town. Your parents may have played music to you as an infant to soothe and calm you before bed. Music is used in many different places to set a certain mood or enhance our environment. Music has a tremendous ability to alter our mood, whether to raise goose bumps, bring tears, or get our feet tapping!

While subjective reports of reduced anxiety and stress with increased sensations of relaxation and calmness are common, it was not until the late 1980s and early 1990s that a biochemical mechanism for music therapy was discovered. Music is processed predominantly in the nonverbal areas in the temporal lobe of the brain. By stimulating these relaxing, nonverbal pathways to the brain, not only is there a direct increase in the relaxation response physically and psychologically, but there is also a balance that is restored to the brain.

Numerous studies have shown a significant decrease in heart rate, skin temperature, and muscle activation, and stress while listening to music. In one study, 43 females and 44 males were exposed to the cognitive stress of preparing for an oral presentation. Half the students listened to Pachelbel's Canon in D major while preparing for their presentation, while the control group worked in silence. Subjective anxiety, heart rate, blood pressure, cortisol, and salivary IgA were measured during rest and after the presentation. The control group demonstrated significantly increased anxiety, heart rate and blood pressure, findings not seen in those exposed to music. This effect was gender independent. Music also increased salivary IgA levels showing an increase in immunity.

Similar results were found in patients awaiting surgical procedures. The results indicated that heart rate and blood pressure dropped significantly in the group that heard music prior to the procedure, while the control group remained unchanged. In addition, the group receiving music intervention required less physician-administered sedation during the procedure than the control group.

Another interesting study looked at the effect of drumming sessions on stress levels in workers at a retirement community. For 1 hour each week over a 6-week trial period, participants used percussion instruments, along with breathing, imagery, and movement. At the end of the trial, 46% reported reduced stress and anxiety and improved mood. Six weeks later this figure was 62%. In addition, over the subsequent year, staff retention was significantly higher.

Music Therapy Strategies

- Try driving to work with soothing classical music — you will be surprised how little traffic and irresponsible drivers bother you!
- Put on some soothing music during your deep-breathing exercises.
- Listen to some relaxing music while wearing headphones and shut your eyes when you get home from work.

Contemporary Music for Relaxation

Enya
Enigma
Sarah McLachlan
Loreena McKennitt
Jan Garbarek and The Hilliard Ensemble — Officium

Classical Music for Relaxation

Rachmaninov (Piano Concerto #2 C-Minor Op.18 — 2nd Movt. Adagio)
Chopin (Nocturnes)
Pachelbel (Canon)
Beethoven (Moonlight Sonata)
Albinoni (Adagio)

Laughter Therapy

From Freud to Patch Adams, the role of laughter in stress and disease has been well recognized. Laughter provides a coping mechanism, an alternative to stress, unpleasantness, or despair. There is truth in the saying, "If I didn't laugh, I'd cry." Trying to see the funny side to a particularly desperate or unfortunate situation is an excellent option and acts to mitigate the stress response.

There is ample evidence to support laughter therapy as a form of stress reduction. A study in 1993 in the *International Journal of Humor Research* found laughter to improve mood in subjects exposed to high levels of daily stress. Interestingly, in those who laughed the most, added stress was actually correlated with better mood, indicating that these individuals were coping better and using stress in a positive manner.

There is also evidence that laughter improves disease outcome, not only through improvement in quality of life but by boosting immunity. A study from Indiana found humor to be one of the most frequently used complementary therapies in cancer patients. Laughter therapy was shown to decrease stress and increase natural killer (NK) cell activity, a factor positively associated with better outcome in other studies.

Stress Relief

Prescription for Laughter

- Spend time with happy people and those who make you laugh.
- Rent or go to a comedy movie rather than an action or horror film.
- Go to a comedy show.
- Try to remember jokes and make others laugh.
- Make a list of funny events/pictures/jokes that you can look at when you are stressed.

Pet Therapy

The husband of a good friend of ours has the perfect stress-management system for his wife. Whenever he senses she has a little tension, perhaps after a long day at work, a sensitive family situation, or a financial deadline, he brings up the topic of their pet kitten, often accompanied by a particularly adorable photo. It always does the trick!

There is ample evidence to support the soothing role of pets in innumerable conditions, including chronic illness, anxiety, panic attacks, depression, and social phobias. Researchers have shown that interaction with a pet can improve outcome in psychological treatment programs. Simply stroking a friendly cat or dog induces physiologic relaxation with lowered pulse, blood pressure, and breathing rate, along with overall muscle relaxation and a feeling of calm. Truly man's best friend!

Counseling

Counseling is a therapeutic technique used to help individuals reorganize their life patterns and thought processes by identifying emotional and mental issues and gaining a new perspective on them. Probably the most basic form of therapy, counseling is the most difficult to give and receive.

Lifestyle Changes

Certain very simple lifestyle changes can and should be made to make your life as stress free as possible.

No Multitasking

Do not multitask. Although you may think this is a time-efficient way to go about things, you will rapidly become overloaded. The more stimuli you impose upon yourself, the greater, the activity of the HPA axis and adrenal glands. Keep your tasks or jobs simple, so do them one at a time, and do them well. When you are finished move on to the next.

Learn to Say 'No'

People often have a problem saying 'no' to others for fear of hurting or upsetting them. They end up saying 'yes' to everything, taking on too much and hurting themselves. Learn what your boundaries are, and how much you can handle. Once you reach that limit, do not take on any more commitments or engagements. Others will understand, for they themselves are probably overloaded, otherwise they would not be asking for your help or involvement.

Avoid Known Stressors

If there are certain parts of your day where you know you will encounter stressors, try to alter your pattern. For instance, if you get upset in traffic try not leave the house at prime time. Get up a little earlier so you can miss the traffic — and possibly go for a workout before you start work. Then you can leave the office sooner and miss the traffic on the way home. If you can't avoid the traffic, then prepare yourself for it. Bring some soothing music to listen to, or a tape of something you want to learn. Then, at least, if you are sitting in traffic, you can enjoy yourself.

Counseling has been likened to the advice of a parent, one who listens completely, gives you full attention, and sees things in a different light. The counselor, like the parent, has complete faith in your ability to change and will help you make decisions and informed choices to explore new goals and directions.

Counseling is used for a wide variety of illnesses, such as depression, grief, anxiety, self-esteem, and stress problems. There are also many different types of counseling, and there is no one right answer for everyone. Individuals are different in their thoughts and how they process them, thus each person will be differ in the most effective way to handle them.

Psychoanalysis

The goal of psychoanalysis is to bring the unconscious feelings and impulses repressed in a person to the forefront of the consciousness. This is done to gain insight into where these feeling may have come from and help the individual realize that they are in the past. Once they understand that their present behavior is due to a 'perceived' threat or stressor from the past, and that this stressor no longer exists in the present, it is easier to let go of those behaviors.

Don't Set Unrealistic Goals

Many of us want to do everything and do it as quickly as possible. We are impatient because society has programmed us to expect results right away, whether they are in health care, career advancement, or via high-speed Internet. Our failure to achieve goals is a major stressor. Reset your goals to be attainable, and attainable within realistic time frames.

Positive Affirmation

Wake up and look in the mirror and take note of one positive thing each day. If you see something you don't like, then look away for now. Don't focus on the negative. Try to find something positive in everything, however hard that may seem. The actual process of looking for 'good' is calming — and finding it will improve your mood and outlook.

Journaling

Write down your feelings, thoughts, and expressions. Too often we keep them bottled up inside. Use your journal as a silent counselor, one through whom you can let out all that you feel. Later on, you can go back and read through and identify why certain feelings may have come up, or specific patterns were set. Identification is half of the process, for once you see where behaviors may arise, you can then concentrate on changing them. Alternatively, you can write down your feelings and then throw them away as a symbol of you letting go of those unnecessary thoughts that may be detrimental to your health and causing stress.

Psychoanalysis

Psychoanalysis is best used to help those with repressed memories from childhood. Whether these are true memories, or perceived memories, psychoanalysis can help to identify those past feelings, bring them to the conscious mind, and help resolve them. It is also useful for identifying unconscious conflicts and motives in the past and present. Often people are unaware of what is bothering them, they simply do not feel 'right' or balanced or calm. Psychoanalysis is one form of therapy that can help this individual identify what is locked in the unconscious mind, so that they can let it go and begin the healing process.

Free Association

Psychoanalysis of one's behavior may be conducted in a variety of different ways. Free association is one method, where the therapist says a word or shows the individual a picture and asks them to verbalize the first word or thought that comes into their mind. For example, if the word spoken by the therapist was "authority" and the patient's response is fear, the therapist can then explore with the patient why they may be fearful of authority. Is it a parent or a job that represents authority now? How can this fear then be diffused? By analyzing the very first word or thought that comes to mind, one can usually disregard the power of the conscious thoughts that like to take over our mental and physical processes. This allows the therapist to get at the unbiased subconscious mind.

Dream Interpretation

Psychoanalysis also uses dream interpretation. Again, as we are not consciously aware, nor awake during sleep, our dreams may provide us with an unbiased view of the subconscious mind. Although our dreams may seem irrational or even ridiculous, they are a representation of our body's mental process when it is not controlled by societal thoughts, pressures, and stressors.

The language of dreams is very different from our day-to-day interpretations of our conversations. For instance, death in a dream does not necessarily mean the physical death of a person. It is usually indicative of the 'death' or breaking of a pattern or belief system. Similarly, each color has a specific interpretation and each person (for example, father, boss, sibling) a specific meaning. What these colors or people represent can be different for each patient. One person may associate the color red with anger, one may view it as love.

Gestalt Therapy

Gestalt therapy is used to help the individual 'own' their feelings. Often people will display abnormal behaviors and thoughts, but are not aware as to where they came from and often blame other people for their problems. Gestalt therapy helps the person become connected again and feel more in charge of themselves, rather than at the 'mercy' of others.

This loss of control may only be perceived; there may not actually be someone in their life controlling their thoughts and/or actions, but it is real to them. Most likely, at some point in this person's life, they did feel that someone or some situation did dictate their actions and that feeling has stayed with them, and transcended into several other areas of their present life. For example, a controlling parent in the past can lead to passive and subservient behavior, a sense of lack of control in any situation where there is authority. Sibling rivalry may lead to extreme competition as an adult and the need to win or control every outcome.

Gestalt therapy is also used for those people who may feel incomplete. Many people in today's society experience episodes of emptiness or feeling as if something is missing. For most of these people, such feelings do not alter behavior greatly, but there are some people who do not feel whole and are chronically searching for something to complete them. More often than not, this feeling of emptiness is coming from a lack of love or respect. Gestalt therapy helps these individuals recognize or 'own' their feelings so as to feel 'whole' again.

Behavioral Therapy

Behavioral therapies encompass a wide variety of techniques or procedures used to retrain thought process or behaviors. The goal of this type of therapy is to help the individual learn a new behavior or thought process and use that instead of a damaging one. They replace a negative or maladaptive behavior with a healthy new one. For instance, when one looks in the mirror and sees only negative images, a false view of one's self quickly builds. This negative behavior can be replaced with a positive one by identifying and verbalizing one positive aspect, whether it is physical or emotional, every time one looks in the mirror. Eventually, this positive behavior replaces the conditioned self-defeating negative behavior, and the individuals' view of themselves begins to change.

This therapy uses techniques such as desensitization, conditioning, and modeling. These are all slightly different ways of exposing the individual to their stressor or fear, and helping to remodel the view of it and therefore their response to it. A simple example of this is in treating the fear of heights. Slowly the individual takes small steps toward the edge of the balcony, looking over without an overcoming fear of death. This process may start by simply looking at photos of balconies, progressing to standing under a balcony, then in a house attached to the balcony, and so forth. With each session, the individual deconditions the response of fear to whatever stage (proximity to the balcony) they are at.

Humanistic Therapy

Humanistic therapy encourages unconditional positive affirmation of the self, using techniques that continually guide the patient back to the present, so that they stop dwelling on the past. We cannot change the past but we have the ability to alter the way we live in the present and therefore affect our

Humanistic Therapy

Humanistic therapy is used to retrain perception, mostly disturbed perceptions of one's self. Some people have a distorted match between their real self and what they think they should be (their 'ideal self'), which diminishes their self worth. These people are usually very shy and insecure, and often have associated disorders, such as anorexia or bulimia. By helping these people focus on only the positive and inhibit the return to their negative self-image, they can foster a realistic perception of themselves.

Cognitive Therapy

Best suited for those who have irrational beliefs or thoughts that are negative and self-defeating, cognitive therapy teaches the person to evaluate each situation and to bring it to the conscious mind. Instead of just reacting quickly with pure emotion, cognitive therapy encourages a slower breakdown of the situation into its logical components. This resolves a situation previously perceived as stressful.

future. Humanistic therapy purposely steers away from most 'why' questions, as they tend to recreate the negative feeling. Rather, humanistic therapy deals with the 'how' and 'what' of a situation. How can we change this thought? What can we do about it? For this reason, the majority of humanistic therapy is verbal.

Most people with mismatched perceptions of self do not engage in stimulating challenges for a fear of failure or inadequacy. Humanistic therapy can help the individual stay in the present, and realize that although they may not have thought they could have done something in the past, they are no longer that same person. They now have the strength and ability to achieve their goals. In doing this, the individual develops a sense of pride and self worth. Humanistic therapy focuses on how to achieve the goals and what can be done to change the negative self-doubt, rather than on why the self-doubt arose in the first place.

Cognitive Therapy

Cognitive therapy is somewhat similar to humanistic therapy in that it works to replace negative thought processes. However, the focus is based on logic. Rather than simply replacing a bad thought with a good one and reconditioning the thought process, cognitive therapy works to identify erroneous ideas or beliefs that individuals may have about themselves or things around them.

For example, a person applying for a new job may believe, "I am stupid, there is no way I could do that job." Rather than dismissing the job and passing on this opportunity, cognitive therapy can be used to analyze the situation. Let's say the job opening is for an office receptionist. Cognitive therapy would break this job down accordingly. This woman applying for the job can answer the telephone — she does so all the time at home. She can organize and file things away — after all, she keeps dishes in one place in their house, linens in another. She has computer skills — she chats on-line, researches vacations spots, and e-mails friends from home. By analyzing each task involved in being an office receptionist, this person recognizes she is capable of being this receptionist. In doing so, she has changed the way she views herself and her perception of herself in the world. This alteration in belief and perception is the basis of cognitive therapy.

Anti-Stress Medications

E merging in tandem with our fast-paced lifestyle is a desire for rapid, easy solutions to almost everything, from meals to malaise. Whether it be weight loss, wrinkles, love, or depression, society is looking for the 'magic pill' that will obviate the need for dieting, exercise, communication, learning, or responsibility. After all, who has time for all that? The same is likely true for stress. If you could take a pill rather than read, digest, and institute even part of the treatment recommendations in this book, would you not be tempted? We need to be able to get our stress management out of the way and get back to our hectic lives as soon as possible!

Antianxiety and Antidepressant Drugs

The pharmacological treatment of anxiety and anxiety-related disorders is an expansive and complex topic that is outside the scope of this book. Indeed, the majority of individuals with chronic stress will not need to resort to such therapy.

CRH-Receptor Blockers (Antalarmin and Astressin)

An exciting new prospect for the treatment of stress-related disorders are the CRH-blockers, a new class of drug that targets the HPA-axis stress system directly.

The overwhelming importance of corticotrophin-releasing hormone (CRH) as the 'master hormone' of the stress response is only paralleled by discoveries of its numerous roles as a communicating molecule throughout the body. Not only does it function as a neurotransmitter within the brain, it is found within the gut, the skin, the immune system, and the uterus, to mention but a few of its many sites of activity. The omnipresence of CRH has spurred research into its precise function throughout the body, acting as it does through receptors on the surface of the variety of cells with which it interacts — CRH-1 and CRH-2 receptors.

Commonly Prescribed Medications for Stress-Related Mental and Mood Disorders

The following table lists some of the commonly prescribed medications for conditions known to be associated with stress. Note that these medications often have significant side effects and interactions with other drugs, so let your prescribing physician know of any other medicines or supplements you are taking.

Drug	Action/Contraindications/Side Effects
Beta-blockers (Inderal, Tenormin)	Block the action of adrenaline to reduce the associated feelings of panic associated with situation-specific anxiety. Used in social anxiety disorder. Not to be used in the presence of asthma, heart failure, artery disease, and hypothyroidism.
Benzodiazepines (Valium, Xanax, Serax)	Enhance the function of GABA within the brain. Used in GAD and panic disorder. May cause drowsiness and depression.
SSRIs (selective serotonin reuptake inhibitors) (Prozac, Paxil, Zoloft)	Influence serotonin concentration and receptor sensitivity in the brain. Used in GAD, panic disorder, OCD, and PTSD. Take 2-6 weeks to be effective. Can cause nervousness, nausea, reduced libido.
MAOIs (Monoamine Oxidase Inhibitors) (Eldepryl, Nardil, Parnate)	Block the action of an enzyme in the brain that breaks down serotonin and noradrenaline, thereby increasing their concentration. Used in panic disorders and post-traumatic stress disorder (PTSD), particularly when other drugs have not been successful. Require dietary controls. Severe drug interactions, affect blood pressure, reduce libido, and cause insomnia.
Tricyclic Antidepressants (Anafranil, Tofranil, Elavil)	Affect serotonin and noradrenaline activity within the brain. Used in panic disorders and PTSD usually as second-line drugs. Take 2-6 weeks to be effective. Side effects include dry mouth, constipation, blurred vision, dizziness, and low blood pressure.
Buspirone	A relatively new psychotropic drug with anxiolytic properties. Relieves anxiety without causing sedation. Unlike the benzodiazepines, Buspirone does not act on the GABA receptor but works through the dopamine and serotonin (5-HT) system.

As a natural step in this investigation, drugs have been developed that block these receptors, thereby preventing the CRH from exerting its influence. The clinical effects of CRH blockers (such as antalarmin and astressin) are the subject of a growing body of research.

Associated Activities

Although CRH, through its stimulation of cortisol production, might be thought of as having an anti-inflammatory role, there is ample evidence that it acts peripherally to enhance the inflammatory response. CRH induces mast-cell degranulation, a process liberating numerous inflammatory chemicals into the involved tissue. In addition, it appears to have a direct pro-inflammatory action on many immune cells, which carry specific CRH receptors. Exciting research using animal models of arthritis has shown CRH-blocking drugs to reduce the pain, swelling, and damage associated with this condition significantly. This offers the possibility of significant therapeutic potential for inflammation-related diseases.

CRH, along with other neurotransmitters within the brain such as CCK, are particularly involved in the regulation of appetite, reward, and anxiety. There is significant recent evidence that point to an important role for CRH in conditions of dependency and addiction, whether the addiction be to drugs, alcohol, or certain foods (those high in glucose or fat). Research using animal models has found reversal of addictive behavior in association with reduced anxiety with CRH-blocker treatment. There may be a future role for these drugs in addiction, alcoholism, and obesity.

The interaction of CRH with the immune system, in particular, the mast cell, implicates this hormone as the link between stress and the development or exacerbation of inflammatory conditions, such as asthma, dermatitis, and inflammatory bowel disease (IBD), as well as migraine and heart attack. Further elucidation of this relationship may reveal a role for CRH-blocking drugs in the prevention or treatment of these conditions.

CRH produced in the endometrium of the uterus has a vital role in both controlling implantation and inducing contractions during labor. The importance of CRH in implantation and early maintenance of pregnancy could lead to a contraceptive role. Studies on sheep have used CRH-blockers to delay labor safely and effectively, offering a potential use in premature delivery.

Effectiveness

The recognition that CRH and cortisol play important roles in depression and anxiety-related disorders has fueled the bulk of research into possible pharmacological roles for CRH-blockers. There is substantial evidence from animal studies that these drugs are effective at reducing or abolishing the stress response, improving anxiety and depression in these models. Interestingly, the drugs were most effective in models of chronic stress where the CRH/cortisol 'tone' was high rather than in normal subjects. Early studies on human subjects are encouraging, with significant antidepressant and antianxiety action without side effects found with traditional medication.

Prescribe with Caution

CRH blockers are currently experimental. The majority of research involves animal models with human clinical trials at only a very early stage. The precise role for these drugs is undetermined at present, their side effects and long-term sequelae unknown. While it does appear that CRH blockers will become a useful addition to the pharmacological armory, particularly in the field of psychiatry, they are unlikely to be the panacea for chronic stress. They may help counteract the actions of CRH in promoting disease, but this should be considered a case of closing the stable door after the horse has not only bolted, but disappeared over the horizon. Our recommendation is to act now, use the suggestions and techniques in this book to reduce and control stress. Prevent problems before they arise and treat the symptoms you have. Do not wait for the 'magic bullet' — it might miss!

8-Week Stress Solution Program

Now that we have seen the individual treatments available for balancing the stress response and avoiding chronic stress, we can put them all together in an easy-to-follow program. This program is designed to restore your body to a balanced state (homeostasis) so you can prevent chronic stress and stress-related diseases and disorders. During an 8-week program of natural biological therapy — diet, nutritional supplements, physical, and psychological relaxation therapies — you should be able to establish lifestyle changes that will help you manage your stress forever. Beware sabre-toothed tigers!

Four Stages

The program is compartmentalized into four stages: the first two stages run for two weeks each, the third for four weeks, the final stage for the rest of your life. Each stage changes slightly as your stress response changes. Stage one introduces a strict naturopathic diet, with more natural supplementation and hands-on physical therapy, but less exercise than subsequent stages. During stage two, as your hormone levels normalize and your stress response lessens, your requirement for natural supplementation to alter hormone levels diminishes. In addition, as your body is more balanced and calm, you will find it easier to do more relaxation exercises, such as deep breathing or yoga at home. Once you have reached a balanced level after 8 weeks, you can maintain your stress response in a healthy state forever.

In most cases, this 8-week program will be sufficient to allow progression to a maintenance regimen. However, in some cases, a more prolonged initial period may be required. Again, in this case, help from your health-care practitioner is recommended. In addition, during times of excessive stress, such as exams, deadlines, or personal crises, a short period of return to stage one or two will be beneficial.

Program Components

Naturopathic Diet

Diet is the central component of all three stages of stress management in order to ensure proper blood sugar level stability at all times. This is achieved through the naturopathic diet with the addition of protein at each meal and the reduction of carbohydrates. Your body still requires carbohydrates, but it is important to eat vegetables and salads as your primary source. High-glycemic carbohydrates, such as sugars or starch (pasta, rice, potatoes), cause rapid swings in blood sugar levels, an added stressor to the body.

The naturopathic diet program for each stage is designed for two different groups. The first is for those who only want to stabilize blood sugar levels and prevent hypoglycemia from being a stressor. The second is for those who also want to lose weight as part of their stress-management program. The diets change over the 8-week period, culminating in a maintenance program, which is a lifestyle change with numerous health benefits in addition to stress reduction.

Natural Supplements

As the symptoms, causes, and problems that result from stress differ so much between individuals, so does the type of supplementation. However, there are a few supplements that are very valuable in all cases of stress that can be taken with no side effects. Be sure to discuss any existing supplement and drug program with your health-care practitioner before integrating any new therapy.

Supplements are primarily used in the earlier stages of the program as a means of reducing stress and cortisol levels. The aim, however, is for diet, exercise, physical therapies, and relaxation therapy to provide the long-term solution.

• Vitamin B complex	100 mg per day, with food
• Essential Fatty Acids (Omega 3, 6, 9)	2000 mg per day, with food
• Calcium-Magnesium	350-175 mg, 2 times per day with food
• Hydrolyzed Milk Peptide	100 mg, 2 times per day, without food
OR	
• Magnolia Bark Extract	250 mg, 2 times per day, without food

Cardiovascular Exercise

Cardiovascular exercise is a great stress reliever. Not only does it divert your mind from work and other angst-inducing thoughts, it increases growth hormone and serotonin, releases pent-up energy, improves sleep, burns fat, and helps control blood sugar levels. The intensity with which you exercise should be about 65% of your maximum heart rate. This translates into exercise where it is hard to speak continuously while exercising, but you could, with a little difficulty, hold a brief conversation. (Of course, this is for the purpose of example only — exercise is your time, not to be interrupted by a chat or cell-phone!) As you get fitter, you can increase the intensity of your workout. If you already exercise regularly, then continue to do so. Just ensure that you are not overtraining. Make sure that you are only doing a maximum of 45 to 55 minutes cardiovascular exercise a day. Remember that increasing your cardiovascular exercise above this limit in order to deal with added stress is unlikely to be successful and may actually make things worse. Individuals in training or maintaining high exercise levels should consult with their trainer or doctor if they are concerned about stress or overtraining.

Ensure that your program incorporates a significant stretching component. Strength training can be used as additional exercise or as an alternative on certain days.

Physical Therapy

Physical therapy or bodywork incorporates massage, aromatherapy, acupuncture, craniosacral therapy, reflexology, Rei-ki and other 'hands-on' therapies. They are a tremendously important part of stress management, especially in the early stages where your body may not actually know how to relax. Individuals vary in their preference and response to different treatments, so use those treatments that seem to work best for you. You can reduce the frequency of physical therapies as the program progresses to a maintenance level, with opportunity for additional treatments as lifestyle dictates.

Relaxation Techniques

You can learn relaxation techniques that you can do at home, at work, in the car — or anywhere stress is likely to strike! These techniques allow you to manage stress on your own on a regular basis, preventing buildup during the day. Such lifestyle changes may be difficult at the beginning of a program, but it is important to keep practicing them. They will soon become second nature.

- Deep Breathing
- Visualization
- Yoga
- Meditation
- Lavender Bath
- Tai Chi

8-Week Program

Stage 1 (Weeks 1 and 2)

Naturopathic Diet

This diet section is divided into two parts. The first is for those who just wish to stabilize blood sugar levels and prevent hypoglycemia from being a stressor. The second is for those who wish to lose weight at the same time.

For Stress Management
- 1 gram of protein per kilogram of body weight divided throughout the day
- Unlimited vegetables and salads
- Maximum of 4 fruits a day (1 glass of juice is one piece of fruit and no bananas)
- Any dressing or condiment
- 2 slices of cheese every day, but not more.
- 5 nuts a day, but not more
- When consuming high-glycemic carbohydrates, such as bread, pasta, rice, potato, squash, corn, popcorn, yogurt, or cereal, ensure that the physical size of these carbohydrates is equal to or smaller than the physical size of the protein.
- No alcohol or sweets/desserts
- Try to only have a maximum of 1 cup of coffee per day. If you consume more than 3 a day, change your cups of coffee to half caffeinated and half decaffeinated, still consuming the same number of coffees a day. Slowly cut back by 1 cup every 3 days.

For Weight Loss and Stress Management
The diet remains unchanged for the full 8 weeks.
- 1 gram of protein per kilogram of body weight divided throughout the day
- Unlimited vegetables and salads
- Maximum of 2 fruits a day (1 glass of juice is 1 piece of fruit and no bananas)
- Any dressing or condiment
- A slice of cheese every other day, but not more
- 5 nuts a day, but not more

- No grains or starches — no bread, pasta, rice, potato, squash, corn, popcorn, yogurt, candy, cereal, or alcohol for these 2 weeks
- Try to only have a maximum of 1 cup of coffee per day. If you consume more than 3 a day, change your cups of coffee to half caffeinated and half decaffeinated, still consuming the same number of coffees a day. Slowly cut back by 1 cup every 3 days.

Natural Supplements

• Vitamin B Complex	100 mg per day, with food
• Essential Fatty Acids (Omega 3, 6, 9)	2000 mg per day, with food
• Calcium-Magnesium	175-350 mg, 2 times per day with food
• Hydrolyzed Milk Peptide	100 mg, 2 times per day, without food

OR

• Magnolia Bark Extract	250 mg, 2 times per day, without food

Cardiovascular Exercise

- 10 minutes stretching daily
- 30 minutes of cardiovascular exercise 3 times a week. The type of exercise is up to you: swimming, jogging, cycling, an aerobics class, or walking very briskly.

Physical Therapies (Bodywork)

- One hour of therapeutic bodywork each week: massage, reflexology, shiatsu, etc. This may be any type of bodywork, but it must be a type that is performed on you, not one that you do on your own.

Relaxation Techniques

- 1 hour of relaxation, such as yoga or meditation a week. This may be done at home with a video, at a gym in a class, or with a personal trainer. This may be split into two 30-minute sessions a week.
- 10 minutes of deep breathing each day. Do not worry if your mind travels at first when you start breathing — simply refocus your thoughts toward your breath and continue. As you progress, you will find it easier to stay focused.
- Take a 15-minute bath with lavender oil, 2 times a week.

Stage 2 (Weeks 3 and 4)

Naturopathic Diet

Once again, the diet section is divided into 2 parts. The first is for those who just wish to stabilize blood sugar levels and prevent hypoglycemia from being a stressor. The second for those who, in addition, wish to lose weight at the same time.

For Stress Management

- 1 gram of protein per kilogram of body weight divided throughout the day
- Unlimited vegetables and salads
- Maximum of 4 fruits a day (1 glass of juice is 1 piece of fruit and no bananas)
- Any dressing or condiment
- 2 slices of cheese every day, but not more
- 10 nuts a day, but not more
- When consuming high-glycemic carbohydrates, such as bread, pasta, rice, potato, squash, corn, popcorn, yogurt, or cereal, ensure that the physical size of these carbohydrates is equal to or smaller than the physical size of the protein.
- Maximum of 1 sweet/dessert every other day (must be consumed with protein)
- Maximum of 1 glass of alcohol every other day (must be consumed with protein)
- Maximum of 1 cup of coffee a day

For Weight Loss and Stress Management

The diet remains unchanged for the full 8 weeks.

- 1 gram of protein per kilogram of body weight divided throughout the day
- Unlimited vegetables and salads
- Maximum of 2 fruits a day (1 glass of juice is 1 piece of fruit and no bananas).
- Any dressing or condiment
- A slice of cheese every other day, but not more
- 5 nuts a day, but not more
- No grains or starches — no bread, pasta, rice, potato, squash, corn, popcorn, yogurt, candy, cereal, or alcohol for these 2 weeks

- Try to only have a maximum of 1 cup of coffee per day. If you consume more than 3 per day, change your cups of coffee to half caffeinated and half decaffeinated, still consuming the same number of coffees a day. Slowly cut back by one cup every 3 days.

Natural Supplements

With any natural supplement program, it is important to continue their use unless directed by your health-care practitioner. The first three supplements on the list should be taken on an ongoing basis. The hydrolyzed milk peptide or magnolia extract will be discontinued at a later date once the hormones in the stress pathway are regulated and symptoms resolved. For these 2 weeks, continue all supplements as you did in the first 2 weeks.

- Vitamin B Complex   100 mg per day, with food
- Essential Fatty Acids   2000 mg per day, with food
  (Omega 3, 6, 9)
- Calcium-Magnesium   175-350 mg, 2 times per day with food
- Hydrolyzed Milk Peptide   100 mg, 2 times per day, without food

OR

- Magnolia Bark Extract   250 mg, 2 times per day, without food

Cardiovascular Exercise

If you were a beginner exerciser during the first 2 weeks, then continue on the same exercise regime. If you have exercised in the past, try increasing the intensity of your workout on 1 day and the amount of time you exercise on the other 2 days.

- 10 minutes stretching daily
- 30 minutes of cardiovascular exercise 1 time a week at an intensity where you could not carry on a conversation through the exercise
- 35-40 minutes of cardiovascular exercise 2 times a week. The type of exercise is up to you: swimming, jogging, cycling, an aerobics class, or walking very briskly with a friend.

Physical Therapy (Bodywork)

If your budget and time permits, try to continue with 1 hour of bodywork a week for this 2-week stage.

- 30-60 minutes of therapeutic bodywork a week

Relaxation Techniques

After the first 2 weeks, your body should be starting to relax a little. However, like anything new, it takes time to integrate these techniques so that you can achieve their full benefit.

During this 2-week stage, try to focus more on your breathing and deepen the calming effect your relaxation techniques achieve. The frequency of the exercises remains the same during these 2 weeks, but the intensity and intention change. Rather than simply stretching or holding a yoga posture, for example, really concentrate on breathing deeply into each pose and relaxing each muscle group. Do the same for the deep-breathing exercises. Rather than extending the time you are deep breathing, ensure that you are making it through the full 10 minutes without your mind wandering off in other directions. If you are still having problems with this, you may find it useful to pick up a guided meditation tape.

- 1 hour of relaxation, such as yoga or meditation, each week. This may be done at home with a video, at a gym class, or with a personal trainer. This may be split into two 30-minute sessions a week.

- 10 minutes of deep breathing a day. Do not worry if your mind travels at first when you start breathing. Simply refocus your thoughts toward your breath and continue. As you progress, you will find it easier to stay focused.

- Take 30 minutes out of your day for yourself, to read a book or magazine, listen to music, knit or write. Do something just for you.

Stage 3   (Week 5 to 8)

Naturopathic Diet

Once again, the diet section is divided into two parts. The first is for those who just wish to stabilize blood sugar levels and prevent hypoglycemia from being a stressor. The second for those who wish to lose weight at the same time.

For Stress Management

- 1 gram of protein per kilogram of body weight divided throughout the day
- Unlimited vegetables and salads
- Maximum of 4 fruits a day (1 glass of juice is 1 piece of fruit and no bananas)
- Any dressing or condiment
- 2 slices of cheese every day (but not more)
- 10 nuts a day (but not more)
- When consuming high-glycemic carbohydrates, such as bread, pasta, rice, potato, squash, corn, popcorn, yogurt, or cereal, ensure that the physical size of these carbohydrates is equal to or smaller than the physical size of the protein.
- Maximum of 1 sweet/dessert every day (must be consumed with protein)
- Maximum of 1 glass of alcohol every day (must be consumed with protein)
- Maximum of 1 cup of coffee a day

For Weight Loss and Stress Management

The diet remains unchanged for the full 8 weeks.
- 1 gram of protein per kilogram of body weight divided throughout the day
- Unlimited vegetables and salads
- Maximum of 2 fruits a day (1 glass of juice is 1 piece of fruit and no bananas).
- Any dressing or condiment
- A slice of cheese every other day, but not more
- 5 nuts a day, but not more
- No grains or starches — no bread, pasta, rice, potato, squash, corn, popcorn, yogurt, candy, cereal, or alcohol for these 2 weeks

- Try to only have a maximum of 1 cup of coffee a day. If you consume more than 3 a day, change your cups of coffee to half caffeinated and half decaffeinated, still consuming the same number of coffees a day. Slowly cut back by 1 cup every 3 days.

Natural Supplements

During this stage, as you begin to see the effects of your lifestyle changes and relaxation techniques, you can begin to decrease the doses of the milk peptide and magnolia. Cut the dose in half. So rather than taking the supplements twice a day, cut back to once a day. Watch for signs of increased stress response, such as palpitations, difficulty sleeping, or anxiety. If they return, then increase your dose back up to twice a day and try cutting back in another 3 weeks. We would recommend seeking advice from your health-care practitioner at this stage.

- Vitamin B complex — 100 mg per day, with food
- Essential Fatty Acids (Omega 3, 6, 9) — 2000 mg per day, with food
- Calcium-Magnesium — 175-350 mg, 2 times per day, with food
- Hydrolyzed Milk Peptide — 100 mg *once* per day, without food

OR

- Magnolia Bark Extract — 250 mg *once* per day, without food

Cardiovascular Exercise

No matter at what level of exercise you started, continue to exercise a minimum of 3 times a week. If your schedule permits, try aiming for 4 to 5 times a week. As in weeks 3 and 4, try increasing the intensity or duration of each workout. Rather than simply doing the same exercise at the same pace, alter it. Walk or run uphill, swim with small weights on the ankles, or attend a more vigorous aerobics class. But whatever exercise you do, make sure you enjoy it!

- 10 minutes stretching daily
- 30 minutes of cardiovascular exercise once a week at an intensity where you could not carry on a conversation through the exercise

- 35-40 minutes of cardiovascular exercise twice a week. The type of exercise is up to you. It may be swimming, jogging, an aerobics class, or walking very briskly with a friend.

Physical Therapy (Bodywork)

Continue a minimum of 30 minutes therapeutic bodywork a week. If your budget does not support this, consider buying an instructional massage book, for example, and try exchanging massages with a friend.

Relaxation Techniques

By now your body should be quite accustomed to the relaxation techniques. Your body will become so attuned to these exercises that it will instinctively calm and relax as soon as you start. Even at work, at your desk, you can sit back and deep breathe for 10 breaths and your body will remember how to relax into that exercise and will calm down almost immediately. During this stage of the program, you can begin to integrate these techniques into your daily life.

- 1 hour of relaxation, such as yoga or meditation, per week. This may be done at home with a video, or at a gym in a class, or with a personal trainer. It may be split into two 30-minute sessions a week.

- 10 minutes of deep breathing twice a day. Try to do this at the beginning and end of the day.

- Sit back and deep breathe for 30 seconds whenever you feel stressed, in traffic, at your computer, at work, or just before bedtime. Watch your body relax, feel the muscles loosen, and then return back to the task at hand. You will be in a much better state of mind to handle whatever stressed you.

- Take 30 minutes out of your day for yourself, to read a book or magazine, listen to music, knit, or write. Do something just for you.

Stage 4 (Maintenance)

Naturopathic Diet

Having completed the initial 8-week program, you can progress to a maintenance phase. The diet is less restrictive and should be considered to be a healthy lifestyle change to your eating habits rather than a 'diet'. Besides the benefits of reduced metabolic stress, this maintenance plan has a number of added health benefits, including prevention of diabetes, high cholesterol, and blood pressure. You can deviate now and then without fear of any catastrophic consequences as long as you stick to the basic principles.

Both groups at this stage can follow the guidelines below. For those who wish to lose more weight, continuing with the stage one guidelines will allow this, although in some cases you may reach a plateau. For more information on this aspect of the diet and details on how to overcome the plateau, see our book, *The New Naturopathic Diet*, or consult with your natural health practitioner.

- 1 gram of protein per kilogram of body weight divided throughout the day
- Unlimited vegetables and salads
- Maximum of 4 fruits a day (1 glass of juice is 1 piece of fruit and no bananas)
- Any dressing or condiment
- 2 slices of cheese every day, but not more
- 10 nuts a day, but not more
- When consuming high-glycemic carbohydrates, such as bread, pasta, rice, potato, squash, corn, popcorn, yogurt, or cereal, ensure that the physical size of these carbohydrates is equal to or smaller than the physical size of the protein.
- 1 sweet/dessert every day (must be consumed with protein) — this does not mean you have to have one, but you can if you wish!
- 1-2 glasses of alcohol every day (must be consumed with protein) — this does not mean you have to consume alcohol, but if you do, try not to exceed these limits
- Try to only have a maximum of 1 cup of coffee a day.

Natural Supplements

For maintenance, use only the B-vitamins, essential fatty acids, and calcium-magnesium. For other specific supplements catered to your needs, it is best to see your health-care practitioner.

- Vitamin B complex   100 mg per day, with food
- Essential Fatty Acids   2000 mg per day, with food
  (Omega 3, 6, 9)
- Calcium-Magnesium   175-350 mg, 2 times per day, with food

Cardiovascular Exercise

No matter what level of exercise you started at, continue to exercise at a minimum of 3 times a week. If your schedule permits, try aiming for 4 to 5 times a week. As in weeks 3 and 4, try increasing the intensity or duration of each workout. Rather than simply doing the same exercise at the same pace, alter it. Walk or run uphill, swim with small weights on the ankles, or attend a more vigorous aerobics class. But whatever exercise you do, make sure you enjoy it!

- 10 minutes stretching daily
- 30 minutes of cardiovascular exercise once a week at an intensity where you could not carry on a conversation through the exercise
- 35-40 minutes of cardiovascular exercise twice a week. The type of exercise is up to you. It may be swimming, jogging, an aerobics class or walking very briskly with a friend.

Physical Therapy (Bodywork)

Most people neglect bodywork once they are feeling better. Do not do this. Ongoing bodywork is very important. However, you can cut back to one session a month. Incorporate it into your schedule, as you would to get your hair cut.

- 1 hour of therapeutic body work a month

Relaxation Techniques

The relaxation techniques should be used as part of your daily routine on an ongoing basis. If you feel your shoulders tightening up at work, sit back, take some deep breaths, stretch, and shake them out before they get painful.

- 1 hour of relaxation, such as yoga or meditation, each week. This may be done at home with a video, or at a gym in a class, or with a personal trainer. This may be split into two 30-minute sessions a week.

- 10 minutes of deep breathing twice a day. Try to do this at the beginning and end of the day.

- Try new techniques that differ from those you practiced in the first 8 weeks. Monitor your heart rate before and after the relaxation exercise to see how much your body is relaxing.

- Rent comedy movies as much as possible (rather than thrillers)

- Sit back and deep breath for 30 seconds whenever you feel stressed, for example, in traffic, at your computer, at work, or just before bedtime. Watch your body relax, feel the muscles loosen, and then return back to the task at hand.

- Try to take 30 minutes out of your day for yourself. Do something you enjoy, such as reading a book or magazine, listening to music, knitting, or writing.

Treating & Preventing Stress-Related Disorders & Diseases

Diabetes

Preventing Diabetes

Heidi is a doctor, a slim 29-year-old who works out daily, combining various forms of cardiovascular exercise and weight training. She eats a balanced diet, high in lean protein, vegetables, and salads with few simple carbohydrates. Despite this healthy lifestyle, Heidi gained 7 pounds in the past year, and although this was not substantial, it was central weight gain around her abdomen. As a doctor, Heidi recognized this as a health concern. She also found that her blood sugar levels were above normal. She had developed pre-Type 2 diabetes. She felt she did not fit the demographic — she exercised, ate well, and was not overweight.

Before beginning any pharmaceutical medications, Heidi tried increasing her cardiovascular exercise and further restricted her diet. However, this was to no avail and her blood sugars remained elevated.

During our consultation, Heidi described how overworked she was at her clinic and the local hospital — she started sacrificing sleep in order to fit everything into her schedule. We rapidly recognized that her central weight gain and diabetes were induced by stress.

Heidi began to decrease her hours at the hospital, started regular massage, and traded in some of her weight-training sessions for yoga classes. She started taking a magnolia extract supplement. Not long after that, she began to see a drop in her blood sugar levels. She continued to improve her lifestyle changes and began taking chromium and calcium-magnesium. Within 2 months, she had lost 4 of the 7 pounds around her waist and her blood sugar levels had returned to normal. Overall, she felt more balanced.

DIABETES MELLITUS IS A DISORDER of carbohydrate metabolism characterized by higher than normal blood sugar levels (hyperglycemia) and the inability of the body to utilize glucose as a fuel source. This results both from impaired insulin release from the pancreas in response to glucose, and, in Type 2 diabetics, from decreased insulin effectiveness at the tissue level (insulin resistance). Most Type 2 diabetic patients retain some insulin secretion but the response to glucose is severely decreased.

Diabetes Basics

There are an estimated 18 million people with diabetes in the United States (2 million in Canada) — 6.3% of the population — with about 5 million of those being undiagnosed. Diabetes was the sixth leading cause of death listed on U.S. death certificates in 2000. Altogether, diabetes contributed to 213,062 deaths. Overall, the risk for death among people with diabetes is about twice that of people without diabetes.

The incidence of diabetes is increasing at an alarming rate. Until 1990, the increase was about 1% per year, but since then it has increased to more than 6% per year (a 76% increase from 1990 to 2003), driven almost entirely by Type 2 diabetes.

Complications of Diabetes

Heart Disease and Stroke
- Heart disease is the leading cause of diabetes-related deaths. Adults with diabetes have heart disease death rates about two to four times higher than adults without diabetes.
- The risk for stroke is two to four times higher among people with diabetes.
- About 65% of deaths among people with diabetes are due to heart disease and stroke.

High Blood Pressure
- About 73% of adults with diabetes have blood pressure greater than or equal to 130/80 millimeters of mercury (mm/Hg) or use prescription medications for hypertension.

Blindness
- Diabetes is the leading cause of new cases of blindness among adults 20 to 74 years old.
- Diabetic retinopathy causes from 12,000 to 24,000 new cases of blindness each year.

Kidney Disease
- Diabetes is the leading cause of treated end-stage renal disease, accounting for 43% of new cases.
- In 2000, 41,046 people with diabetes began treatment for end-stage renal disease.
- In 2000, a total of 129,183 people with diabetes underwent dialysis or kidney transplantation.

Nervous System Disease
- About 60% to 70% of people with diabetes have mild to severe forms of nervous system damage. Damage includes impaired sensation or pain in the feet or hands, carpal tunnel syndrome, and other nerve problems.
- Severe forms of diabetic nerve disease are a major contributing cause of lower-extremity amputations.

Amputations
- More than 60% of nontraumatic lower-limb amputations in the United States occur among people with diabetes.
- From 2000 to 2001, about 82,000 nontraumatic lower-limb amputations were performed among people with diabetes.

Diabetes Prevention
The most important fact about pre-diabetes is that with appropriate treatment, including weight-loss, dietary change, exercise, and stress management, it is unlikely to progress to Type 2 diabetes.

Types of Diabetes

Diabetes mellitus is divided into three types. Type 1 or insulin-dependent, Type 2 or non-insulin dependent, and temporary, pregnancy-related, gestational diabetes. Type 1 accounts for 10% of all diabetes cases and individuals must inject extra insulin to help lower blood sugar levels. Type 2 individuals retain some insulin secretion, but may need oral medication and occasionally injected insulin to augment it.

Type 1
• Formerly called insulin-dependent diabetes or juvenile onset diabetes.
• Pancreas stops producing insulin.
• Comprises about 10% of people with diabetes.

Type 2
• Formerly called non-insulin-dependent diabetes or adult onset diabetes.
• Pancreas produces insufficient insulin and the tissues become resistant to its effects.
• Comprises about 90% of people with diabetes.

Gestational
• Temporary condition during pregnancy.
• Affects about 3% of pregnancies.
• Increased risk of future diabetes in mother and infant.

Dental Disease
• Periodontal or gum diseases are more common among people with diabetes than among people without diabetes. Among young adults, those with diabetes are often at twice the risk of those without diabetes.
• Almost one-third of people with diabetes have severe periodontal diseases with loss of attachment of the gums to the teeth measuring 5 millimeters or more.

Pregnancy
• Poorly controlled diabetes before conception and during the first trimester of pregnancy can cause major birth defects in 5% to 10% of pregnancies and spontaneous abortions in 15% to 20% of pregnancies.
• Poorly controlled diabetes during the second and third trimesters of pregnancy can result in excessively large babies, posing a risk to the mother and the child.

Other Complications
• Uncontrolled diabetes often leads to biochemical imbalances that can cause acute life-threatening events, such as diabetic ketoacidosis and hyperosmolar (nonketotic) coma.
• People with diabetes are more susceptible to many other illnesses and, once they acquire these illnesses, often have worse prognoses than people without diabetes. For example, they are more likely to die with pneumonia or influenza than people who do not have diabetes.

Treating & Preventing Stress-Related Disorders & Diseases

Causes of Diabetes

Type 1 diabetes remains of uncertain etiology, although recent research indicates that it is an autoimmune disease in which the body's immune system mounts an attack on the insulin-producing islet cells of the pancreas. It generally develops in children or young adults. There are inheritable risk factors that must come from both parents.

While Type 2 diabetes runs in families, indicating a possible genetic risk factor, this condition is strongly influenced by lifestyle and diet. Individuals not living in Westernized modern society do not tend to develop Type 2 diabetes, even if they have a strong family history. Obesity is a significant risk factor for the development of Type 2 diabetes and is most influential in young people. The past 10 years have seen a frightening increase in childhood obesity and the early onset of this disease, previously only prevalent in middle age. In fact, 80% of patients with this disease are overweight or obese. Labeled teenage-onset-diabetes, this epidemic of Type 2 diabetes in children and young adults is a product of the weight gain seen in this demographic. A gain of only 11 to 18 pounds doubles the risk of developing Type 2 diabetes.

Pre-Diabetes
Pre-diabetes is a condition considered a precursor to Type 2 diabetes. Characterized by higher than normal glucose levels, but not high enough to be called diabetes, this condition affects more than 20% of the U.S. population aged 40 to 74. There is evidence that even this early stage of diabetes increases cardiovascular, kidney, and other disease risks.

Age Onset of Diabetes

	Type 1	Type 2
Age of Onset	< 30 years	Formerly >30 years, now any age
Insulin secretion in response to glucose	Almost absent	Delayed and decreased
Diet causally related	No	Yes
Require insulin	Yes	Not initially
Response to oral medication	None	Good
Associated conditions (retinopathy, neuropathy vascular disease, nephropathy, etc.)	Yes	Yes

Role of Stress in Diabetes

Type 1 Diabetes

Currently, there is no clear link between stress and the development of Type 1 diabetes. Although there is some evidence that the effect of chronic stress on the immune system can increase the incidence and severity of autoimmune disease, no research has identified a specific connection with diabetes. Risk factors or triggers such as viruses or cold weather and the protective effect of breastfeeding may indicate further influence of the immune system. It is possible that in the future a more definite association will be made.

With respect to blood sugar control, although stress management is recommended as part of an overall Type 1 diabetes control program, there are no studies clearly demonstrating improved blood sugar control with such therapy. Available research, however, does reveal improvement in mood and diabetes 'coping skills.' While stress is known to adversely affect diabetes management, it is unclear as to whether this results from HPA-axis overactivity or poorer management by the patient.

✔ **STRESS FACT** **Diabetes Treatment**

Stress management can be recommended for both treatment and prevention of Type 2 diabetes and may be valuable in Type 1, at least from a psychological perspective.

Type 2 Diabetes

Because of its effects on insulin resistance, obesity, and the metabolic syndrome, chronic stress plays a central role in the development of Type 2 diabetes. Although dietary influences, such as fast food, increased carbohydrate consumption, and 'super-sizing', have played an important role, the association of stress has only added fuel to the fire.

There is ample evidence to support a role for stress management in the prevention and treatment of Type 2 diabetes. This form of therapy is appropriate at any stage, whether you are completely healthy, pre-diabetic, or suffer clinical Type 2 diabetes. In most cases, when combined with dietary modification and exercise, blood sugar control can be restored to normal, obviating the need for medication and significantly reducing the risk of diabetes-related disease.

Treatment Program for Stress-Related Diabetes

Note: Ensure that you consult with your doctor before starting any new program or supplement.

1. **Naturopathic Diet**

2. **Cardiovascular Exercise**

3. **Physical and Relaxation Therapies**
   - Deep Breathing
   - Meditation
   - Yoga
   - Massage Therapy

4. **Stress Supplements**
   - Lavender Oil (topical)
   - Milk Peptide
   - Magnolia Bark
   - B Vitamins

5. **Diabetes Supplements**
   - Colosolic Acid
   - Chromium
   - Antioxidants (vitamin C, vitamin E, selenium)

Cardiovascular Disease

Lowering Stress, Lowering Blood Pressure

Mary is a 36-year-old mother of two small children, ages 18 months and 3 years old. She used to work as a receptionist at a very busy hair salon and was accustomed to multitasking. After the birth of her second child, Mary stopped working, and decided to stay at home with her children. Her second child has had sleep difficulties, and Mary has had to wake up several times a night with her child for the past 18 months. As a result, Mary is sleep deprived, and continually wakes exhausted. She is usually unable to nap during the day, since she has to watch over both children and maintain the household.

Since leaving her job, Mary has struggled with the guilt of not working, despite working harder and longer hours now than she did at the hair salon. She also misses the adult interaction and stimulation that she used to get at work. All of this led to an internal emotional struggle. Mary also suspected that her blood pressure was elevated because she would often feel pounding sensations in her head and frequent flushes in the cheeks.

At Mary's last physical, her doctor noticed that her systolic blood pressure was 170, though her diastolic was only 84, so she was not medicated at that point. Mary was instructed to lose a little weight, exercise, and relax. If this did not bring her blood pressure back down, she would have to start medication.

At this point, Mary sought out our help to learn how to 'de-stress'. We began by regulating her diet and stabilizing her blood sugar levels with the introduction of protein at each meal and the temporary removal of grains, starches, and sweets. This alone dropped her blood systolic pressure by 11 points, and she reported feeling more balanced and in control.

Following this, Mary enrolled in yoga classes and starting counseling sessions to help her manage her guilt and feelings of loss of work. In these sessions, she was also taught several relaxation exercises, such as deep breathing and visualization. Within 3 weeks, Mary's blood pressure was stabilizing at 134/81.

Mary then introduced multi-B vitamins and passionflower into her daily supplement regime. This small addition of nutritional supplements, in conjunction with the lifestyle changes she made, dropped her blood pressure to 118/79. Thrilled with the results and feeling much healthier and stronger, she was no longer short tempered with her children. Mary had the strength and energy to support them all day long without tiring herself.

THE ASSOCIATION OF STRESS with both high blood pressure and cardiovascular disease has long been a topic of discussion. The Type-A personality sustaining a heart attack at an early age is a commonplace stereotype that is based on fact. Although there are numerous factors influencing susceptibility to these diseases, including family history, the role of stress appears to be substantial — and largely correctable.

1. Narrowing of the blood vessels. It requires more pressure to force the blood through tighter tubes.
2. Increasing total fluid within the blood vessels. If you increase the volume within a closed container, then the pressure inside increases.

Hypertension (High Blood Pressure)

Hypertension or high blood pressure is defined as blood pressure consistently equal to or over 140/90. The top number in a blood pressure reading is called the *systolic* reading and, in general, this number fluctuates mostly with stress levels, caffeine, and salt intake. The bottom number is the *diastolic* reading, and this number alters more when there is a change in the overall tone or control of the cardiovascular system – heart, arteries, and veins. Although stress primarily affects systolic blood pressure, when this occurs frequently or for prolonged periods, it induces changes in the heart and arteries that produce a rise in diastolic pressure as well. This combination is harmful to our cardiovascular health, increasing the risk of stroke and artery disease.

Hypertension Basics

Normal blood pressure is considered 120/80. Blood pressure measures the force the blood exerts on the walls of the blood vessels, in particular, the arteries. The measurement is dependent on the amount of circulating fluid in the blood vessel and the size of the vessel. As a blood vessel tightens or vasoconstricts, its size decreases. Because the amount of fluid it contains remains constant, the pressure increases. However, if the size of the vessel increases or vasodilates, then the blood pressure drops since the same amount of fluid now has a larger space through which to flow. Similarly, if the amount of fluid in the vessel changes, then the pressure will change correspondingly. It makes sense that if there is more fluid in the same space, or in this case a blood vessel, the pressure will go up. And if the amount of fluid in an enclosed space decreases, the pressure will drop. Thus, the two major factors in blood pressure are the amount of circulating fluid and the size of the vessels themselves.

Role of Stress in Hypertension

The appearance of high blood pressure in metabolic syndrome has been likened to persistent stimulation of the 'alarm reaction'. The initial stage of the fight-or-flight response involves activation of the sympathetic nervous system and the secretion of adrenaline and noradrenaline. This has a profound effect on blood pressure, constricting arteries and increasing heart rate and contraction force within seconds. In chronic stress, the increased cortisol levels heighten the sensitivity of tissues to adrenaline and noradrenaline, producing a more vigorous and prolonged response, and generally increasing the overall 'tone' or set point of the system.

STRESS FACTS Hypertension

Several studies have confirmed the association between stress and hypertension. Studies on animals show that frequent or chronic mental challenges are enough to stimulate hypothalamic centers of the brain affecting blood pressure regulation and endocrine metabolism. Observational data has shown that psychosocial stress, socioeconomic handicaps, lack of exercise and personality traits all cause an alteration in neuro-endocrine patterns leading to chronic hypertension. In time, this greatly increases the risk and development of heart disease and stroke.

Blood Pressure and Cortisol

There are several mechanisms by which stress and cortisol increase blood pressure. Cortisol increases heart contractility and the reactivity of blood vessels to stimuli that cause contraction, such as sympathetic nerve stimulation, adrenaline/noradrenaline, and angiotensin (a hormone produced by the kidneys). In addition, the impaired feedback between the adrenal glands and the hypothalamus and pituitary results in an effective increase in activity of other hormones produced in the adrenal glands, the mineralocorticoids, predominantly aldosterone. This hormone promotes retention of sodium and water, increasing the volume of circulating fluid. A 10% to 15% increase in volume translates into approximately a 15 to 25 mm/Hg rise in blood pressure.

Some patients with elevated blood pressure have a deficiency in the enzymes 11 beta-hydroxylase or 11 beta-hydroxysteroid dehydrogenase type 2. This then leads to an increase in mineral corticoids. Similarly, patients with increased weight and/or hyperglycemia may have elevated levels of 5 alpha-reductase and therefore increased glucocorticoids. The combination of increased mineral corticoids and glucocorticoids is shown to greatly increase blood pressure and cardiovascular risk. This may be a further factor in the development of metabolic syndrome and hypertension in some individuals.

Cortisol and Insulin

There is a definite link between insulin and hypertension. The association is apparent in diabetics and in those with hyperinsulinemia and metabolic syndrome. While insulin appears to have a direct effect to reduce vessel constriction, other factors are likely to be responsible for the increase in blood pressure. These include an effect on the kidneys to increase salt and water retention, increased intracellular calcium, and increased tone of the sympathetic nervous system.

Decreased intracellular nitric oxide synthase (NOS) in the arterial walls secondary to insulin resistance results in constriction of these vessels as NOS normally promotes

Hypertension Treatment
The effect of cortisol on hypertension has been shown to be correctable through dietary changes, such as decreased intake of fats and high-glycemic foods.

High Blood Pressure Stress Cascade

Overactivity of fight-or-flight sympathetic response and release of adrenaline.

Cortisol increases heart contraction and blood vessel sensitivity.

Cortisol increases aldosterone activity.

Cortisol increases renin-angiotensin activity.

Increased insulin affects blood pressure and arterial thickness.

Cortisol increases blood clotting and artery disease.

Stress increases endothelin, which causes vessel constriction and damage.

vessel relaxation. In addition to this short-term mechanism, prolonged hyperinsulinemia, high cholesterol, and high cortisol increase blood vessel wall damage and enhance atherosclerosis (hardening of the arteries), which, in itself, will increase blood pressure.

Patients with insulin/cortisol-related obesity have increased levels of various blood factors that contribute to clotting and coagulation of blood. These blood factors include plasma fibrinogen, plasminogen activator inhibitor, and factor VII. Together these hemostatic abnormalities have a profound effect on blood clotting, viscosity or thickness, and blood flow.

Further research has shown that more than 50% of patients with essential hypertension have some degree of insulin resistance despite the fact that under normal circumstances insulin induces vasodilation (reducing blood pressure). The combination of insulin resistance, obesity, and sympathetic stimulation (both from stress and being overweight) may be another factor by which overactivity of the fight-or-flight response affects blood pressure.

Renin-angiotensin

The renin-angiotensin hormone system of the kidneys is one of the most important blood pressure control mechanisms in the body. Reduced blood flow to the kidneys results in renin production, which promotes formation of angiotensin in the blood. Angiotensin increases blood vessel constriction and promotes retention of salt and water by the kidneys.

Angiotensin also promotes release of aldosterone by the adrenal glands, adding to the salt and water retention. Cortisol increases the amount of angiotensin directly, by stimulating production of the hormone precursor in the liver. In addition, the raised insulin associated with hypercortisolemia and insulin resistance also stimulates the renin-angiotensin system.

These numerous interactions contribute to the hypertension seen in chronic stress and metabolic syndrome. The effectiveness of angiotensin blocking drugs in the control of blood pressure in these individuals further supports this hypothesis.

Endothelin

Endothelin is a small molecule that has a potent effect on arteries, in particular the arteries around the heart. It is produced by cells in the walls of blood vessels and causes constriction through both a direct action on the smooth muscle in artery walls and via central stimulation of the sympathetic system. In addition, endothelin increases the cardiac work rate and stimulates release of aldosterone from

Treating & Preventing Stress-Related Disorders & Diseases

the adrenal glands, which increases blood pressure through salt retention. Endothelin, however, does appear to be an important factor in blood pressure regulation.

Studies on hypertensive patients have found increased levels of endothelin. It is suggested that not only is endothelin an important regulator of blood pressure, its high levels in hypertension may mediate some of the arterial damage that contributes to the increased risk of heart disease in these patients.

 STRESS FACT Psychological Link

Acute mental stress raises endothelin levels, and chronic mental stress has been shown to induce dysfunction of arterial wall cells via the same molecule. This provides a potentially important link between psychological factors and hypertension.

Stress Management of Blood Pressure

There is ample evidence to link stress and high blood pressure. Certain individuals may be at higher risk, showing increased cardiovascular responsiveness to stress and other emotional factors. In subjects who underwent 24-hour heart monitoring, those showing higher emotional responsivity demonstrated greater increases in heart rate and blood pressure than calmer individuals.

One study evaluated men and women, 28 to 75 years of age, with blood pressure above 140/90. Some were randomly assigned to undergo immediate stress management, while the others were offered it later on. The treatment group showed significant reduction in blood pressure (average 134/86), while that of the control group remained unchanged. When the controls subsequently completed their stress management program, they too showed similar reductions. In other randomized clinical studies, transcendental meditation has been shown to be effective at reducing blood pressure.

 STRESS FACT Controlling Blood Pressure

The role for stress management in the control of blood pressure is supported by both hormonal and biochemical research and by clinical studies. The long-term association of stress and hypertension appears to be borne out by hormonal interplay and dysfunction. Fortunately, controlling stress is easily within our grasp and will likely offer far more benefit to our health than just a reduction in blood pressure.

Treatment Program for Stress-Related Hypertension

Note: Ensure that you consult with your doctor before starting any new program or supplement.

1. Naturopathic Diet

For all individuals, start stage one of the naturopathic diet, even those who do not need to lose weight, for a minimum of 4 weeks. If you do not need to lose weight, then increase the amount of fruit in the diet so that weight loss is minimized. It is important to follow this to ensure that your insulin levels are very low. Remember insulin increases blood pressure and cholesterol production. For those who need to lose weight, continue on stage one of the diet for a minimum of 8 weeks and slowly integrate into stage two.

2. Cardiovascular Exercise

3. Physical and Relaxation Therapy

- Yoga
- Tai Chi
- Deep Breathing
- Accupuncture

4. Stress Supplements

- Vitamin B Complex
- Theanine
- Milk Peptide

5. Cardiovascular Supplements

- CoQ-10
- Calcium-Magnesium
- Policosinals (for high cholesterol)
- Hawthorn (not to be taken if on other antihypertensive medication)

Heart Attack

A study from Florida published in the journal *Circulation* in April 2002 evaluated a group of heart disease patients who, on testing, demonstrated marked reduction of blood flow to the heart during acute mental stress. At their 5-year follow-up, these patients were three times more likely to have died from a heart attack than other patients with coronary artery disease who did not show the same response to stress.

Heart Attack Basics

A heart attack, also called a myocardial infarction, occurs when there is injury to the heart muscle due to insufficient blood supply. More than a million people in the United States suffer a heart attack each year, and although advances in medical care, public awareness, and emergency treatment have reduced the number of deaths, the morbidity and disability is persistent.

The factors that increase your risk of suffering from coronary artery disease and heart attack are well established. They include high blood pressure (above 140/90), as well as high cholesterol and LDL (low-density lipoproteins). Diabetes and obesity increase risk by a number of factors. Cigarette smoking is well known to significantly promote heart disease. Family history is very important, acting through influence on a number of different risk elements.

Causes of Heart Attack

1. An artery supplying blood to the heart (coronary arteries), already narrowed by disease (atherosclerosis or cholesterol-related hardening), is completely blocked. This is thought to be the most common scenario.

2. A blood clot from elsewhere breaks off and lodges in one of the narrowed or even one of the normal artery coronary arteries.

3. A coronary artery spasm creates a sudden constriction of one or more of the coronary arteries.

Role of Stress in Heart Attack

Stress and heart attacks have always had a strong association. Stress is listed as a risk factor in most information packages about coronary artery disease and heart attack, and most post-infarction treatment regimens will incorporate stress management along with exercise, diet, and medication.

Psychological traits such as anxiety and depression produce chronic mental stress shown to be an independent risk factor for heart attack. A study following more than 73,000 people in Japan found that those suffering from high levels of chronic psychological stress had over twice the risk of dying from a heart attack. Acute mental stress also increases risk. For example, the rate of heart attacks in Tel Aviv went up significantly during Iraq's bombing of Israel in the 1991 Gulf War. Both chronic and acute stress appear to influence cardiac disease. A greater understanding of the mechanisms behind this risk factor can only help in both the prevention and treatment of heart attack.

We have seen how chronic stress affects blood pressure. This has an additive effect on the increase induced by the metabolic changes related to cortisol and insulin resistance. Add in the increased damage to the blood vessel walls, high cholesterol, and enhanced blood clotting, and the stage is set for a major assault on the vessels of the heart.

Endothelin

The release of endothelin is likely the major cause of stress-related coronary artery spasm and myocardial ischaemia (heart damage related to insufficient blood supply). This spasm occurs in up to 85% of patients with coronary artery disease and is measurable and reproducible.

Risk Factors for Heart Attack
- High Blood Pressure
- High Cholesterol/ Low-Density Lipoprotein (LDL) Levels
- Obesity
- Diabetes
- Lack of Exercise
- Cigarette Smoking
- Family History
- Stress

✔ STRESS FACT Endothelin and Hardening of the Arteries

Chronic mental stress has been shown to induce changes in the walls of blood vessels that are a prelude to the development of atherosclerosis (hardening of the arteries). This effect seems to be mediated by the same molecule, endothelin.

Mast Cells

Mast cells are present in tissues throughout the body. They contain granules of highly active chemicals that promote inflammation, which are released when the cell is triggered to 'degranulate'. There are numerous triggers, including allergens (such as pollens in asthma or certain proteins in atopic dermatitis), chemicals from other immune cells, and, most recently recognized, CRH, the body's master stress hormone.

Mast cells are known to be present within the cardiac muscle of the heart, located in close proximity to the nerves supplying this organ. They have been found in the walls of arteries damaged by atherosclerosis and are implicated in coronary artery spasm. Research on rat heart muscle has demonstrated stress-induced mast cell degranulation, a process dependent on CRH and prevented by CRH-receptor blocking drugs.

 STRESS FACT CRH Links

Corticotropin-releasing hormone, through its interaction with mast cells, may be the link between stress and the exacerbation of inflammatory conditions such as asthma, dermatitis, and bowel disease. It may also be responsible for inducing migraine. This recent evidence points to an important role for stress in triggering angina and sudden cardiac arrest.

Vagus Nerve

The vagus nerve is part of the parasympathetic system, responsible for slowing the heart. This is a converse effect to the fight-or-flight sympathetic system that increases heart rate. The influence of the vagus nerve can be felt by taking a deep breath while monitoring your pulse. Inhalation and lung expansion causes centers in the brainstem to increase output to the vagus and the heart rate can be felt to be slowing down. This normal physiologic phenomenon is called sinus arrhythmia.

There is some evidence to indicate that a poorly functioning vagus with impaired sinus arrhythmia (reduced heart-rate variability) is associated with an increased risk of cardiovascular disease and increased probability of death after a heart attack. Investigators believe the vagus plays an important protective role, particularly during times of cardiac stress, in particular as it relates to the fight-or-flight response.

Treating & Preventing Stress-Related Disorders & Diseases

Researchers have found that children with greater vagal control were less likely to suffer emotional or societal dysfunction as they got older. In adults, the inability to regulate heart rate without triggering the stress response leads to increased blood pressure and heart rate without substantial increase in blood circulation during challenging times. This response is not only ineffectual in achieving the goals of the fight-or-flight response, but leads to vessel damage and cardiovascular disease. There appears to be a strong correlation between anger and hostility as a personality trait, impaired vagal braking, and the risk of heart disease.

Estrogen

It is well known that the protective effect of estrogen is responsible for the lower rates of coronary artery disease and heart attack seen in women. Nevertheless, heart disease is the leading cause of mortality in women, accounting for 250,000 deaths a year in the United States. This effect is diminished after menopause. Low levels of estrogen before menopause, however, result in a dramatic increase in risk. Animal studies show this risk to be as high as four times the normal rate.

 STRESS FACT Reduced Estrogen Levels

Chronic stress is associated with a marked reduction in estrogen levels, which again is demonstrated in animal studies. This may be one further factor whereby stress affects heart attack risk.

Stress Management of Heart Attack

Only an estimated 10% to 20% of heart disease patients receive any stress management treatment, a factor related to both insurance coverage and medical practice. However, the evidence above indicates that this type of therapy may be beneficial to most and crucial to others.

Available studies do show substantial benefit from stress-management programs. A 1997 study at Duke University evaluated 107 patients with coronary artery disease. They were randomly assigned to a 4-month program of exercise or stress management. While the exercise group did show some long-term benefit at reducing the incidence of cardiac events, it was not significant. The stress-management group, however, reduced their risk by 75%. A similar study published in 2002 by the same author found not only significant reductions in cardiac events, but far lower medical costs than regular care and exercise treatments.

Vagal Brake
A reduction in vagal output may act as a subtle form of fight-or-flight, allowing an increase in heart rate without the many other complex and often disruptive endocrine reactions associated with the fully fledged stress response. Being able to modify this 'vagal brake', as it has been termed, may confer a greater coping ability upon an individual in today's society.

Treatment Program for Stress-Related Heart Attack

Note: Ensure that you consult with your doctor before starting any new program or supplement.

1. Naturopathic Diet

For all individuals, start stage one of the naturopathic diet, even those who do not need to lose weight, for a minimum of 4 weeks. If you do not need to lose weight, then increase the amount of fruit in the diet so that weight loss is minimized. It is important to follow this to ensure that your insulin levels are very low. Remember insulin increases blood pressure and cholesterol production. For those who need to lose weight, continue with stage one of the diet for a minimum of 8 weeks and slowly integrate into stage two.

2. Cardiovascular Exercise

Any exercise needs to be discussed with your cardiologist.

3. Physical and Relaxation Therapy

- Yoga
- Tai Chi
- Deep Breathing
- Visualization

4. Stress Supplements

- Vitamin B Complex
- Magnolia
- Milk Peptide

5. Cardiovascular Supplements

- CoQ-10
- Calcium-Magnesium
- Policosinals (for high cholesterol)
- Gingko
- Essential Fatty Acids

Gastrointestinal Disorders

Controlling Stress Levels Before They Control You

Mark is a successful 47-year-old actor who has been working in the entertainment industry for 12 years. Unfortunately, his mother was recently diagnosed with cancer, and Mark began taking her to chemotherapy treatments each week. He has a very close relationship with her. It distressed him to see her get so very thin and weak. The possibility of losing her kept him up at night.

During this difficult time, Mark received news that he had secured a significant role in a large-budget film. Having had several major roles before, Mark did not feel nervous. However, the morning of his first day on set, he started getting painful cramping in his bowel. Very quickly, he found himself rushing to the washroom with diarrhea. Assuming he had food poisoning, he tried to think back on what he ate the night before. Nothing particular came to mind, and as his bowel was feeling slightly better, he decided not to do anything about it. He left for work, but when he got there, the same thing happened again — and most days thereafter. Soon, he began to notice mucus in his stools. He was in chronic discomfort from gas and bloating.

Mark went to his family physician, who diagnosed him with irritable bowel syndrome, likely a result of the accumulated stress triggered by his concern for his mother, lack of sleep, and the excitement of his movie.

On his doctor's advice, Mark sought naturopathic input. Following our consultation, we recommended taking milk peptide extracts, 5-HTP, and a multi-B vitamin daily for stress, along with slippery elm, cabbage extract, and L-glutamine to help repair his bowel. In addition, Mark started deep breathing before bed every night and meditation when he got home from work or from the hospital after visiting his mother. He did not have time for massage therapy, but invested in a 'thumper', a home electronic massager, and used this on his shoulders whenever they started to tighten.

One year later and Mark's movie is a box-office hit. He has learned how to control his stress levels — before they control him. Every time he neglects his health or increases his workload too much, he feels twinges in his bowel. Mark now listens to these twinges, as small reminders to take a deep breath and relax.

WE HAVE ALL EXPERIENCED the loss of appetite and possibly nausea associated with a stressful situation such as an important interview or exam. We have felt 'butterflies in our stomach' and the gurgling and rumbling that prove so embarrassing in a quiet waiting room. Some of us may even experience painful spasms or diarrhea at times of stress.

The association of stress and gastrointestinal symptoms is not surprising given the connection between our central nervous system and the gut. There are extensive nervous connections through the autonomic nervous system, which control blood flow and gut muscle activity. In addition, many of the hormones found in the gut have been discovered to be neurotransmitters in the brain — for example, cholecystokinin (CCK) and vasoactive intestinal peptide (VIP). Although other factors are now recognized as important, the association of stress and stomach ulceration has been recognized for many years. Increasingly, the role of our mood and levels of stress and anxiety are being identified as crucial factors in the development, progression and severity of diseases of the stomach and intestines.

Irritable Bowel Syndrome

Irritable bowel syndrome (IBS) is an extremely common disorder affecting approximately 20% of the American population. Studies have shown that upwards of 35 million Americans have IBS. It ranks as one of the major causes of lost work. It accounts for more than three million visits to the doctor in the United States each year.

The symptoms of IBS are frequently intermittent, with patients experiencing prolonged periods with essentially normal bowel function. Women are twice as likely as men to suffer from IBS and their symptoms frequently appear or become more severe around the time of the menstrual period.

 STRESS FACT Unknown Cause

IBS is a condition of unknown cause. It should not be confused with inflammatory bowel disease, such as Crohn's disease or ulcerative colitis, because there are no inflammatory changes in the bowel itself. IBS does not appear to result from, or cause any damage to the intestines. Although patients may pass mucus with their bowel movements, there is no blood. There is no increased risk of developing cancer.

IBS Basics

Symptoms of IBS can be severe enough to markedly interfere with lifestyle. Patients may be unable to attend social events or go out to dinner or even spend any prolonged time at the workplace. Although absorption is unchanged, the development of symptoms 30 to 60 minutes after food with acute pain, spasm, and loose bowel movements may cause individuals to significantly reduce their diet. This in itself may result in malnutrition.

The diagnosis of IBS is based on symptoms and the exclusion of other diseases in the bowel, such as inflammatory bowel disease. Following a history and physical examination, laboratory tests will be carried out, including a stool sample to test for evidence of bleeding. Bowel radiographs, such as a barium enema or direct evaluation with use of fiberoptic endoscopy, may be ordered. In the absence of any identifiable bowel disease, a diagnosis of IBS can be made.

IBS Symptoms
- Recurrent abdominal pain
- Cramping
- Bloating
- Gas
- Alternating Diarrhea and Constipation

Role of Stress in Irritable Bowel Syndrome

The functional distress associated with IBS gives rise to a chicken or egg question. Is the stress responsible for the IBS or is the IBS causing the stress? Personal experience with patients in our practice strongly suggests an association between stress and the development of symptoms. Certainly, individuals with a tendency toward symptoms of IBS experience a marked exacerbation in pain, cramping, and diarrhea at times of increased stress and resolution of symptoms during times of relaxation, such as holidays. In addition, the fact that the condition is so rare in children indicates the presence of a factor that exists predominantly during adulthood — stress. This observation is supported by clinical research, which finds lifestyle and stress levels to be a strong predictor of disease progression and severity.

Autonomic Nervous System

The autonomic nervous system exerts a powerful influence over the function of the bowel. In addition, we have seen that the autonomic nervous system plays a pivotal role in the fight-or-flight response that initiates the stress reaction. Studies have shown evidence of a central nervous system abnormality with dysregulation of the autonomic nervous system and overall increased excitability of the brain associated with anxiety.

The association of IBS with chronic fatigue syndrome and psychiatric disorders, including panic disorder (panic attacks), anxiety disorder, and depression, has led to a theory based on brain-gut interaction. CRH is thought to be the principal

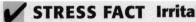 **STRESS FACT Irritable Bowel Syndrome**

Research has recognized the association of IBS and abnormalities of the hypothalamus-pituitary-adrenal (HPA) axis, stress, and cortisol. A number of studies have shown that patients with IBS have increased levels of adrenalin, noradrenalin, and cortisol in the resting state. In addition, IBS patients with a predominantly diarrhea-type pattern showed increased levels of cortisol and excessive autonomic stimulation following a meal when compared to normal subjects.

stimulator of anxiety and panic attacks. It also has a potent effect on the bowel, increasing motility and promoting release of histamine from mast cells, which augments its stimulatory effect. Patients with IBS have a heightened response to CRH, indicating dysregulation of the hypothalamus-gut control mechanism in these subjects.

IBS demonstrates no clear immune response as is seen in inflammatory bowel disease (IBD). However, IBS patients do have reduced natural killer (NK) cell number and activity when compared to healthy individuals. Whether this is a reflection of increased stress in these individuals or part of an overall irregularity of the neuro-endocrine axis of the gut and the immune system remains to be elucidated.

✔ STRESS FACT IBS Treatment

With increasing recognition of the role stress and anxiety play in the development and recurrence of IBS, treatment is beginning to include stress-relieving therapy. This includes counseling, biofeedback, regular exercise, and other musculoskeletal therapies, such as yoga and massage, meditation, deep breathing, and hypnosis.

Stress Management of IBS

In the absence of any clear cause of IBS, treatment is based on control of symptoms. Changes in diet and bowel activity modifiers (such as fiber or constipating agents) are used in the initial stages. In more severe cases, tricyclic antidepressants and serotonin re-uptake inhibitors, such as Fluoxetine (Prozac), can be prescribed. A number of other drugs aimed at controlling activity within the bowel are under investigation.

In a review of treatments for gastrointestinal diseases, in particular IBS, 19 controlled studies showed a statistically significant superiority of psychological over conventional therapies. Importantly, the gains made during the cognitive training and relaxation therapy lasted beyond the duration of treatment. A one-year follow-up study from New York found 'relaxation response meditation' to reduce symptoms of pain and bloating significantly, as well as diarrhea and flatulence.

Treatment Program for Stress-Related IBS

Note: Ensure that you consult with your doctor before starting any new program or supplement.

1. Naturopathic Diet

Follow stage two or the maintenance phase of the naturopathic diet. This will ensure a stable blood sugar level and a drop in stress hormones without weight reduction. It is important that you eliminate wheat, gluten, and corn for a minimum of 6 weeks and up to 4 months. Thus, even in maintenance, no wheat products, like breads, bagels, etc., should be included

in the diet. These foods are very hard on the bowel and can easily cause further irritation. Instead, opt for such grains and starches as whole grain rice, oatmeal, and potatoes. These carbohydrates are broken down and absorbed with little irritation to the bowel.

2. Cardiovascular Exercise

3. Physical and Relaxation Therapy

- Massage: Once a week over the abdominal area to help relax the abdominal muscles and regulate bowel patterns. Ensure that this is balanced with massage over the lower back area.
- Yoga
- Deep Breathing
- Meditation

4. Stress Supplements

- 5-HTP
- Magnolia

5. Gastrointestinal Supplements

- Slippery Elm
- L-glutamine
- Digestive Enzymes
- Acidophilus
- Essential Fatty Acids

Inflammatory Bowel Disease (IBD)

Crohn's disease (CD) and ulcerative colitis (UC) are the two most common forms of IBD, affecting more than 1 million Americans. With onset usually before the age of 30, these diseases are characterized by chronic relapsing inflammation and ulceration of the small and large intestines. UC is more common than CD and its effects are restricted to the colon and rectum. CD may affect any part of the digestive tract. Women and men are equally affected, but there is a strong genetic risk with 15% of IBD patients having at least one affected first-degree relative.

IBD causes recurrent abdominal pain, diarrhea with blood and mucus in the stools, fatigue, weight loss, and fever. In severe disease, there may be 10 to 20 episodes of diarrhea a day. IBD may result in anemia, malnutrition, mouth ulcers, and obstruction of the bowel. The disease may affect areas away from the gut, such as the eyes, liver, and bones.

IBD Basics

The immune response appears to be triggered by an as-yet unidentified environmental factor and is directed at the gut bacteria. There is a vigorous and aggressive inflammatory response, which destroys the architecture of the intestinal wall, severely affecting its digestive function. This leads to malabsorption, vitamin and mineral deficiencies, and anemia. Scarring may result in strictures and adhesions that block the bowel, resulting in a surgical emergency. IBD results in a significant increase in the risk of developing bowel cancer over the lifetime of a patient.

 STRESS FACT Idiopathic Forms

Ulcerative colitis (UC) and Crohn's disease (CD) are often termed 'idiopathic' forms of IBD, which means that no one is quite sure of the true underlying cause. The disease was originally thought to be entirely psychosomatic, but most current research indicates a malfunction of the immune system in a genetically susceptible individual.

Role of Stress in Irritable Bowel Disease

The two major systems that appear to be dysfunctional in IBD are the immune system and the autonomic nervous system. These two systems are themselves interrelated through the hypothalamus and fight-or-flight stress response. Studies have demonstrated disruption of the hypothalamus-coordinated mechanism that normally activates the sympathetic system and the adrenal-cortisol axis simultaneously in healthy individuals. For example, IBD patients show sympathetic activation *without* increased cortisol. In addition, UC patients show greater sympathetic nerve activity in the lower bowel.

Immune System Activity

The effects of chronic stress on the immune system likely have profound influence on the development and progression of IBD. The interaction between the immune system and the HPA axis is a two-way street. The immune system and chemical mediators of inflammation, such as the cytokines, exert a similar influence on the hypothalamus and adrenal glands.

Stress appears to alter the balance or threshold of response to the numerous neuro-endocrine factors that control gut function and play such an important contributory role in IBD. Neurotensin and substance-P are neurotransmitters, chemicals that allow nerve cells in the brain to communicate. They are also important transmitters in the gut, mediating the inflammation, increased motility, and greater permeability seen in IBD. CRH, the hypothalamic hormone at the start of the cortisol stress response, also acts on the gut and has an analog produced locally by cells in the intestinal wall that increases permeability and secretion of mucus and enzymes. Cortisol itself has a direct effect on permeability and also influences the balance of immune cells within the gut wall. In addition, mast cells in the wall of the intestine are activated by stress and mediate the effects of CRH on tissue inflammation.

Autonomic Nervous System

Chronic stress affects intestinal permeability and alters enzyme secretion. Acute stress increases protective mucus production (part of the protective fight-or-flight response), whereas chronic stress depletes mucus cells and reduces gut wall protection. Stress has also been shown to alter the normal bacterial flora of the gut, reducing the numbers of healthy lactobacilli in favor of more aggressive organisms. These factors, in association with alterations in autonomic and neuro-endocrine responsiveness, likely cause increased antigen (foreign protein) invasion. The combination of this assault in the presence of a dysfunctional immune response (also caused by the chronic stress) may set the stage for the development or reactivation of IBD in a genetically at-risk population.

Psychological Factors

There have been a large number of studies looking *prospectively* at the relationship between psychological factors and IBD. One found social and emotional dysfunction to be one of the best predictors of disease activity, worsening over time. Animal studies have shown that stress can promote the more rapid development of induced colitis and can reactivate it once in remission. Rats demonstrate a four-fold increase in the number of inflammatory cells in the gut wall in response to stress and gibbon monkeys develop severe colitis in response to social upheaval.

✔ **STRESS FACT Inflammatory Bowel Disease**

Although recognized as a disease of immune dysfunction, there is ample evidence to support the role of stress in the development and progression of the disease. The initial presentation often follows an acutely stressful event and relapses frequently following periods of emotional upheaval. One study showed long-term 'perceived' stress to be a major influence on disease severity and recurrence rate. There is also a strong association between IBD and obsessive-compulsive disorders, anxiety and perfectionism.

The importance of central nervous system input in IBD is exemplified by the strong placebo effect in these patients. Not only will the placebo effect improve perception of disease and symptoms, it will also reduce clinically measured and observed gut inflammation.

Stress Management of IBD

Despite the increasing body of evidence linking stress and IBD, there have been few studies evaluating stress management and psychological treatments in UC and Crohn's patients. An older study from 1969 showed benefit of psychotherapy in chronic UC patients and a 1986 randomized study of the value of stress management in IBD patients demonstrated significant benefit in both physical and psychosocial well-being.

Other studies, however, have found little impact on symptoms of IBD, even though patients overall felt and coped better with their illness. It is likely that renewed interest in the neuro-endocrine effect on the immune system in IBD will prompt further evaluation of these treatments.

Treatment Program for Stress-Related IBD

Note: Ensure that you consult with your doctor before starting any new program or supplement.

1. Naturopathic Diet

Follow stage two or the maintenance phase of the naturopathic diet. This will ensure a stable blood sugar level and a drop in stress hormones without weight reduction. It is important that you eliminate wheat, gluten, and corn for a minimum of 6 weeks and up to 4 months. Thus, even in maintenance, no wheat products, like breads, bagels, etc., should be included in the diet. These foods are very hard on the bowel and can easily cause further irritation. Instead, opt for such grains and starches as whole grain rice, oatmeal, and potatoes. These carbohydrates are broken down and absorbed with little irritation to the bowel.

2. Cardiovascular Exercise

3. Physical and Relaxation Therapy

- Massage: Once per week over the abdominal area to help relax the abdominal muscles and regulate bowel patterns. Ensure that this is balanced with massage over the lower back area.
- Yoga
- Deep Breathing
- Visualization

4. Stress Supplements

- 5-HTP
- Magnolia
- Theanine

5. Gastrointestinal Supplements

- Slippery Elm
- Cabbage
- Zinc
- L-glutamine
- Digestive Enzymes
- Acidophilus
- Essential Fatty Acids

Peptic Ulceration (Stomach and Duodenal Ulcers)

For many years, the association between stress and ulcers of the stomach and duodenum (the first part of the intestine) appeared clear-cut and was well accepted by the medical community. However, with the discovery of the organism Helicobacter pylori (H. pylori), the role of stress was rapidly discarded and continues to be ignored in the majority of treatment regimes. Physicians suddenly had an identifiable and tangible cause of the disease, one that was eminently treatable. Previous research alluding to personality traits and psychological factors was dismissed, as peptic ulcer disease became regarded simply as an infectious condition.

Despite widespread acceptance of H. pylori as the sole cause of peptic ulcer disease, closer scrutiny reveals there are likely other factors at play. There is ample evidence in statistics associated with peptic ulceration. While it is estimated that 60% of Americans become infected with H. pylori, only 5% to 10% of the population will develop peptic ulceration during their lifetime. Further, 10% of patients with non-NSAID (anti-inflammatory drug)-related peptic ulcers show no evidence of H. pylori infection. Blinkered thought processes and simplification of treatment have steered peptic ulcer theory toward this 'single' cause theory. What may be more reasonable is to consider peptic ulcer disease a multi-factorial condition with numerous etiologies working in conjunction with H. pylori to produce or exacerbate the disease.

Peptic Ulcer Basics

A peptic ulcer occurs when the acid and digestive enzymes normally present in the stomach or duodenum break through the protective lining of these organs and start to damage the underlying tissue. Under normal circumstances, the aggressive and damaging forces of the acid and proteolytic enzymes are balanced by the defensive forces of mucus and bicarbonate secretion, the regenerative capacity of the surface cells, the action of local prostaglandins, and blood flow through the walls of the stomach and intestines.

Development of an ulcer is thought to occur in the presence of impaired defenses or increased aggression.

Peptic Ulcer Symptoms

The classic symptoms of a peptic ulcer include pain and discomfort in the upper abdomen. Pain affects 70% of people with duodenal ulcers and 50% with stomach ulcers. Duodenal ulcers are the more common, developing from around age 25

Factors Leading to Peptic Ulceration

Impaired Defense
- Reduced or poor quality mucus
- Reduced bicarbonate secretion
- Poor blood flow
- Impaired cell regeneration
- Low levels of prostaglandins

Increased Aggression
- H. pylori infection
- Aspirin/anti-inflammatory medication
- Alcohol and cigarettes
- Impaired acid regulation

Potential Role of Stress in Peptic Ulceration

- Persistent cortisol secretion weakens gastric and duodenal wall defenses
- Reduced immunity against H. pylori
- Reduced glutamine availability
- Increased acid production
- Alteration in rate of gastric emptying
- Impaired healing of gut wall
- Abnormal melatonin secretion
- Factors associated with stress, such as smoking and alcohol

with a peak at 45 years of age. Stomach ulcers tend to occur later in life and in particular in individuals over the age of 60. Men are more susceptible than women.

The pain associated with ulceration can be gnawing or burning, often with radiation through to the back. It can come on anywhere from 30 minutes to 2 hours after a meal and can last minutes to hours. The pain is often relieved by eating more food or by taking antacids. The pain can occur at night and this is more common with duodenal ulcers.

The pain may be associated with nausea and vomiting and occasionally with loss of appetite. Ulcers can sometimes be painless and present with symptoms such as weight loss or anemia (caused by blood loss through the surface of the ulcer). On occasion, the presentation may be a catastrophic bleed if a previously unrecognized ulcer erodes into a large blood vessel.

H. Pylori

H. pylori is a contagious bacterium generally considered to be the most important factor in the development and persistence of peptic ulceration. Previous theories regarding genetic susceptibility are now thought to be due to cross infection. The organism has the ability to damage the protective mucus layer that covers the cells lining the stomach and duodenum. Once this occurs, the acid and peptic enzymes are able to inflict further damage on the area, resulting in development of an ulcer.

One interesting paradox is the fact that although most ulcers occur in the duodenum, H. pylori infection is essentially limited to the stomach. Studies have suggested a role of a down-regulated immune response in the duodenal wall as being partially responsible for the development of ulcers in this area.

H. pylori provides the basis of certain tests for peptic ulcer disease. It can be detected using blood and breath tests, and also via sampling at endoscopy, a procedure in which a telescopic tube is passed from the mouth down into the stomach. Research work is currently aimed at developing an effective vaccine against H. pylori in an attempt to prevent or control peptic ulcer disease.

Role of Stress in Peptic Ulcer Disease

There are a number of ways in which stress may contribute to the development, progression, or increase in symptoms of peptic ulcer disease.

Cortisol

A number of studies have indicated the importance of cortisol in the maintenance of gastric and duodenal defense mechanisms and the prevention of peptic ulceration. While this initially might appear to negate any potential role for stress in the development of ulceration, closer examination reveals a differential response. Short-term high levels of cortisol are effective at stimulating the production of the prostaglandins that provide protection for the stomach and duodenum.

In addition, increased levels of local cortisol are needed to maintain blood flow, which also reduces the risk of damage. This would fit with the important evolutionary role of cortisol in the vital fight-or-flight response as a protective and stabilizing hormone. However, it appears that prolonged, lower levels of cortisol stimulation inhibit the production of the protective prostaglandins. There is also a reduction in the number of cortisol receptors. It appears possible, therefore, that chronic stress associated with abnormalities in the vital fight-or-flight response and rhythm of cortisol secretion may well contribute to a weakening of the gastric and duodenal defenses.

Reduced Immunity

The effect of chronic stress and prolonged stimulation of the cortisol response is known to have a profound effect on the immune system. Cortisol impairs the function of the cells and chemicals responsible for attacking invading organisms. The profound effect of cortisol and chronic stress on the immune response is likely to play an important role in allowing H. pylori to commence its attack or increase its activity resulting in increased ulceration.

✔ STRESS FACT Glutamine Therapy

Chronic stress reduces the population and activity of natural killer (NK) cells and generally impairs the cellular immune response. Of particular interest, with respect to peptic ulcer disease, is a reduction in the availability of the amino acid glutamine. Not only is this amino acid essential for the cellular immune response, it is also the principal source of energy for cells lining the stomach and intestine. Preliminary studies have indicated an important therapeutic role for glutamine in the prevention and treatment of stress-related ulceration.

Acid Production

A number of clinical studies have clearly demonstrated a link between psychosocial and physical stress and increased acid production in the stomach. The fact that other studies have refuted this finding, likely indicates the possibility of an 'at-risk' population in which stress results in a significant increase in hydrochloric acid production and a potentially increased risk of stomach ulceration. A secondary factor is the variable effect of stress on stomach emptying. Delaying the emptying of the stomach contents may result in an increased risk of stomach ulcer. Increased mobility and rapid release of acid into the duodenum could increase the risk of ulceration here, both by direct effect and by providing a more appropriate environment for H. pylori.

Healing

Healing of skin and other soft tissues is impaired by stress. This has been shown in a number of clinical studies, one of which found a 40% slower healing rate in students approaching an important exam. This appeared to be related not only to a direct effect on local cellular activity and prostaglandin production, but also to reduce growth hormone production.

Melatonin

Melatonin is a hormone produced by the pineal gland of the brain. Its primary role appears to be control of the daily cycle of waking and sleeping. Levels are reduced during daylight and increased substantially with the onset of darkness. Levels peak at between 2:00 and 4:00 a.m., but appear to decrease long before dawn indicating overall timing control by the hypothalamus. Recent studies have attributed significant ulcer healing potential to melatonin. Infusion of melatonin prior to stress in an animal model resulted in reduced acid secretion, improved blood circulation to the gastric tissue, and markedly reduced incidence of stomach ulceration.

Abnormalities in sleep patterns associated with stress and feedback abnormalities within in the hypothalamus might feasibly result in impaired defenses in the wall of the stomach and duodenum.

Other Contributing Factors

Other factors well recognized for potentiating gastric ulceration are smoking, alcohol intake, anti-inflammatory use (for musculoskeletal pain or headaches), and dietary irregularity. An increased incidence of these contributing factors in subjects with chronic stress likely contributes significantly to

✔ STRESS FACT Peptic Ulceration

There is certainly sufficient evidence to conclude that stress is at least a contributing factor to the development and progression of peptic ulcer disease. There is a strong association between catastrophic events, such as war or earthquake, and the development of peptic ulceration. In addition, a number of animal models have been developed in which stress produces ulceration in the absence of H. pylori. It is also well recognized that acute physical stress to the body, including major burns and surgery, greatly increase the risk of developing peptic ulcers.

the development of ulcers in some individuals. There is, however, ample evidence that even when these factors are accounted for, stress alone has a very important role.

Stress Management of Peptic Ulceration

Peptic ulcer may represent an excellent example of the interplay of numerous etiologic factors, including stress, in the development and recurrence of a disease. Rather than being considered mutually exclusive causes, infection and stress may represent synergistic factors that influence pathology. A recent controlled study has shown benefit from an integrated stress management program with subjects in the treatment group experiencing mental and physical improvements in addition to improved ulcer healing. A study in *The Lancet* from 1988 found that combining hypnotherapy with drug treatment was more effective than drug treatment alone in preventing recurrence in duodenal ulceration. Studies looking at the effect of psychotherapy alone have not found significant benefit, indicating that a stress-management approach with true lifestyle change may be the most effective direction to pursue treatment.

Treatment Program for Stress-Related Peptic Ulceration

Note: Ensure that you consult with your doctor before starting any new program or supplement.

1. Naturopathic Diet

Follow stage two or the maintenance phase of the naturopathic diet. This will ensure a stable blood sugar level and a drop in stress hormones without weight reduction. It is important that you eliminate wheat, gluten, and corn for a minimum of 6 weeks and up to 4 months. Thus, even in maintenance, no wheat products, like breads, bagels, etc., should be included in the diet. These foods are very hard on the bowel and can easily cause further irritation. Instead, opt for such grains and starches as whole grain rice, oatmeal and potatoes. These carbohydrates are broken down and absorbed with little irritation to the bowel.

2. Cardiovascular Exercise

3. Physical and Relaxation Therapy
- Massage
- Yoga
- Deep Breathing
- Acupuncture

4. Stress Supplements
- Milk Peptide
- Magnolia
- Theanine

5. Gastrointestinal Supplements
- Slippery Elm
- Cabbage
- Olive Leaf Extract
- L-glutamine
- Digestive Enzymes
- Acidophilus

Immune System Disorders and Allergies

Boosting Immunity, Beating Stress

Jane is a 19-year-old college student who came to our office complaining of frequent colds and bouts of influenza that lasted much longer than normal. She usually ended up taking antibiotics to recover fully from most of her infections.

A typical college student, she burned the candle at both ends by studying and staying out late with her friends. Her diet was the typical student pasta diet, complemented by coffee and beer. After 2 years of this lifestyle, Jane started catching colds, flus, and chest infections every other month. It got to the point where there was only 1 or 2 weeks between each infection.

Apart from further antibiotic use and more sleep, she did not know what else to do. We began by altering Jane's diet greatly, increasing her protein content to give her body the ingredients it needed to start producing more antibodies. We then balanced this with increased vegetable, fruits, and fluids. We also started Jane on an antioxidant supplement to reduce the free radical inflammation from smoke-filled bars, alcohol, and general pollution. Jane also began plant sterols to increase her interleukin and tumor necrosis factor production. In addition, we temporarily put Jane on olive leaf extract to help further decrease viral replication. All of this greatly helped Jane. Her body began to strengthen and fight infections on its own.

However, each time exam period came around, Jane would still get quite ill and need to postpone some of her exams. At this point, she knew that her stress levels were affecting her immune system to the point of illness. She then began to take magnolia extract and high dose B vitamins during this period. She also used lemon balm before bed to help her relax. She remained on this regime for a week past her exam period and then came off the extra supplements.

Since learning how to handle her stress and support her body through stressful times, Jane has graduated college with honors and made it through the last year-and-a-half without any illnesses at all.

IT IS NOT JUST COINCIDENCE that you seem to get ill during the stressful times of your life. Just when you are at your busiest with way too much to do, you get sick, and it slows you down even more. You don't have time to stay home in bed and recover, so you keep working, which makes the cold or flu last twice as long as it normally would. When you are tired, stressed, and run down, your body does not seem to have its usual resilience to fight infection. Your mom used to say that if you didn't slow down and give your body time to recoup, it would force you to do so. And you know what? Mom was right!

Stress, and its associated hormonal disruption have a profound impact on the immune system. Not only is it energetically costly to keep the fight-or-flight system stimulated all the time, the increased exposure to cortisol actually impairs our ability to fight disease.

Immunity Disorders

In order to understand how stress can affect the immune system, we need to comprehend how the body fights different types of illness.

The immune system is comprised of millions and millions of cells distributed throughout the body. The blood contains red cells to carry oxygen, platelets to assist with blood clotting, and white cells, the immune component. Besides the immune cells circulating in the blood, there are large numbers clustered in specific areas that comprise the lymphoreticular organs. These organs include the lymph nodes, spleen, bone marrow, lymphoid tissue, thymus, and groups of cells in the gastrointestinal and respiratory tracts.

The two populations (the blood and the lymph organs) are in a constant state of exchange and equilibrium. All immune cells originate from the bone marrow where they 'grow up' or differentiate into their destined immune cell type. This includes lymphocytes, monocytes or macrophages, mast cells, and eosinophils. Lymphocytes are the most populous, making up 1% of total body weight, and are found predominantly in the spleen and intestine.

Immune System Organs

Bone Marrow
The cavity in the middle of most bones contains marrow. This tissue provides the basic immune cells capable of maturing into all the different cell types.

Thymus
Organ in the upper chest that produces lymphocytes in the growing fetus. Allows maturation of T-cells after birth. Shrinks after puberty.

Lymph Nodes
Nodules at the junction of major lymphatic tracts. Filter foreign material and present it to the immune system. If stimulated, lymphocytes proliferate here to enhance immune response.

Spleen
Like a giant lymph node in the upper left abdomen. It performs other functions, such as blood filtration and removal of damaged cells.

Peyer's Patches
Lymph glands in the gut predominantly responsible for the development of B-cells. Similar patches are found in the airways of the lungs.

Infection Response Mechanisms

One of the most common immune responses occurs when you develop a small skin infection following a scratch, for example. The tissue trauma results in inflammation, increased blood flow (the redness), and leakage of fluid and cells, particularly granulocytes and monocytes into the area (the swelling). They release chemicals, including histamine and prostaglandins, which amplify the inflammatory process (itching and swelling). Within minutes, local macrophages in the tissue recognize the foreign material and bacteria introduced by the scratch and start to engulf it.

Further release of chemicals attracts increasing numbers of granulocytes and monocytes, which also attack the foreign material. These chemicals include the complement system, which is activated by non-specific stimuli in this phase of the immune response. The complement molecules perform a number of functions, including attraction of immune cells and potentiating their lethal action on bacteria. The chemical mediators secreted into the blood from the inflamed tissue stimulate the bone marrow to release even more granulocytes — the reason your white cell count goes up during infection. These chemicals also cause a rise in body temperature and make you feel sick.

White Blood Cells (Leukocytes) of the Immune System

Lymphocytes

T-lymphocytes: Provide cell-mediated immunity to viruses, bacteria, yeast and parasites, as well as foreign cells and cancer. Includes T-helper cells that regulate much of the immune response via interferon and lymphokines production, cytotoxic T-cells that directly attack foreign, cancerous or infected cells, and suppressor T-cells that inhibit immune response.

B-lymphocytes: Produce antibodies in response to stimulation directly or via stimulation by T-cells.

Natural Killer (NK): Powerful and specialized cells targeting cancerous and virus-infected cells. They act independent from T-cells.

Granulocytes

Neutrophils: Cells that eat and kill bacteria and other particles.

Basophils: Histamine-bearing cells similar to mast cells found in tissues.

Eosinophils: Histamine-bearing cells active in parasite infections.

Monocytes/Microphages

Specialized cells that engulf foreign material such as bacteria. They can present this foreign material to the T-cells in order to stimulate an immune response.

Mediators in the Immune System

Antibodies

Also called immunoglobulins. They comprise 5 classes of molecules (IgA, IgE, IgG, IgM, IgD) that are able to recognize foreign substances (antigens) and stimulate the inflammatory and immune response.

Complement

A combination of chemicals in the blood that amplify the inflammatory and immune response.

Prostaglandins and Leukotrienes

Two families of inflammatory chemical mediators that promote and maintain the inflammatory response. Both groups are manufactured from arachidonic acid by the enzymes cyclo-oxygenase (COX) and 5-lipooxygenase respectively.

Cytokines

Proteins secreted by lymphocytes that regulate the magnitude of the inflammatory response. They include the interleukins, tumour necrosis factor (TNF) and interferon.

Helper T-Cells

Fluid draining from the area of inflammation travels in the lymph vessels to the lymph nodes. Here, the foreign material is presented to helper T-cells, which institute a second line of attack. The response to the infection thus far has been non-specific, a standard response to any foreign assault regardless of type. It provides a first line of defense and, in most cases, is all that is required to resolve the attack on the body. If the stimulus continues, however, it helps contain the infection until the specific immune response is able to build strength, a process that may take several days.

The antigen-specific immune response is mounted by the T and B cells of the immune system. As opposed to the nonspecific response, this phase involves cells that specifically recognize the foreign proteins of the invading organism. There are two prongs to this attack. One involves B-cells and antibodies, the other cytotoxic T-cells.

Both antigen-specific responses require the assistance of helper T-cells (CD4 cells). The organisms ingested by the macrophages are presented to the helper T-cells in a form they recognize as foreign. These helper T-cells (CD4 cells) produce cytokines in response to this recognition. In turn, the cytokines stimulate B-cells and CD8 cells to defeat the infection.

Once the attack is over and the organism defeated, the macrophages and fibroblasts tidy up, removing the debris and creating scar tissue. Suppressor T-cells wind down the immune reaction, leaving some of the activated B and T cells as 'memory cells' in the circulation, ready to mount a more rapid response should the same organism attack again.

Viruses and Other Invaders

Viruses and other invading organisms are recognized in much the same way as described earlier. They may be identified in the blood stream, the airways, or the gut, depending on how they gain access to the body. Once again, the macrophages in these areas provide the initial response and recognition, ingesting the invader and presenting it to the lymphocytes (T and B cells) at the nearest lymph node in order to start the immune response.

Tumor Cells

Currently, it is thought that roaming cytotoxic T-cells, natural killer (NK) cells, and macrophages defend against tumor cells. These cells have the ability to recognize the altered proteins on the surface of these mutated cancer cells and mount a response against them. NK cells appear to be the most important initial line of defense and somewhat less specific in their recognition of tumor cells.

Cytotoxic T-cells and macrophages require the assistance of helper T-cells, which release cytokines, including interferon and tumor necrosis factor (TNF), empowering these tumor-killing cells.

Immune System and Adrenal Gland Interaction

There is a rapidly growing body of research documenting the interaction of the immune system, the brain (particularly the hypothalamus), and the adrenal glands. Inflammation and activation of the immune system stimulates central and adrenal stress mechanisms with resulting increases in CRH and cortisol. These stress hormones then have a regulatory

Cytokine Action

Cytokines are able to stimulate the two prongs of the attack on infections:

1. B-Cells

B-cells are covered with antibody molecules (immunoglobulins), which have the ability to recognize specific foreign proteins. Once the B-cell binds the invading organism, it has the potential to start multiplying to form a clone of cells capable of producing large amounts of the same antibody. However, it cannot do this without the CD-4 cytokine stimulation.

The antibodies produced by the B-cell (now called a plasma cell) interact with the foreign organism (antigen) making it more sensitive to attack by granulocytes. The antibody-antigen complex also activates the complement system, which results in lethal damage to the invading organism.

2. CD8 Cells

Cytokines act on other T-cells (CD8 cells), inducing them to become cytotoxic T-cells capable of directly killing foreign organisms or infected cells. They also enhance the function of natural killer (NK) cells and macrophages, both of which are capable of killing cells infected with viruses, bacteria, or fungi, and tumor cells.

effect on many aspects of the immune response. The principal controlling elements of the immune system are the cytokines, particularly interleukin-6 (IL-6) and TNF. IL-6 is a powerful stimulator of cortisol release through both the hypothalamus and CRH and by direct action on the adrenal gland.

The importance of this feedback mechanism has been identified in numerous diseases, including rheumatoid arthritis and inflammatory bowel disease. It has even been hypothesized that during growth, immune stimulation of the stress response in susceptible individuals may lead to abnormal development of the brain-adrenal-immune axis. The resulting alteration in the relationship between these components may predispose an individual to physical and psychological disease.

Effects of Stress on Immune System

1. Immune Reaction Impairment
Cortisol and the hypothalamus-pituitary-adrenal system, along with the fight-or-flight sympathetic mechanism, impair the function of cells and messengers within the immune system.

2. Feedback Impairment
The overstimulated and less responsive stress mechanism in the chronically stressed individual fails to respond adequately to control inflammation and hyperactivity of the immune system.

Role of Stress in the Immune Response
With a basic understanding of the cells, chemicals, and interactions of the immune response, we can look at how stress and cortisol undermine the efficiency and integrity of the system to increase our risk of disease.

The link between stress and the immune system has always been suspected, but over the past few years there has been an enormous increase in research to document this interaction. The connection between the brain and hypothalamus, the neuro-endocrine system, the cortisol axis, and the immune response is clearly complex. The field is expanding and promises to produce new avenues of treatment for diseases as diverse as cancer and the common cold.

For the time being, the effect of chronic stress appears to be highly detrimental to the function and control of our immune system through two mechanisms. First, there is a cortisol-induced suppression of a number of important elements of the immune response. Second, impaired feedback leads to a lack of control over the immune reaction and subsequent inappropriate overactivity of certain elements.

Cellular Immunity

It is likely that chronic stress and overstimulation of the cortisol system has its most profound effect on cellular immunity, our primary defense against viruses and cancer.

Stress-Related Impairment of the Immune Reaction

Cortisol has been shown to have a significant effect on cell populations within the immune system. For example, acute stress appears to cause a temporary rise in the numbers of natural killer (NK) cells, while more prolonged exposure to high cortisol results in a fall in their population and activity, with levels dropping by as much as 50% in some studies.

Cortisol also promotes death and absorption of T-lymphocytes, impairs their proliferation, and inhibits their production of interleukin-2, one of the cytokines responsible for stimulating the immune response. In addition, stress reduces levels of glutamine, an amino acid essential to the functioning and sustenance of the cellular immune response.

Cortisol impairs the inflammatory response, which reduces the efficacy of both the nonspecific and antigen-specific immune reactions. Cortisol directly inhibits the cyclooxygenase 2 enzyme (COX-2) — the same enzyme targeted by the new anti-inflammatory arthritis drugs, such as rofecoxib or Vioxx and celecoxib or Celebrex. This reduces prostaglandin production and thus dampens the inflammatory cascade. Cortisol induces lipocortin production, a chemical that inhibits the enzyme phospholipase-A2, responsible for the manufacture of both prostaglandins and leukotrienes and is also known to inhibit the function of neutrophils, eosinophils and monocytes, important cellular components of the initial assault force on foreign organisms. Although a reduction in the inflammatory reaction may be desirable in diseases such as arthritis, its suppression may increase the likelihood of infection gaining a foothold.

Cortisol interferes with the production of cytokines by T-cells. It reduces the production of most pro-inflammatory, immune-boosting cytokines, including interleukin-2, interleukin-6, TNF-alpha and interferon.

Low CG Syndrome

The combination of low plasma levels of the amino acids cysteine and glutamine with reduced NK-cell activity is termed low CG syndrome and is found in numerous disease

---

✔ STRESS FACT Viral Infections

The old wives' tale that associates stress and fatigue with an increased risk of a cough or cold may actually not be too far from the truth. Certainly, there is a strong association between the impaired immunity seen in overtrained athletes and the frequency and severity of viral infections such as influenza. The association of stress and the appearance of cold sores (herpes virus) is well documented and is not just a coincidence. Both these observations may be a reflection of reduced cellular immunity resulting from prolonged cortisol exposure.

Activated Whey Protein

Chronic stress and cortisol reduce levels of cysteine and glutamine, amino acids essential for the manufacture of glutathione, an antioxidant vital to immune function. Use of an activated whey protein isolate can be used to counteract this effect until other stress management measures are implemented.

Activated whey protein is a purified milk whey protein isolate that is high in the amino acid cysteine – the limiting factor in glutathione production. It increases glutathione production in the body.

IMMUNOCAL (www.immunocal.com) and HMS-90 (www.immunotec.com) are pharmaceutical-grade milk serum protein isolates that increase cysteine available to cells for normal metabolic processing.

states, including sepsis, major injuries, HIV infection, cancer, Crohn's disease, ulcerative colitis, chronic fatigue syndrome, and overtraining syndrome. There is associated muscle wasting and fatigue, as well as increased urea production (a protein breakdown product).

Stress and Viral Infection

The effect of stress on potential viral infection has been studied recently. Studies on astronauts have indicated that the stress of space flight results in the reactivation of viruses, such as herpes and CMV (cytomegalovirus), through the down-regulation of cellular immunity associated with stimulation of the cortisol pathway. Another study observed the immune system of astronauts during space missions. They were chosen because of the tremendous stress associated with space travel and the relatively controlled environment.

The objective of the study was to determine the effects of stress on the levels of adrenaline, noradrenaline and cortisol, and their relationship to levels of antibodies specific to the Epstein-Barr virus (EBV) and the EBV antigen itself. This virus has been implicated as one contributing factor in the development of disorders such as chronic fatigue syndrome. Compared to baseline samples taken at their annual medicals, significant increases in EBV levels were found in their blood 10 days before flight, landing day and 3 days after landing. Associated with this were decreased levels of anti-EBV antibodies indicating that the physical and psychological stresses associated with space flight resulted in decreased virus-specific T-cell immunity and subsequent reactivation of the Epstein-Barr virus.

Stress and Cancer

The cancer surveillance system of the body involves cells of the immune system detecting and eradicating mutated cells with the potential to form tumors. These cells are also part of the immune response activated against existing tumors to prevent their spread both locally and via the bloodstream. The

Role of Glutathione

Glutathione is the major endogenous antioxidant of all cell types.

- Protects cells from 'free-radical' damage.
- Helps recycle other antioxidants, such as vitamin C and E.
- Aids in the removal of toxins from the body
- Controls balance of oxidation in the cell during protein synthesis, DNA replication or repair, and enzyme activity.
- Allows lymphocytes to multiply.
- Vital to 'killer' activity of immune cells in attacking cancer or virus-infected cells.

most important front-line cells appear to be the natural killer (NK) cells, and we know the number and potency of these cells is reduced by prolonged stress and high cortisol.

A study involving 104 women with metastatic breast cancer were observed for circulating cortisol levels and its relationship to their disease outcome. Women with abnormal daily cortisol patterns who lacked the 6:00 to 8:00 a.m. morning peak and showed irregular peaks and troughs throughout the day (typical of chronic stress) had a shorter lifespan than those with more normal cortisol cycles. This was independent of other lifestyle or environmental factors. In addition, the patients with these abnormal cortisol patterns had fewer and less active NK cells.

Direct Effects of Cortisol on the Immune System

1. Suppresses production of pro-inflammatory cytokines, IL-1, IL-6, and TNF.
2. Inhibits prostaglandin and leukotriene synthesis by suppressing the enzymes that manufacture them.
3. Reduces cysteine and glutamine levels, amino acids essential for T-cell function.
4. Induces lipocortin production. Lipocortin inhibits phospholipase-A2 and thus reduces prostaglandin and leukotriene production. It also inhibits the function of neutrophils, eosinophils and monocytes.
5. Promotes T-lymphocyte death, inhibits their proliferation, and suppresses their interleukin-2 production.
6. Impairs activity of monocytes and macrophages.
7. Prolonged stress decreases NK-cell number/activity.

Chronic Stress Impairment of Normal Immune Feedback

Under normal circumstances, inflammation and activation of the immune system results in the production of numerous chemical mediators or cytokines that stimulate the stress response. IL-6 induces cortisol release from the adrenal gland and also CRH from the hypothalamus, both of which modulate the immune response. Thus, there is feedback control that limits the ferocity and extent of the immune attack and subsequent inflammation.

As we have seen, in chronic stress the overall responsiveness of the hypothalamus-pituitary-adrenal system is diminished, being readjusted to a higher 'set point' with regards to feedback. This appears to affect the ability of inflammatory cytokines to control the system as well. Rheumatoid arthritis patients show a markedly diminished cortisol response to IL-6, a factor which is positively correlated with inflammation. The reduced sensitivity of the system may be one mechanism whereby chronic stress increases susceptibility to diseases that involve unchecked activation of the immune reaction, such as inflammatory bowel disease and rheumatoid arthritis.

Sympathetic Nervous System

Besides modulation by the central nervous system through hormones, including cortisol, the sympathetic fight-or-flight nervous system also appears to influence immune cells and inflammation directly. The production and function of granulocytes, white blood cells involved with inflammation and attack of foreign organisms, is stimulated by the sympathetic nervous system. Granulocytes have receptors on their cell surface that respond to adrenaline and cortisol, allowing a direct effect of these hormones. This may be part of the body's protective mechanism during times of acute stress. However, when the sympathetic system and cortisol axis are consistently stimulated through chronic stress, the immune system produces an abnormally large number of granulocytes. This has been associated with the onset, development, and recurrence of many different diseases, such as inflammatory bowel disease, collagen disorders, and cancers.

Boosting Immunity
Relieving stress is an important first step to improving our immune health and both fighting and preventing disease.

Treatment Program for Stress-Related Immunity Disorders

Note: Ensure that you consult with your doctor before starting any new program or supplement.

1. **Naturopathic Diet**
   Increased protein to stabilize blood sugar and provide material to rebuild the body.

2. **Physical Therapies**
   - Massage
   - Lymphatic Drainage
   - Yoga

3. **Psychological/Relaxation Therapies**
   - Meditation
   - Counseling

4. **Natural Supplements**
   - Magnolia Bark
   - Lavender
   - Activated Whey Protein
   - Plant Sterols
   - Antioxidants (vitamins A, C, E and selenium)
   - Zinc
   - Olive Leaf Extract
   - Oregano Oil

Type 1 Allergic Reactions

Allergic Asthma
Allergic Rhinitis
Allergic Bowel Disease
Atopic Dermatitis
Hives (urticaria)
Anaphylaxis (life-threatening allergic reaction)

Allergic Response

Most people who suffer from allergies, skin rashes, or asthma experience a worsening of their symptoms during times of stress. Indeed, an acutely stressful event may initiate a rapid onset of hives or asthma in some individuals. Many people simply believe that stress aggravates the situation by making them *feel* worse, rather than actually being physically worse. However, there does appear to be a connection between stress and increased allergic symptoms, the result of the interaction between the HPA-axis, cortisol, and the immune system.

CASE STUDY

'Primed' by Stress for Allergies

A 28-year-old female came to the office with a full body, itchy, warm rash. Apart from the rash, Jolene was in no acute distress, with no breathing difficulties and no swelling of the tongue. The rash appeared very suddenly and had lasted 5 days.

This is longer than a typical allergic reaction. What was more interesting was that she had no known allergies, and tested negative to everything except blueberries. She reported that she had previously enjoyed blueberries quite regularly without even the slightest allergic symptom.

Careful history revealed that she had been under a great deal of stress for the past 4 to 6 months. After further investigation, we concluded that this stress had affected her immune response such that she was 'primed' for a hypersensitivity reaction. Her cortisol response was blunted, causing her to lack the necessary feedback to control such a reaction. When she ate blueberries, to which she was so mildly allergic that she had never previously reacted, the stage was set for a catastrophic reaction. The blueberries were the trigger, but the underlying problem was stress.

Primed by chronic exposure to CRH and cortisol, a vigorous and prolonged reaction resulted in a massive release of histamine by mast cells in the skin. Inadequate response by the adrenal glands to control this reaction exacerbated its severity.

Along with her medical doctor, we decided her initial treatment would include antihistamines and a short course of oral steroid therapy to resolve the rash and itching. We supported her with quercetin, vitamin C, stinging nettle extract, zinc, and calamine (topically). Subsequent allergy testing revealed only a very mild sensitivity to blueberries, and although Jolene now avoids them, stress management has been the mainstay of her preventive treatment.

Allergic Response Basics

Allergies are over-reactions of the immune system. They are termed hypersensitivity reactions since they are an exaggeration of an otherwise normal response. They can result in potentially harmful tissue inflammation and damage. The clinical features of a specific allergic reaction relate to the immune process that mediates it, rather than the environmental stimulus that caused it. The most common of these reactions result from stimulation of mast cells and immunoglobulin-E (IgE) and are called type 1 reactions.

Mast Cells and IgE

Our immune system mounts a response to any foreign substance when it enters the body, through the gut, the lungs, or the skin. The main purpose is to determine whether the body recognizes this substance and whether or not it is harmful. If unrecognized, it will be treated as foreign and therefore dangerous. The immune system will then attempt to immobilize or destroy it. This incoming foreign substance is termed an antigen.

The key feature of type 1 allergic reactions is the direct stimulation of mast cells by the antigen. Mast cells are very similar to the white blood cell type, the basophil. However, rather than being located mainly in the bloodstream, they are found in tissues, such as the walls of bronchioles (breathing tubes in the lung), the gut, blood vessels, and skin. These cells contain numerous granules of active chemicals that promote inflammation, accumulation of excess fluid in tissues, muscle spasm and vessel constriction. They are covered by a special type of antibody, IgE. When an antigen attaches to the IgE antibody, it stimulates the mast cell to release the active chemical mediators and synthesize new ones. These released chemicals cause the *immediate phase* allergic response, which varies according to site.

Anaphylaxis

Anaphylaxis is the simultaneous occurrence of immediate phase reactions mediated by IgE throughout the body in numerous systems. It can lead to shock, obstruction of the throat and airways, and generalized skin rash (urticaria). It can be fatal if untreated — those with known risk carry injectable adrenaline as a first-line treatment.

Atopy

Atopy is an inherited propensity to suffer from allergic reactions. An estimated 10% to 30% of individuals in developed countries are considered atopic, although there is no specific diagnostic test. The most common presentations are allergic rhinitis and asthma.

Both genetic and environmental factors are thought to play a role in the development and realization of atopy. Atopic individuals generally have higher than normal levels of IgE and produce these antibodies to a wider range of environmental stimulants. They also appear to have larger numbers of mast cells, with those cells being covered with more IgE.

One theory of atopy is that an imbalance or dysfunction of helper T-cells results in an inordinate number of B-cells being converted to IgE producing plasma cells. This conversion is mediated by cytokines. Cortisol and chronic stress affect both T-cell function and cytokine production, possibly increasing the risk of developing allergic diseases, such as asthma in genetically susceptible individuals.

Immediate Phase Allergic Response

Lung: constriction of airway, increased fluid/mucus

Nose: runny nose, teary/itchy eyes, sore throat

Gut: cramping, nausea, gas/bloating, diarrhea

Skin: red, itchy, raised rash

An important clinical study carried out in Finland and published in 2002 set out to determine whether the onset of various allergic diseases, such as asthma, allergic rhinitis, conjunctivitis, and atopic dermatitis, were associated with stressful life events. The researchers concluded that there was a strong association between stressful life events and the risk of development of atopic disease, as well as the exacerbation of symptoms in existing disease.

✔ STRESS FACT Parasympathetic Overactivity

The sympathetic system dilates bronchioles in the lungs, improving ability to breathe, whereas the parasympathetic system causes constriction. Asthmatics seem to have a relative overactivity of the parasympathetic system with impaired response to adrenaline stimulation. A similar imbalance is seen in chronic stress and overtraining in athletes, likely due to exhaustion of the sympathetic fight-or-flight response. This may be one of the ways stress can influence the allergic response.

Role of Stress in Allergies

There is an increasing body of evidence associating stress with the development and progression of allergic diseases, including asthma and dermatitis. There are a number of theories as to why this occurs.

Autonomic Nervous System

The role of the autonomic nervous system in atopy may be important as it influences both the presence and activity of immune cells and the responsiveness of tissues to the chemicals released by the mast cells. An autonomic imbalance in favor of the parasympathetic system (the system that opposes the sympathetic fight-or-flight system) may result in a tendency to hypersensitivity. It would increase numbers of histamine-producing basophil cells and heighten sensitivity of the tissues.

Cortisol

One of the most important ways in which chronic stress can influence the immune system is through a reduction in the ability of the adrenal glands to mount an adequate response to immune stress. Cortisol would normally be released in response to a number of stimuli and act to moderate the immune response and degree of inflammation. In chronic stress, this feedback control mechanism is impaired, allowing the immune system to overreact to stimulation. Patients with atopic dermatitis are found to have significantly attenuated cortisol and ACTH responses to stressful stimuli.

CRH

One further factor that may be important in the association between stress and the allergic reaction is the role of corticotrophin-releasing hormone (CRH), the stress hormone released from the hypothalamus as the initial stage of the stress response. CRH has a potent effect on mast cells, causing them to release histamine and other active inflammatory chemicals. Other neurotransmitters, notably neurotensin and substance-P, which are linked to the hypothalamus and found in the peripheral nervous system, also exacerbate the allergic response.

Hypothalamic stimulation resulting from acute stress will cause release of these messengers and may provide one pathway to explain stress-related reactivation on asthma, dermatitis, and possibly inflammatory bowel disease. In the presence of impaired pituitary and adrenal response to CRH, there will be less cortisol to counteract the process, potentially making the reaction even greater.

 STRESS FACT Histamine Levels

Histamine levels show a daily variation with a peak around 1:00 to 2:00 a.m., a time when asthma sufferers often experience an exacerbation of symptoms. This just happens to coincide with the lowest levels of cortisol. Studies have also shown an association between chronic stress, reduced morning cortisol levels, and exacerbation of asthma.

Psychosocial Stress

The immune changes induced by stress have been studied to determine the impact of acute psychosocial stress on the immune function of those suffering from atopic dermatitis. Thirty-six patients with atopic dermatitis were compared to 37 controls (non-atopic individuals) and exposed to a standardized stress test involving mental arithmetic tasks and free speech in front of an audience. Blood samples of all the participants were collected, under resting conditions, 10 minutes before, then 1, 10, and 60 minutes, and finally 24 hours after the stress test. Analysis revealed elevated lymphocytes, monocytes, neutrophils, and basophils 10 minutes after the stress test with no significant difference between the allergic and non-allergic groups. However, when the researchers looked at eosinophils (the cells most associated with histamine and the allergic response), they found greatly increased numbers only in those patients suffering from atopic dermatitis. In addition, at 24 hours, these patients showed a significantly raised level of IgE antibody (also associated with the allergic response), a finding not observed in normal subjects. The study concluded that this stress-induced immune system modulation may be one of the factors behind the aggravation of symptoms in atopic individuals.

Atopy and the allergic diseases are intimately linked to the immune system. Stress affects immune system function by altering the delicate balance of cellular interaction and disabling the body's ability to keep the immune reaction in check. It comes as little surprise, therefore, to find that stress can influence the development, progression, and severity of allergies and their associated diseases of skin, lungs, nose, and possibly intestine. Fortunately, recognition of the role of stress has prompted exploration of stress management techniques as another method with which they can be treated.

Stress Management of Allergies

Research has gone some way in explaining the clinically observed association of allergic reactions and stress. It has also opened the door to treatments that address psychological issues, such as chronic stress and anxiety, in patients.

One recent study evaluated the benefit of a self-administered stress management intervention for individuals with asthma. A 4-week program was compared to a matched placebo intervention (similar format but without effectively treating stress). Both groups reported that they felt the treatments were credible and compliance was excellent. However, the group performing the stress-management program reported significantly greater improvement of lung function compared to those with the placebo.

Treatment Program for Stress-Related Allergies

Note: Ensure that you consult with your doctor before starting any new program or supplement.

1. **Naturopathic Diet**
   Increased protein to stabilize blood sugar and provide material to rebuild the body.

2. **Physical Therapies**
   - Massage
   - Lymphatic Drainage
   - Acupuncture

3. **Psychological/Relaxation Therapies**
   - Lifestyle Changes:
     - new pillows and bed sheets
     - air purifier in bedroom
     - do not exercise in midday heat and humidity
   - Visualization:
     - visualize your mast cells and basophils stabilizing

4. **Stress Supplements**
   - Magnolia Bark

5. **Allergy/Immune Supplements**
   - Quercetin
   - Stinging Nettle
   - Plant Sterols
   - Antioxidants (vitamins A, C, E and selenium)
   - Olive Leaf Extract
   - Oregano Oil
   - Zinc

Musculoskeletal Disorders

High Stress, Low Back Pain

When George first came to our office, he was 45 years old and had been plagued by recurrent episodes of low back pain for the past 10 years. His job involves a great deal of walking, bending, and lifting, but he has noted that his back pain often flares up at times of stress rather than with extra workload.

Once we completed a careful examination and a number of tests to rule out any significant damage or pathology in George's spine, we explained the role stress plays in this condition. We then formulated a comprehensive treatment plan that included postural and ergonomic education, core conditioning, and stress management. Milk peptide and valerian root at night were added to his low back pain supplements, which included calcium/magnesium, boron, and a full-spectrum antioxidant. Deep-breathing exercises were introduced, along with massage and acupuncture.

George has been back-pain free for 3 years and reports an overall improvement in his health.

THE ASSOCIATION OF STRESS with musculoskeletal disorders is well established in the field of sports medicine where overtraining syndrome has long been recognized as the deterioration of physical functioning from excessive exercise stress. However, recent research also finds that more common disorders, such as osteoporosis (thinning of the bones), arthritis, and low back pain, are influenced by both acute and chronic stress.

Overtraining Syndrome (OTS)

Overstimulation of the stress response in athletes leading to reduced performance, exhaustion, suppression of the immune system, and poor motivation has been recognized for many years and has been termed overtraining syndrome (OTS). The hormonal and biochemical abnormalities seen in OTS share many similarities with chronic stress and metabolic syndrome. OTS involves physical, behavioral, and emotional components persisting for weeks to months, recognized initially as 'burn out'.

- Plateaued or reduced
  performance
- Fatigue
- Altered mood and/or
  irritability
- Altered/poor sleep
  pattern
- Poor motivation
  and reduced
  competitiveness
- Reduced appetite and
  associated weight loss
- Persistent muscle
  soreness
- Increased injury rate,
  poor healing and
  recovery
- Increased incidence
  of viral illness

Overtraining Syndrome Basics

"No pain, no gain." To improve performance, you have to work hard, we've been told. You also need to rest. The rest periods between exercises are what make you stronger. Beneficial changes in cardiovascular and muscular systems, including improved efficiency, increased energy stores, and higher enzyme levels, occur during the periods of rest and recovery following vigorous exercise.

Overtraining syndrome is not a result of training too hard — it is a result of training without adequate rest and recovery periods. An overtraining athlete will eventually reach the point at which sufficient damage and deterioration have been done that even increased periods of rest are insufficient to provide adequate recovery.

The incidence of OTS is more common than generally appreciated. Some studies show rates of up to 50% for elite athletes in individual sports. The incidence in individual sports is significantly higher than team sports and less demanding sports. It is estimated that more than 60% of distance runners suffer OTS at least once in their career and 50% of soccer players during a 4-month season.

It appears that emotional and psychosocial stressors contribute to the problem in addition to pure overtraining.

Diagnosis of Overtraining Syndrome

The specific diagnosis of OTS has proved to be difficult, notably because of the presence of essentially normal biochemical and hormonal markers in many athletes with symptoms typical of OTS. Currently, the most reliable test for OTS is a reduction in sports-specific performance.

Stress Hormone Levels

The early stages of OTS are often considered 'overreaching' where increased resting plasma concentrations of noradrenalin have been identified. In established OTS, decreased nighttime urinary excretion of adrenalin and noradrenalin has been identified and may represent the late-stage parasympathetic phase of OTS with collapse of the sympathetic system. Absolute serum cortisol levels do not show consistent irregularity but, as we have noted previously, this measure is an unreliable indicator of the state of the stress response. What is more important is the reduced responsiveness of the adrenal glands to stimulation by ACTH and the impaired feedback on the hypothalamus and pituitary seen in these individuals.

Mood Change

Attempts at subjective measurement of mood state may be useful in identifying psychological and motivational disturbances associated with OTS. Deterioration in mood appears to precede deterioration in performance by a considerable period of time. In addition, high-level athletes are often able to mask the psychological component of their condition for fear of being dropped from the team.

Immune Impairment

Impairment of the immune system is well recognized in OTS and increased incidence of viral infection is one of the diagnostic features. The persistent cortisol secretion resulting from vigorous exercise causes a decrease in circulating lymphocytes and impaired release of inflammatory cytokines and prostaglandins. A reduction in interleukin production is known to impair the cell-mediated immune response. Increased cortisol in association with exercise causes a reduction in glutamine and cysteine levels, essential amino acids for the manufacture of glutathione, the body's major endogenous antioxidant and free-radical scavenger. Further studies have demonstrated a reduction in natural killer (NK) cell population and activity following vigorous exercise.

Under normal conditions, recovery following exercise is rapid and the changes in the immune system temporary. However, in OTS there appears to be a cumulative effect with failure of the immune mechanism to return to normal. This is thought to result in decreased resilience in particular to viral infections.

Role of Stress in Overtraining Syndrome

Autonomic Imbalance

Two types of autonomic imbalance as related to OTS have been identified. One involves sympathetic hyperactivity with increased blood levels of noradrenalin and increased resting heart rate and blood pressure. A second involves a parasympathetic form with decreased noradrenalin secretion, reduced heart rate and blood pressure, and lowered muscle sensitivity.

There is some evidence that the sympathetic form is more common during team sports and sprint events, with the parasympathetic form being more common in endurance athletes. The parasympathetic form represents a collapse of the sympathetic system due to overstress and may possibly be considered as the final stage in Hans Selye's adaptation theory. This collapse is associated with impaired signaling to the periphery and reduced response when there is an attempt at exercise. In effect, 'you step on the gas' and nothing happens.

Dysfunction of the Cortisol Response

Overtrained athletes show a higher pituitary response to CRH, subsequent increased ACTH release, but impaired response of the adrenal glands to the ACTH, resulting in impaired cortisol secretion. This may be an adaptive mechanism to maintain the ratio of testosterone to cortisol and thus prevent excessive muscle breakdown.

Cytokine Hypothesis

A unifying theory has been proposed in which the cytokines (inflammatory chemicals), released as a result of vigorous training, induce changes in mental status, metabolism, immune function, and muscle recovery. We know that in chronic stress there is an impaired adrenal response to cytokine stimulation, with subsequent reduced cortisol release to control inflammation. This may also occur in OTS, the cytokine buildup and level of inflammation going unchecked due to exhaustion of the adrenal response.

Stress Management of OTS

One of the difficulties of preventing OTS is the inability to identify it in its early stages. Even overreaching and staleness, the first steps on the pathway to OTS, have proven difficult to detect. Further complicating the picture is the overall stress experienced by the athlete, including emotional and psychosocial factors.

One factor to be considered in avoidance of OTS is the concept of 'intensity versus volume'. In one study, two separate groups of runners were subjected to increased training: one group simply increased weekly distance, while the other group increased speed and intensity with only a slight increase in distance. The group that increased training only by distance failed to show improvement in performance and began to demonstrate symptoms of OTS. The group with increased intensity demonstrated a marked increase in performance and results without the appearance of OTS features.

The treatment for established OTS is essentially rest. The longer the period of overtraining, the longer the rest period required. Three to 4 weeks of overtraining will usually require a complete cessation of training with associated rest and recuperation for 3 to 5 days. Following this, training can be commenced, but it is recommended that it be carried out on alternate days. Overall volume must be reduced, but intensity can gradually be increased.

In more prolonged cases where overtraining has been present for many weeks or months, a long period of rest may be required before returning to training. Overall recovery may take many months. In general during this period, in order to prevent 'exercise withdrawal', the athlete is encouraged to train in sports other than the one that caused the overtraining in the first place.

Treatment Program for Stress-Related Overtraining Syndrome

Note: Ensure that you consult with your doctor before starting any new program or supplement.

1. Rest
- 3 to 4 days of rest for each 3 to 4 weeks of overtraining
- For longer periods, train using other sports
- Return with alternate day training

2. Relaxation
- Meditation
- Yoga
- Breathing Exercises
- Massage

3. Counseling
- Sports Counseling/Psychology

4. Nutrition and Supplements
- Adequate intake of balanced protein and carbohydrates. Calorie- or protein-restricted diet increases cortisol and reduces muscle mass.
- Ingestion of food during the recovery phase
- Cysteine and Glutamine (activated whey protein)
- Phosphatidylserine may reduce cortisol levels post-exercise
- Antioxidants (vitamins A, C, E and selenium)
- Calcium/Magnesium
- Glucosamine Sulphate
- Magnolia Bark or Trypsin Milk Peptide

Osteoporosis

Osteoporosis or thinning of the bones is a condition that affects 10 million Americans, of which 68% are women. It refers to a condition in which bone loss leads to weakening of bones and increased risk of fractures particularly of the hip, spine and wrist. Fifty percent of women and one in eight men over the age of 50 will sustain a fracture related to osteoporosis at some point in their life.

Osteoporosis Basics

Bone is an active living tissue comprised of a structural framework made mostly of collagen fibers with protein and calcium phosphate to provide strength. It contains cells predominantly of two types: osteoblasts that lay down new bone and osteoclasts that absorb it. The combination of the protein fibers of collagen and the hard calcium phosphate mineral give bone its unique characteristics of strength and flexibility.

Bone is continually turning over, being resorbed by the osteoclasts and laid down by the osteoblasts. Up to approximately age 30 more bone is laid down than resorbed. This point represents peak bone mass, a time at which there is maximum bone density and strength. Thereafter, the resorption of bone exceeds creation. In the first few years after menopause in women, the degree of resorption is extremely rapid. Osteoporosis occurs when bone is resorbed too quickly, resulting in a reduction of bone density below a critical level, which increases risk of fracture.

Risk Factors for Osteoporosis

- Female
- Post-menopause
- Smoking
- Anorexia/Malabsorption/ Underweight
- Lack of Exercise
- Steroid Use
- Kidney/Liver Problems
- Family History (by far the greatest additional risk factor)

Role of Stress in Osteoporosis

Cortisol

High levels of cortisol or other steroids are associated with osteoporosis. This is most clearly demonstrated in Cushing's disease (abnormal secretion of high levels of cortisol) and in certain diseases, such a rheumatoid arthritis, where prednisone (a medicinal form of cortisol) is administered orally for prolonged periods. Even subjects with mildly increased cortisol levels are found to have significantly increased bone loss compared to normal.

Major depressive disorder is associated with a disruption of the hypothalamus-pituitary-adrenal (HPA) axis and chronically elevated cortisol levels not responsive to endogenous or exogenous suppression or feedback. These individuals are at significantly higher risk of osteoporosis.

One mechanism behind the osteoporotic effects of cortisol is thought to be its influence on the sensitivity of bone cells to chemical messengers (cytokines). Bone mass is a reflection of the balance of activity of osteoblasts, which lay down bone, and osteoclasts, which absorb it. Cortisol appears to affect the sensitivity of these cells to their normal chemical modulators, swinging the balance in favor of the osteoclasts.

Kinds of Osteoporosis

Osteoporosis arises when bone is not replaced as quickly as it is resorbed. This can happen in two situations:

1. **High-turnover Osteoporosis:** resorption is occurring at an excessively high rate such that new bone formation (remodeling) fails to keep up.
2. **Low-turnover Osteoporosis:** new bone formation is impaired in the presence of normal resorption.

Osteoprotegerin

Osteoprotegerin is an important bone cytokine that has the ability to bind the chemical messenger that normally induces bone cells to form new bone-absorbing osteoclasts. By this means, it acts to reduce bone resorption. Cortisol significantly reduces the amount of osteoprotegerin, resulting in an increase in osteoclast formation and a shift in favor of resorption.

Osteocalcin

Osteocalcin is a protein molecule produced by osteoblasts during production of bone. It provides a marker for bone activity and is generally increased in osteoporosis associated with high-bone turnover and reduced in the low-turnover type, such as malnutrition-associated osteoporosis. Cortisol impairs production of new bone by osteoblasts and thereby reduces levels of osteocalcin.

Osteocalcin, in fact, shows a daily rhythm of activity similar to that seen with cortisol. Studies of patients with anorexia and Cushing's disease, in which cortisol levels are elevated, reveal a marked reduction in osteocalcin levels. Osteoporosis is common to both these conditions.

Cortisol induces osteoporosis through both high- and low-turnover mechanisms.

Leptin

Leptin is a hormone produced by fat tissue, one of a group of adipokines that signal the body's nutritional status to the brain. Its primary effects are to reduce appetite and increase energy expenditure, part of the body's control mechanism to maintain a steady weight. During starvation, it allows conservation of energy by reducing metabolic rate, whereas in the well-fed state, it's increased production by fat cells promotes calorie burning. Its daily cycle incorporates a peak at night, ensuring we continue to burn calories yet don't feel hungry. Leptin resistance within the hypothalamus may be one of the factors behind the development of obesity.

Leptin also appears to have a role in bone metabolism, acting centrally within the brain via the sympathetic system to inhibit bone formation. The pathways by which leptin affects bone mass and obesity are different, perhaps explaining why, in starvation, a state with low leptin, osteoblast activity is reduced (as measured by osteocalcin), and, in obesity, associated with high leptin, osteoporosis is unusual. Both of these clinical observations point to a role for leptin in the maintenance of bone mass. Further research is ongoing to elucidate the role of this important hormone so as to develop new treatments for osteoporosis.

Estrogen and Testosterone

Stress results in a reduction in gonadotropin-releasing hormone (GnRH) from the hypothalamus, with subsequent effects on the reproductive hormone levels in men and women. A reduction in estrogen or testosterone has a profound effect on bone mass and this likely represents another avenue through which cortisol increases osteoporosis risk.

Effects of Cortisol on Bone

- Reduces osteoblast function and bone formation
- Increases osteoclast activity and bone resorption
- Reduces calcium absorption from the gut.
- Increases calcium loss from the kidney
- Reduces estrogen and testosterone levels

 STRESS FACT Osteoporosis Treatment

While there have been no definitive studies linking chronic stress and osteoporosis, there is clearly a connection between bone mass, bone cell activity, and the production of cortisol. Reduction of stress is certainly one way of reducing your risk of osteoporosis and should be combined with other treatments listed below.

Treatment Program for Stress-Related Osteoporosis

Note: Ensure that you consult with your doctor before starting any new program or supplement.

Prevention of Osteoporosis

Maximum bone mass is attained by age 30 and starts to decrease thereafter. Prevention aims to make sure your bones are as strong as possible at this stage and helps slow subsequent loss.

1. Calcium: required amount varies with sex and age
2. Vitamin D: if not adequate from diet and sunlight
3. Exercise: stimulates bone formation
4. No Smoking: smoking increases bone loss
5. Limited Alcohol: in excess, increases osteoporosis risk

Treatment of Osteoporosis

May be employed as a preventive measure in 'at risk' individuals or in established cases.

1. Nutrition: adequate protein, calcium, vitamin D
2. Exercise: remains important at any age
3. Medication:
   - Biphosphonates (Alendronate/Fosamax, Risedronate/Actonel)
     – act to reduce bone resorption
     – may increase osteoblast activity
   - SERMs (selective estrogen receptor modulators) Raloxifene/Evista
     – used after menopause only
     – reduce resorption
   - Calcitonin (injectable/nasal spray form of bone hormone)
     – acts to reduce bone resorption
     – may increase osteoblast activity
     – useful for pain control
   - Teriparatide (Forteo) Injectable Parathyroid Hormone
     – act to increase bone formation
   - Hormone Replacement Therapy
     – acts to reduce bone resorption
     – may increase osteoblast activity
     – recent evidence cautions use due to side effects
4. Fall Prevention: balance training and home-proofing

Stress Management in Osteoporosis

1. Exercise
2. Massage, Yoga, Tai Chi
3. Deep Breathing and Meditation
4. Supplements: Magnolia Bark

Arthritis

Arthritis accounts for more impairment of function among middle-aged and older adults than any other disease category. Twice as many people are limited in their mobility by arthritis than by heart disease. Arthritis is the leading cause of physician visits over age 65. But arthritis is not a disease confined to the middle-aged or the elderly. Arthritis causes debility and pain that can have a significant impact on our enjoyment of life at any age.

Arthritis Basics

The word 'arthritis' literally means inflammation of a joint. Arthritis, however, is perhaps best considered as a symptom. It describes an inflamed, stiff, swollen joint, which is the end result of a number of disease processes. While inflammation may be the principal underlying process that has resulted in the symptoms of pain and swelling, its cause may be quite varied. In addition, the disease causing arthritis may affect other tissues in close proximity, or in some cases, at some distance from the joint.

By attaching other descriptions to the word 'arthritis', we can more closely identify and distinguish the different disease processes and patterns, for example osteoarthritis or rheumatoid arthritis. However, the classification of arthritis has become increasingly difficult in recent years as research into the immunology and biochemistry of disease processes has revealed similarities between conditions previously considered separate entities. The classic division between noninflammatory or osteoarthritis and inflammatory (typically rheumatoid) arthritis has become particularly blurred as more and more inflammatory chemicals, such interleukin-1 (IL-1) and tumor necrosis factor (TNF), are discovered as playing an important part in the development and progression of all forms of arthritis. No longer does it appear that osteoarthritis is purely the result of wear and tear, or that rheumatoid arthritis is purely the result of immunological overactivity.

The Role of Stress in Arthritis

The central role of inflammation in the development and progression of arthritis has prompted investigation into its association with the immune system and the effects of stress. Numerous anecdotal reports that link stressful events with the onset or exacerbation of arthritis are increasingly supported by clinical observations and laboratory studies.

Cortisol

A study of chronically stressed individuals (parents of children with cancer) found that the degree of immune and inflammatory suppression (measured by IL-6) produced by injection of cortisol was significantly diminished compared to nonstressed control subjects.

Another study confirmed the relative underactivity and reduced responsiveness of the cortisol system in patients with rheumatoid arthritis and polymyalgia rheumatica (a painful rheumatic disease of the muscles). A further study indicated that it was reduced sensitivity of the adrenal glands to stimulation by the stress hormone ACTH. A simulated stress reaction actually resulted in a decrease in cortisol levels, a possible explanation for the flare of arthritis and inflammatory symptoms seen with stress.

Arthritis Prevalence
The self-reported prevalence of arthritis is 25% in the 45 to 65 age group and 50% in the over-65 age group. For individuals over 63, at least 10% have knee arthritis significant enough to cause pain and disability; the figure is 5% for hip arthritis.

Pregnancy

A study from the National Institutes of Health found that the symptoms of rheumatoid arthritis eased or even disappeared during the third trimester of pregnancy. Following birth, symptoms returned and were often more severe. This was associated with increasing levels of cortisol and noradrenaline. Even in women without any history of joint pain or swelling, there was a strong association between pregnancy and the development of rheumatoid arthritis in the year following birth.

CRH, the master stress hormone produced by the hypothalamus in response to stress, is secreted by the placenta during pregnancy. This is what causes the increased cortisol secretion and the suppression of inflammation with subsequent reduction in arthritis symptoms. However, after the birth of the child, CRH is no longer produced by the placenta, and it takes the hypothalamus 12 weeks to get its own production back to normal. During this period there is a huge drop in CRH and cortisol with a rebound in IL-12 and TNF-alpha. This is likely responsible for the sudden resurgence of inflammation.

Autonomic Nervous System

There is evidence that sympathetic nerve function is reduced in rheumatoid arthritis. This may represent part of the disturbance in the fight-or-flight stress response more easily identified through the hypothalamus-pituitary-adrenal (HPA) axis.

Stress Management of Arthritis

The associations between stress, cortisol, the immune system, and inflammation appear to have significant impact on the development and progression of arthritis. Most research relates to the inflammatory arthritides, more closely linked to autoimmunity. However, the lines dividing different types of arthritis are becoming blurred, and this research likely has equal relevance to all forms of arthritis, including osteoarthritis.

A randomized, controlled study from New York evaluated the benefit of a written stress-management program on patients with rheumatoid arthritis or asthma. Control patients with the same diseases wrote about daily life. Nearly 50% of those writing about their stress had clinical improvement in symptoms compared to 24% of controls; 22% of those in the control group actually got worse compared to only 4% of the study patients. At 4 months, the rheumatoid arthritis patients showed a 28% reduction in disease activity.

The availability of such treatment programs for arthritis is currently limited and research sparse. However, as numerous authors have indicated in subject papers over the past few years, the increasing body of evidence linking the neuro-endocrine and immune systems to arthritis should stimulate interest in this direction.

Treatment Program for Stress-Related Arthritis

Note: Ensure that you consult with your doctor before starting any new program or supplement.

1. Naturopathic Diet

For those who need to lose weight, following stage one of the naturopathic diet is crucial. Try to avoid the deadly nightshade foods, such as tomatoes, eggplant, and peppers. In addition, try to choose more fish as your protein sources to help reduce inflammation. If you do not need to lose weight, start in the maintenance phase, still avoiding the nightshade foods.

2. Exercise

A combination of cardiovascular exercise and strength training is indicated. Try to choose non-impact exercise, such as cycling, swimming, or water aerobics. Strengthening the muscles around a joint can help reduce impact forces and pain.

3. Physical and Relaxation Therapy

- Massage
- Yoga
- Tai Chi
- Acupuncture

4. Stress Supplements

- Milk Peptide
- 5-HTP

5. Arthritis Supplements

- Glucosamine Sulfate, MSM, Chondroitin Sulfate, and Hyaluronic Acid. A combination formula of these supplements (Arthrimin effervescent powder is the most effective) provides ingredients that the body requires to synthesize cartilage and collagen within the joints. It will also act as a natural anti-inflammatory agent and inhibit destructive enzymes.
- Ginger Extract (note precautions and interactions)
- Essential Fatty Acids

Note: For a more comprehensive review of arthritis and its numerous natural and traditional treatments, see the book Healing Arthritis *by Stephen Reed and Penny Kendall-Reed.*

Low Back Pain

Studies show that 90% of individuals will, at some point in their life, experience low back pain. Fortunately, only a small number of us will go on to develop recurrent or chronic pain, but for those individuals, the condition can become debilitating and disruptive to many aspects of their lives.

Role of Stress and the Psyche in Low Back Pain

While we all have the same nerve receptors, nerve fibers, and pain pathways, some of us 'feel' pain more than others, and some of us seem better able to cope with it. Individuals with exactly the same pathologic process, the same size disc pressing on the same nerve, will have completely different experiences and outcomes. One person may be back at work in a week, while another remains disabled for years, unable to recover, plagued by the accompaniments of chronic pain, such as

The role of stress as a significant risk factor in the development and recurrence of low back pain is becoming increasingly recognized. A study published in *The American Journal of Public Health* in 2001 found that individuals who experienced significant psychological stress in their early twenties were over two-and-a-half times as likely to develop low back pain in their thirties as similar stress-free subjects. This finding accounted for other factors, such as smoking and social status.

depression, anxiety, and fatigue. While there are undoubtedly innumerable factors at play, the role of stress and the psyche has become increasingly recognized as a contributing factor.

The experience of pain relates to two areas of the brain, the sensory cortex and the frontal lobe. The sensory cortex is where pain is identified, its location on the body mapped, and its nature determined. The frontal lobe is where the emotional component of pain is registered. Through connections with the limbic system, the emotional component interacts with memory and the fear/stress response. Patients lacking frontal lobes can identify pain but do not 'suffer'.

Recent studies examining brain activity with MRI scanning have revealed that individuals with chronic pain, such as fibromyalgia or low back pain, showed a marked increase in activity in the frontal cortex and cingulate gyrus (the initial communication point with the limbic system) compared to normal subjects. The cingulate gyrus is also responsible for switching attention; it is thought that an abnormality here leads to individuals 'focusing' on their pain.

Genetic factors combined with developmental emotional trauma have been shown to have a significant influence on the development of both psychological and chronic pain conditions, such as fibromyalgia. Post-traumatic stress disorder, for example, is thought to arise from an inadequate cortisol response to a stressful event in a genetically susceptible individual. It is likely that a similar susceptibility exists for back pain, causing some individuals to develop chronic symptoms and experience more profound disability.

Central Sensitization

Chronic stress appears able to influence the degree of central sensitization within the spinal cord. This is a heightened state in which even normally pleasant sensations are interpreted as pain. A reduced level of the calming neurotransmitter serotonin in stress and chronic pain allows increased activity of the excitatory transmitter, glutamate. Serotonin acts to inhibit pain message transmission within the brain, so there is less control over the incoming pain messages. In addition, a high concentration of the pain transmitter substance-P has been found in the spinal cord of chronic pain sufferers. This will increase pain fiber firing and induce sensitization within the cord.

Stress and Recurrent Back Pain

Psychological factors appear to be better predictors of low back pain than MRI findings. Stress in day-to-day life, especially in the workplace, increases risk of both the development and recurrence of low back pain. In one study, subjects were required to perform a lifting task with or without additional psychological stress. Shear and compression forces across the spine increased substantially in the presence of mental stress, a finding the authors propose might be due to reduced muscle coordination and impaired ergonomics.

Stress Management for Low Back Pain

A stress reduction program is a valuable adjunct to other treatments for low back pain. In addition to weight loss (if needed), posture and ergonomic training, an exercise plan, supplements, deep breathing exercises, yoga, meditation, acupuncture and massage all can have a profound effect on pain through reduction in stress and cortisol.

Yoga, in particular, has been shown to be very beneficial in the treatment of back pain and in the prevention of reinjury in the workplace. A study performed at Berkley in California showed that short interludes of Yoga at work helped to teach important stress management techniques and relieve muscular tension in the back. This led to statistically fewer back injuries and a more rapid recovery from existing back problems with a non-specific origin.

Treatment Program for Stress-Related Low Back Pain

Note: Ensure that you consult with your doctor before starting any new program or supplement.

1. Naturopathic Diet

For those who need to lose weight, following stage one of the naturopathic diet is crucial. Try to avoid the deadly nightshade foods, such as tomatoes, eggplant, and peppers. In addition, try to choose more fish as your protein sources to help reduce inflammation. If you do not need to lose weight, start in the maintenance phase, still avoiding the nightshade foods.

2. Exercise

A combination of cardiovascular exercise and strength training is indicated. Try to choose non-impact exercise, such as cycling, swimming, or water aerobics. Flexibility of the hamstrings along with a core-conditioning program is essential. Core conditioning to improve strength and tone in the abdominal muscles and spine helps support the spinal elements, reducing forces across them, relieving pain, and preventing reinjury.

3. Physical and Relaxation Therapy
- Massage
- Yoga
- Tai Chi
- Acupuncture

4. Stress Supplements
- Milk Peptide
- 5-HTP

5. Low Back Pain Supplements
- Glucosamine Sulfate, MSM, Chondroitin Sulfate, and Hyaluronic Acid.
- Ginger Extract (note precautions and interactions)
- Essential Fatty Acids
- Calcium-Magnesium
- Boron
- Antioxidants (vitamins A, C, E and selenium)

Note: For a more comprehensive review of low back pain and its numerous natural and traditional treatments, see the book The Complete Doctor's Healthy Back Bible *by Stephen Reed and Penny Kendall-Reed.*

Reproductive Disorders

Reducing Stress, Conceiving Children

Anne owns her own small business. She is 32 years old with one child, aged two-and-a-half years old. She and her husband have been trying to conceive for the past 17 months without success. The couple had no trouble getting pregnant with their first child, so this new experience of infertility has been upsetting both of them. Their sex life has since turned into an accurately timed science experiment, despite their efforts to make it spontaneous!

After 5 months, Anne saw both her general practitioner and her gynecologist, both of whom reassured her after extensive testing there was nothing wrong. However, despite these words, Anne was not comforted. If nothing was wrong, then why could she not get pregnant?

When Anne came to our office, she was quite discouraged and upset. She had been working long hours, running home after work to put her child to bed, and then falling asleep herself. She was trying to maintain a healthy diet, but time constraints meant she was frequently turning to sugar and starchy snacks. Her exercise regimen was rushed and inconsistent. Although tired, Anne's sleep was disturbed, and she would awake frequently at 3:00 a.m. with her heart pounding, would toss and turn thinking about work and her inability to get pregnant. Anne's menstrual cycle was irregular with cycles varying from 28 to 34 days in length.

Anne decided to change her diet. After eating balanced meals with protein and nutrient dense carbohydrate to stabilize her blood sugar levels, Anne's energy returned. She also began a series of massage therapy sessions to help relax her body. She started a supplementation course of theanine, B vitamins, and passionflower at nighttime. Within 3 months, Anne became pregnant.

HOW MANY COUPLES DO YOU KNOW that have been trying to conceive for a long time without success, yet as soon as they stop trying they get pregnant very quickly? Infertility affects as many as 10 million women in North America. In 10% to 15% of infertile couples, no cause can be found. The importance of stress as a factor in infertility and miscarriage is being increasingly recognized and treatment programs aimed at stress management have met with marked success.

Infertility

Reproduction Basics

The menstrual and reproductive cycle, albeit very important to us, is not considered an essential function for our immediate survival. Although it is necessary for the survival of a species or race, when faced with other threats like famine or disease, reproduction has always taken a back seat to other aspects of health.

Whenever a change in the menstrual cycle occurs, it is usually a good indicator that some type of stress is affecting the body. During evolution, the inability to have a child during times of stress and hardship may have been protective in that the child would have been unlikely to survive and would have been a further drain on sparse resources.

In order to understand how stress can have an impact on the menstrual cycle and therefore fertility and reproduction, it is necessary to understand the sequence of hormonal events that occur every month in the body.

Female Reproductive Cycle

Control of the female menstrual cycle originates in the brain, specifically the area we have seen as orchestrating the stress response, the hypothalamus. It releases a hormone called gonadotropin-releasing hormone (GnRH). This hormone begins to develop in mid-fetal life, and is released in a pulse-like fashion. The pulses continue to build in strength and size until age 10 to 13 when it initiates the onset of puberty. The specific reason as to why the hypothalamus does not secrete sufficient GnRH to stimulate ovulation and menstruation until this age is unclear. It is likely related to maturation in other areas of the brain, along with other environmental and hormonal factors.

GnRH Secretion

GnRH is secreted in pulses lasting 1 to 3 minutes occurring every 1 to 3 hours. This pulsatile secretion is essential to proper function of the system. Artificial *continuous* infusion fails to induce the normal release of gonadotropins (LH and FSH) from the pituitary gland. After being released from the hypothalamus, GnRH travels to the pituitary gland, where it stimulates the release of the two gonadotropins or sex hormones, luteinizing hormone (LH) and follicle-stimulating hormone (FSH). These are the hormones responsible for coordinating the reproductive cycle, including egg maturation, ovulation and menstruation. The secretion of these hormones is also pulsatile, acting on the ovaries to stimulate ovulation.

Estrogen and Progesterone

The developing egg or follicle secretes the estrogen and progesterone responsible for buildup of the uterine lining in preparation for implantation of a fertilized egg or, in the absence of this event, menstruation. Estrogen and progesterone also act on the pituitary and hypothalamus, reducing LH and FSH secretion, thereby providing a feedback mechanism (like cortisol does in the stress response).

In the event of fertilization, the developing placenta produces human chorionic gonadotropin (HCG), which prevents the demise of the corpus luteum despite falling FSH and LH. HCG is present in maternal blood and urine 8 to 10 days after fertilization and provides the basis of tests for pregnancy. The corpus luteum continues to produce increasing amounts of progesterone, supporting development of the lining of the uterus and placenta to nourish the fetus.

✔ **STRESS FACT Reproductive Cycle**

This complex interaction of brain, ovaries, and uterus involved in the reproductive cycle, with numerous hormones, cycles, and feedback loops, works surprisingly well most of the time. However, this cycle is very sensitive to stress due to the controlling influence of the whole system by the hypothalamus processes and acts on all stressful stimuli.

Infertility Diagnosis

An estimated 10% to 15% of North American couples are infertile. Infertility is defined as the failure to conceive after one year of unprotected sex: 90% of fertile couples will be successful in this period. This time frame can often seem very long, particularly as many of today's couples are already in their thirties and, having decided to start a family, are anxious to get pregnant as soon as possible.

Fertility Testing

Screening for infertility involves evaluation of the couple together and includes tests on both. A history and physical exam will evaluate for health problems, current or in the past, which may adversely affect fertility. This includes medications (prescription and over-the-counter) and herbal supplements. Sexual history and current practice is important to assess as these factors account for up to 5% of infertility cases. Clinical exam will assess for abnormalities of the anatomy and may be backed up if there are concerns with tests such as an ultrasound scan. Blood tests for hormone levels in both men and women are essential. Other tests include sperm count, motility and immunology in the man, and ovulation monitoring,

Treating & Preventing Stress-Related Disorders & Diseases

Reproductive Cycle

1. Follicular Phase
GnRH induces FSH and LH release from pituitary.
FSH and LH stimulate development of follicles (eggs) in the ovary.
One follicle outgrows the others producing large amounts of estrogen.
Estrogen stimulates uterus lining to develop.
Estrogen inhibits GnRH, FSH, and LH release from the hypothalamus and pituitary.

2. Ovulation
Surge of LH release 10 to 12 hours before ovulation.
LH promotes androgen (male hormone) production, which stimulates libido.
LH stimulates prostaglandin secretion causing rupture of the follicle and egg release.
Follicle is now called corpus luteum.

3. Luteal Phase
Ovary (corpus luteum) produces progesterone and estrogen.
Progesterone induces maturation of uterine lining.

4. Menstruation
Progesterone and estrogen from ovary inhibit GnRH, FSH, and LH release from hypothalamus
and pituitary.
FSH and LH levels fall over 12 days.
Low FSH and LH cause corpus luteum to shrink with rapid drop in estrogen and progesterone.
Lack of progesterone induces menstruation.

biopsy (taking a specimen for microscopic analysis) of the uterus lining and evaluation of the tubal system by dye test or laparoscopy (looking into the abdomen with a tiny camera) in the woman.

The causes of infertility are well recognized and are usually diagnosed by your family doctor or gynecologist and possibly an endocrinologist (physician specializing in hormone disorders). In some cases, the cause may remain elusive and termed 'undiagnosed infertility.' Recent research indicates that a large number of these cases may be due to the effect of stress on the reproductive cycles of both men and women.

Role of Stress in Infertility: Women

CRH
The main effect of stress on the reproductive cycle is mediated through corticotropin-releasing hormone (CRH), the hormone released by the hypothalamus in response to stress. CRH is responsible for initiating the cascade of hormonal events that result in cortisol secretion.

CRH acts locally in the hypothalamus to inhibit release of GnRH, the hormone released in pulse-fashion from the

CAUSES OF INFERTILITY

Male (30-40%)

1. Reduced Sperm Count
- age
- varicocele (distended veins in the testes)
- medications
- smoking and alcohol
- heat (tight underpants!)
- undescended testicles
- hormonal abnormalities (e.g., low thyroid)

2. Reduced Sperm Motility
- age
- medication
- high immunity

3. Obstruction of Sperm Ducts
- resulting from infection or unusual anatomy

Female (60%)

1. Impaired Ovulation (10% to 15%)
- age
- inadequate body fat leading to hormone deficiency
- polycystic ovary syndrome
- absence of follicular rupture

2. Abnormalities of Anatomy (40% to 55%)
- tubal obstruction (infection, endometriosis, surgery)
- polyps or fibroids

hypothalamus to act on the pituitary. The reduction in GnRH results in impaired LH and FSH secretion and thus disruption of the reproductive cycle. The effect of CRH is mediated by cells secreting the morphine-like chemical beta-endorphin and explains the effect of chronic morphine use on reproductive function. The resulting amenorrhea (lack of menstrual period) and loss of ovulation is typically seen in high-level athletes (where there is also an effect of low body fat), anxiety, and depression.

Prolactin

Prolactin (the hormone responsible for lactation) is also affected by stress. Prolactin is released from the pituitary gland upon stimulation from the hypothalamus, with an increase during pregnancy and milk production. This hormone is a potent inhibitor of GnRH — hence the partially contraceptive effect of breast-feeding. Stress appears to *increase* prolactin production, which, in the non-pregnant woman, will result in alteration of the menstrual cycle and ovulation.

High Cortisol

Women with mild to moderate hypercortisolemia (high cortisol levels or Cushing's disease) show marked disruption of their reproductive cycle along with infertility. The higher the cortisol levels, the lower the levels of LH and FSH.

The term 'functional hypothalamic amenorrhea' or FHA has been used to describe this syndrome of unexplained infertility associated with disruption of the hormonal control mechanism by stress and associated dietary abnormalities. Affecting up to 5% of women in their reproductive years, FHA is associated with highly irregular or absent periods.

Other Factors

There are also some other factors related to stress that have an impact on fertility. Stimulation of the fight-or-flight response and the sympathetic nervous system leads to spasm in the fallopian tubes (the tubes from the ovaries to the uterus) and the uterus through direct nerve supply. This may affect egg transport and the ability to implant.

Stress also reduces libido, an effect thought to be primarily due to overactivity of CRH in the hypothalamus. This is most apparent in depression and anorexia where CRH levels are markedly elevated.

Stress associated with poor diet and extreme weight loss can also have a profound effect on the reproductive cycle.

Exercise-induced amenorrhea occurs when women athletes fall below a critical weight and likely involves a combination of factors, including the stress of excessive training. Low

Treating & Preventing Stress-Related Disorders & Diseases

levels of GnRH, LH, and FSH are seen, a result of raised CRH and endorphin release (morphine-like chemical released in the brain). In addition, low levels of the fat hormone leptin will result in reduced GnRH secretion, an evolutionary mechanism ensuring pregnancy only proceeds in the presence of adequate nutrition. It is feasible that the 'leptin resistance' seen in chronic stress may mimic this scenario, even in the absence of significant weight loss.

Stress is associated with increased risk of miscarriage and is related to reduced levels of the LH required to maintain the pregnancy and increased production of prostaglandins by the placenta induced by CRH.

Role of Stress in Infertility: Men

Just like women, men also have a reproductive cycle, mediated by GnRH from the hypothalamus and secretion of LH and FSH by the pituitary. LH stimulates the Leydig cells of the testes to produce testosterone. The testosterone, in combination with FSH, acts on the Sertoli cells in the testes, causing them to produce sperm. The timing of the cycle is more variable than that in women but may be associated with similar mood changes.

Chronic stress in men causes a reduction in GnRH, LH, and FSH, much as it does in women. This has a profound effect on sperm production, with reduced counts and motility. In addition, stress lowers testosterone levels, which reduces libido. Overactivity of the fight-or-flight sympathetic system can result in impotence and problems with ejaculation, although this can also result from any number of emotional and physical factors, including the stress and anxiety of infertility in a couple.

Stress Management of Infertility

An increasing number of studies have addressed the issue of stress and unexplained infertility. Using counseling and relaxation techniques to alleviate stress, significant numbers of couples have been able to get pregnant.

One study used cognitive behavioral therapy to help women identify their stressors and discuss ways to cope with them. The women were individually counseled by an endocrinologist to help them understand how stress affects their

Stress-Related Infertility Cascade

Stress increases CRH, which inhibits release of GnRH from the hypothalamus.

↓

Low GnRH decreases pituitary LH and FSH secretion in both men and women.

↓

In women, altered ovulation and menstrual cycle (FHA) results. In men, sperm production and motility is reduced.

↓

Stress induces fallopian tube spasm.

↓

Stress reduces libido in men and women.

↓

Stress increases risk of miscarriage.

↓

Stress is increased by infertility.

 STRESS FACT Infertility

It appears that not only can stress cause infertility, the whole experience of infertility can be extremely stressful to the couple. This 'vicious cycle' only exacerbates the overall effect of stress on the hormonal and sexual function of both men and women.

reproductive hormone. After 20 weeks, all women in the study had increased levels of reproductive hormones, and 80% had sufficient levels to ovulate.

Another investigation performed at the Mind-Body Institute at Harvard Medical School revealed that stress reduction can increase fertility. In this study, 300 women diagnosed with unexplained fertility (no physical barriers to conception) underwent a 10-week program of stress reduction. The program was not designed to discuss and manage infertility, but simply to focus on stress patterns and breaking negative behaviors. The program was based on coping skills, shifting thought processes from stress reaction to relaxation, nutrition, exercise, yoga, and visualization. Most of the women reported feeling significantly better, calmer, and more relaxed. Within 6 months of completing the program, nearly 60% of these women became pregnant.

Treatment Program for Stress-Related Infertility

Infertility is often a complex and highly individualized subject. It entails a more in-depth analysis of clinical findings and, in addition, patients may already be on a variety of hormone replacements and supplements. Therefore, we would recommend that your fertility program be designed by a health-care practitioner. Here are some simple starting points:

1. Detoxification
Cleansing the liver to help it recycle hormones more effectively is a key component in fertility treatment.

2. Supplements
Supplements to reduce inflammation in the lining of the uterus such as essential fatty acids, willow, or baby aspirin are useful.

3. Adrenal Hormones
Stabilizing adrenal hormone output is essential since it will affect the levels of active estrogen and progesterone in the body.

Irregular Menstruation

Traditional thinking is that variability in the length of a menstrual cycle occurs during the first 2 weeks of a 28-day cycle, the time leading up to ovulation. After ovulation, there is a set 14 days until bleeding occurs, the first day of menstruation.

CRH, produced by the hypothalamus in response to stress, decreases the release of GnRH, the hormone responsible for stimulating FSH and LH production by the pituitary gland. FSH and LH are required to stimulate development of the egg so lower levels of these hormones will delay egg maturation and release, effectively lengthening the first phase (follicular phase) of the menstrual cycle.

Treating & Preventing Stress-Related Disorders & Diseases

Although stress may result in overall reduced estrogen levels, as a result of the prolonged follicular phase, the uterine lining is under the influence of estrogen (from the developing follicle) for a longer period. Estrogen builds the lining of the uterus in preparation for potential implantation of a fertilized egg, so this extended exposure results in a thicker and more vascular tissue. When, in the absence of pregnancy, this lining is shed at the end of the luteal phase as progesterone falls, the resulting period is often heavier, prolonged, and contains more clots.

Prolonged estrogen exposure during the first half of the cycle depletes B vitamins and subsequently production of serotonin. This can result in heightened moodiness or PMS, as well as increased craving for chocolate! Estrogen can also deplete calcium, required to prevent cramping during the early stages of menstruation, and essential fatty acids, important to reduce inflammation, cramping, and bloating.

In addition to its effect on the first phase of the menstrual cycle, stress may also affect the second phase by reducing the amount of progesterone produced by the corpus luteum. This will delay feedback inhibition on the pituitary of FSH and LH, increasing the time from ovulation to menstruation. It will also influence uterine-lining maturation.

Stress Management of Irregular Menstruation

Stress appears to have inconsistent influence on the menstrual cycle. In our practice, we have found numerous patterns, including absence of periods all together for several months, alternating early and late periods, and regular cycles with increased symptoms. Common to all is moodiness and poor sleep for several nights leading up to the period, along with increased cramping and bloating.

Although numerous other factors are involved — including poor diet, excessive exercise, medication, peri-menopause, and smoking — stress management, in appropriate cases, certainly improves both period regularity and symptoms.

Menopause

Menopause is defined as not having had a menstrual period for at least 1 year — somewhat of a retrospective diagnosis. The average age of onset is 51, but menopause occurs naturally any time after 40. Onset is usually heralded by altered hormone levels, irregular or light periods, and a number of systemic symptoms, including hot flashes, night sweats, fatigue, irritability, headaches, vaginal dryness, poor bladder control, and pain during sex.

Menstrual Irregularity
While there are numerous types of menstrual irregularity with various different causes, stress can cause variations in cycle length and frequency.

Stress cannot only increase cycle time by an effect on both phases of the cycle, it can increase perimenstrual symptoms and the severity of cramps and bleeding.

Menopause occurs primarily due to a drop in estrogen and progesterone production by the ovaries and is considered a natural part of aging. There have been few factors found to influence this. Smoking appears to promote earlier menopause, as does having no children and having a history of epileptic seizures.

Premature Menopause

Along with other practitioners, we have noted an alarming increase in patients presenting with symptoms of menopause in their early forties or even late thirties. Hormonal tests show typically low estrogen/progesterone and high FSH/LH. They have no history of surgery or radiation and have been investigated for autoimmune disease (another possible cause of early-onset menopause).

Our evaluation of this group of premature menopause patients has found evidence of chronic stress with signs and symptoms common to other patients with this condition. Furthermore, their response to stress management and 'cortisol-lowering' therapy gives far better results with respect to their menopause symptoms than standard menopause treatment.

The effect of chronic HPA-axis stimulation on the reproductive hormones is clear. Premature menopause may represent yet another deleterious effect of persistent CRH/cortisol secretion. Further research into this phenomenon is warranted.

Treatment Program for Stress-Related Menopause Symptoms

Note: Ensure that you consult with your doctor before starting any new program or supplement.

1. Standard Natural Menopause Therapy
- Soy Isoflavones
- Black Cohosh
- Vitamin E
- Evening Primrose Oil

2. Stress Management
- Trypsin Milk Peptide
- Magnolia Bark
- Vitamin B complex
- Massage Therapy
- Meditation/Deep Breathing

Sleep Disorders

Lower Stress, Better Sleep

Joe works as a stockbroker and enjoys heading out for a drink with his friends after work to unwind. He's 42 years old. Lately, Joe has found that the glass of wine that used to help him relax and sleep does not seem to work any longer. He now has difficulty falling asleep, and when he does, he always wakes around 2:30 a.m. Once he wakes up, he is unable to shut off his racing thoughts, tossing and turning until his alarm clock goes off at 6:00 a.m.

Not wanting to use sleeping pills for fear of becoming dependent upon them, Joe sought out our help. After an initial consultation, it was evident that his stress levels were affecting more than just his sleep. His chronic sleep deprivation had led to a decreased immune system as seen through his continual low-grade coughs and colds. In addition, he had found himself less able to concentrate at work, resulting in less productivity and more errors.

When all tests came back clear, we proceeded with natural management of his stress hormone. Joe began a combination of magnolia and theanine to inhibit the release of cortisol from his adrenal glands. In addition, we boosted Joe's immune system with plant sterols and olive extract. To help Joe sleep until the other measures took full effect, we used valerian root and lemon balm at night.

Within four nights, Joe was sleeping much better and felt more rested during the daytime. He remained on this regime for 4.5 weeks until his hormonal levels had stabilized, sleep patterns were regular, and his immune system was strong again.

Joe then began massage treatment every other week, a balanced diet, and regular exercise in the late afternoon. Joe is now off all supplements and uses them only on an as-needed basis (only during very busy or stressful times at work). Using the supplements this way helps to maintain a low cortisol level and prevent his body form 'crashing' again.

HOW MANY NIGHTS have you lay awake in bed worrying about the exam you have the next day or the early flight you have to catch? Despite feeling exhausted when you got into bed, you are now wide awake unable to relax, and definitely unable to sleep. Your mind starts racing, going over the day, yesterday, tomorrow or any day. You begin to review and preview almost everything, except the stress-management techniques you learned last week in yoga class. Unfortunately, you can't remember them because you were preoccupied during the instruction, mentally preparing for your lunch meeting that day.

Your time-saving strategies, developed to cope with an overwhelming number of tasks, are now catching up with you. If you don't change this pattern, not only will your time management techniques become less successful, they will begin to have an impact on your stress level, your health, and your sleep.

Sleep Basics

"If sleep does not serve an absolutely vital function," it has been said, "then it is the biggest mistake the evolutionary process has ever made." Despite extensive human and animal research, the function of sleep remains unknown. In animal models, sleep deprivation results in a marked deterioration in mental and physical health, followed eventually by death. In humans, physical and mental function fail and psychotic symptoms develop. It appears that the brain is the only organ that requires sleep, and once deprivation has ended, it will catch up all the non-REM deep sleep and half the missed REM sleep.

 STRESS FACT Sleep Deprivation

Sleep deprivation does not just refer to months of medical-intern-style scheduling! A decrease of only one hour a night can have a detrimental effect on us.

Just as a person cannot run or swim continuously for days on end, the brain cannot function uninterrupted. It requires rest. If the brain does not receive breaks, it begins to shut down for periods of microsleep. This is essentially several seconds of actual sleep: delta waves (stage 3 and 4 of deep sleep) interrupt the regular EEG of an awake person. This will significantly impair function and is a major cause of motor vehicle accidents in tired drivers.

Physiologically, increased protein generation with reduced rate of breakdown in the brain during sleep may be part of an important regenerative state. Impaired sleep results in a weakened immune system with reduced white blood cell numbers and activity. Levels of growth hormone are reduced and the ability to metabolize sugar is impaired leading to greater storage as fat.

The number of hours of sleep each person needs is variable, but the majority of us need 7 to 9 hours.

Role of Stress in Sleep

Cortisol Cycle

Several studies have shown a direct link between sleep deprivation and cortisol production.

One such study looked at 42 women, 20 of whom were on estrogen replacement therapy and 22 who were not. Their urine cortisol levels were measured and sleep patterns recorded on polysomnographs (sleep monitoring machines). This study revealed a direct correlation between increased

Stages of Sleep

Although sleep may seem like one continuous event, it actually consists of several different stages. These stages are differentiated by variations in brain-wave activity (frequency and amplitude). One complete sleep cycle, including all stages lasts between 90 and 100 minutes. Thus, the average person will go through 4 to 5 complete cycles a night. The stages begin with 4 non-REM (rapid eye movement) stages that are characterized by slow-wave activity, then one REM stage characterized by fast waves. The amount of time spent in each stage varies as the night progresses. In the beginning, more time is spent in slower-wave sleep. Then as the body rests and rejuvenates, more time is spent in the faster dream-wave REM sleep.

NON-REM
Stage 1 (5to 10 minutes)

The transition from wakefulness to this first stage of sleep generally occurs within minutes. During this stage, the person is less aware of their surroundings, yet may still wake with a whisper or noise. They are relaxed, breathing is regular but slower, and there is some rolling eye movement. During this stage of sleep people may have hypnotic experiences, such as sensations of falling, hearing voices or seeing flashes of light.

Brain-wave activity is slow, and fairly regular suggesting mental relaxation. There are two types of waves here, theta and alpha. Most of the waves are theta waves, with brief periods of alpha waves. Alpha waves are similar to those seen when people are awake but relaxed. During stage 1, progressively fewer alpha waves are seen.

Stage 2 (30 minutes)

Stage 2 is the first true stage of sleep: 50% of our sleep is said to be in this stage. During this stage, people are even less aware of their surrounding environment. This is still considered a transitional stage. Light noises and movements can still wake you easily.

The wave pattern of stage 2 sleep is different from that of stage 1. The peaks of brain-wave activity become higher (sleep spindles) and then have larger troughs (K complexes). Theta waves are still present, and once again, as this stage progresses theta waves are replaced by more spindles and K complexes.

Stages 3 and 4

Stages 3 and 4 are very similar in wave types. They are the deepest levels of sleep, also known as slow-wave sleep. Stage 3 comprises approximately 7% of our total sleep time and stage 4 around 11%. In these stages, relaxation deepens, the heart rate slows, and the respiratory rate begins to decrease. In addition, if people are woken up during these stages, they will be very confused and groggy.

There are two types of waves that characterize these stages. In stage 3, only 20% to 40% of the waves are delta waves and the remaining time is spent in theta-wave sleep. Delta waves are characterized by much larger waveforms and deeper sleep. In stage 4, more than 50% of the time is spent in delta-wave sleep. Stage 4 is thought to be the most essential and rejuvenating stage of sleep.

REM (RAPID EYE MOVEMENT) SLEEP

The final stage of sleep is probably the best known. As the name suggests, in this sleep stage people's eyes move in a rapid, flickering motion while their eyelids are closed tightly. Dreaming occurs during this stage and may be important from a psychological perspective. However, it is not as important to regeneration as stage 3 and stage 4 sleep.

cortisol levels and decreased sleep on several levels. First, when cortisol levels were elevated, all the women woke much earlier in the morning. Second, raised cortisol not only affected the number of hours of sleep, but also the *quality* of sleep. The study showed that when cortisol levels rose, the women spent less time in stages 2 through 4 and more time in REM. This indicates a less restful, less rejuvenating, and a more disturbed sleep pattern when cortisol or stress levels are elevated.

Another sleep study not only revealed an association between increased cortisol and decreased sleep, but also noticed a difference in sleep patterns between genders. Men demonstrated higher cortisol levels than women when exposed to the same stress. This resulted in a greater disruption in sleep patterns and a decreased depth of sleep in the male members of the study.

 STRESS FACT Vicious Cycle

There is a direct relationship between stress, increased secretion of cortisol and impaired sleep patterns. To compound this effect, decreased sleep hours or decreased quality of sleep both lead to an increase in cortisol. If the body spends insufficient time in stage 4 sleep, the normal diurnal rhythm of cortisol secretion is disrupted. Cortisol levels do not fall sufficiently overnight. In addition to the extra cortisol produced in response to a stressful and restless night, this results in a gradual increase in overall cortisol levels in the body. This increase further disrupts our sleep pattern, creating a vicious cycle.

Cortisol Clock

When sleep deprivation occurs frequently, there is a change in the daily cortisol secretion pattern. Cortisol should have its maximal output around 6:00 to 8:00 a.m. in the morning in order to wake us for the upcoming day. With inadequate sleep, our cortisol levels do not have sufficient time to drop to a low enough level for this controlled peak to occur. We awake feeling groggy in the morning, drowsy, not refreshed, and ill prepared to face the rigors of the day ahead. Despite overall higher cortisol levels during the day, we feel tired and may need to nap once or twice (if we have the opportunity).

The next night, raised cortisol levels and our unresolved stress keep us awake, further perpetuating the disruption of the cycle. The altered sleep-wake cycle and periodic naps eventually lead to a shift in our 'cortisol clock', and we now find that we have a new peak in cortisol around 2:00 to 4:00 a.m. in the morning. From a physiological point of view, our body is now hormonally in fight-or-flight mode at this time.

Treating & Preventing Stress-Related Disorders & Diseases

Sleep is impossible and the wakefulness is associated with anxiety, racing heart, and an overactive mind. As we lie there, staring at the alarm clock, exhausted yet unable to relax and sleep, our body is giving us a warning. We need to get our cortisol under control.

The after-effect of cortisol release is an increase in hunger, which, in the case of a 2:00 a.m. to 4.00 a.m. peak, will result in the 'midnight munchies' and a trip to the fridge in the early hours, another cause of lost sleep.

Low Growth Hormone Level

A low level of growth hormone is associated with reduced energy, weight gain, decreased immunity, weakness and impaired endurance, poor libido, high cholesterol, and many other symptoms and signs found as we age. In addition, there is a strong correlation between low growth hormone levels and altered sleep pattern. There is also a strong relationship between sleep deprivation and reduced growth hormone production. When our body is not allowed to sleep approximately 8.5 hours a night, our levels of growth hormone decrease significantly. One double-blind trial on eight healthy men demonstrated that reduced sleep over only a 2-day period significantly reduced the production of growth hormone as compared to controls.

Blood Pressure

Elevated blood pressure is a common cause of insomnia. Studies have demonstrated that patients with elevated evening blood pressure suffered much more from insomnia and disrupted sleep patterns than those with lower evening blood pressure readings. Following a 10-day administration of a drug used to lower blood pressure, all patients improved significantly with respect to sleep patterns.

Blood Sugar Levels

Poor blood sugar control is a result of both the hormonal abnormalities associated with chronic stress and a diet with excessive high-glycemic carbohydrates (sugars and starches) and insufficient protein. This is exactly the diet most common to our society and favored by chronically stressed individuals.

Low blood sugar levels at night promote increased cortisol secretion, which, as we have seen, interferes with our sleep. The cortisol raises blood sugar, which then, as a result of our insulin resistance, causes a large release of insulin. The insulin stores the sugar as fat, dropping our blood levels once more and stimulating our fight-or-flight reaction, again not conducive to a restful or rejuvenating sleep.

Low Growth Hormone and Chronic Stress
Recent studies have revealed striking similarities between symptoms associated with low growth hormone and those of chronic stress syndrome (metabolic syndrome with elevated cortisol and insulin). Poor sleep associated with high cortisol has an adverse effect on the level and function of growth hormone and possibly on the process of aging.

Exercise

Exercising in the evening can increase cortisol levels. People often think that exercise will tire them out and ensure a good night's sleep. While this may be true for some, the increased activity of the sympathetic system, circulating adrenaline and noradrenaline, along with cortisol, will be a stimulant rather than a sedative in most individuals.

Treatment Program for Stress-Related Sleep Disorders

1. Reducing Cortisol Levels
- Deep Breathing
- Massage Therapy
- Aromatherapy
- Magnolia Bark

2. Setting a Pattern
Our body loves routine. Providing it with a rehearsed setting for sleep is a valuable step toward programming a successful night. This means getting into bed at the same time each night, particularly during the initial retraining period.

3. Controlling Light and Melatonin
Once we fall asleep, our body starts to produce melatonin, our sleeping hormone. It changes our brain waves from the active beta waves to the calm theta waves of deep sleep. Production of this hormone is also linked to light and darkness. Our body will increase the production of melatonin when it is dark and suppress its production in the light. So try to make your room as dark as possible to mimic nighttime and increase production of your sleeping hormone. It is also wise not to spend your last hour before getting into bed under bright lights. This will hinder the secretion of melatonin and make sleep more difficult.

4. Exercise
Try to avoid vigorous exercise in the evening, as this is likely to increase cortisol and other stimulatory hormones, which will make relaxation difficult.

5. Food and Drink
Avoid a large meal late in the evening as it is likely to result in a higher than normal peak in glucose levels due to the inactivity that follows as you head to bed. This will increase insulin, dropping blood glucose dramatically and stimulating cortisol release. A light protein and carbohydrate snack before bed can help stabilize your blood sugar levels and prevent hypoglycemia during the night. This snack should be 1.5 parts protein and 1 part carbohydrate.

Alcohol is also known to increase CRH and cortisol levels, so avoid it if you are having trouble sleeping. Caffeine in tea, coffee, or soda can have a long-lasting stimulant effect, interfering with restful sleep. Try to avoid it after lunchtime and certainly during the evening.

Chronic Pain Disorders

Reducing Stress, Ending Pain

Paula is a 35-year-old accountant, who, until the past year or so, had rarely suffered from headaches. However, soon after starting work with a new firm, she began to notice increasingly frequent headaches, severe enough to require a strong painkiller, and occasionally so bad she had to stay in bed. Interestingly, the most severe attacks would often occur on the weekend, preventing her from enjoying time with her family.

After seeing her family doctor, having her eyes checked, and consulting with a neurologist, Paula was diagnosed with migraine headaches and prescribed medication to help control their frequency.

Paula brought the subject up when she next visited us. We discussed the possibility that stress was, in part, responsible for her headaches. Certainly, the pressures of a new job, a young family for whom she was the principal bread-winner, and some worries about her husband's health had markedly increased her feelings of anxiety and inability to cope. The appearance of headaches at the weekend when she was trying to wind down was also a clue.

We instituted a program of dietary change to stabilize blood sugar, increased her hydration with water, reducing her use of coffee and alcohol. We added supplemental 5-HTP, theanine, calcium/magnesium, a B vitamin complex, and essential fatty acids. Paula began weekly reflexology and acupuncture treatments. She also started a home relaxation program of deep breathing and meditation.

Paula has been headache-free for 6 months. She maintains her diet and relaxation program, along with regular reflexology treatments and acupuncture at times of increased stress.

THE NUMBER OF INDIVIDUALS suffering from chronic pain conditions, including migraine, fibromyalgia and chronic fatigue syndrome (CFS), has risen dramatically over the past 20 years. While some of this increase can be attributed to better diagnosis, there appears to be an emerging link to chronic stress. Research has revealed striking similarities between affected individuals, while the role of stress in development and stress management in treatment is expanding.

An additional factor to be considered is the influence of pain on the hippocampus, that part of the limbic system responsible for coordinating the fight-or-flight stress response. Chronic pain is associated with altered responsiveness of the stress pathway, reduced cortisol, and impaired secretion of corticotropin-releasing hormone (CRH) from the hypothalamus. This is thought to be partially due to cell death and shrinkage of the hippocampus, a finding also seen in chronic

- Stress
- Light/Noise
- Sleep Deprivation
- Hunger
- Hormone Levels (e.g., menstrual cycle)
- Food (nuts, chocolate, cheese and other dairy, MSG and other additives)
- Drinks/Drugs (coffee, alcohol, red wine)

stress. Not only does this affect the way the individual handles new stress, it also has a profound influence on all tissues and systems of the body, leading to the development and progression of illness, both physical and mental.

Migraine

There are an estimated 28 million migraine sufferers in America, with the condition affecting 20% to 25% of all women and 5% to 8% of men. Migraine headaches account for millions of lost workdays and billions of dollars in productivity and health costs.

Migraines are severe headaches, characterized by their association with nausea, vomiting, and sensitivity to light. They are preceded by an 'aura', symptoms that occur just before the headache. These include flashing lights, stars, blind spots, or 'zig-zags'. While associated with stress, unlike tension headaches, migraines usually occur during a period of relative rest following stress, for example, on the weekend after a busy week. Migraines have a number of well-recognized triggers besides stress, including meal irregularity, hormone levels (there is a strong association with ovulation and the menstrual cycle), foods, and drinks.

Migraine Basics

Most migraine sufferers report stress to be the most important trigger for their headaches. A study from Boston in 2001 found the most common precipitating factors in both migraine and tension headache to be stress/tension, not eating at regular times, fatigue, and lack of sleep. A similar review of factors influencing migraine development noted that 76% of participants reported stress as a trigger. Other triggers noted were sensory stimuli, such as light and sound (75%), sleep deprivation (49%), and hunger (48%).

Theories of Migraine

The specific cause of migraine headaches remains elusive. Originally, it was thought that the problem was purely vascular, that is, related to the blood vessels. Constriction caused the aura, and dilation the headache. Current research, however, points to a 'migraine generator' in the brainstem, which stimulates sensory nerves (particularly the trigeminal nerve supplying sensation to the face and head). These nerves then release active chemicals, including nitrous oxide, responsible for inducing constriction and dilation in the cerebral arteries. This generator may be unbalanced by a combination of genetic factors, environmental influences, and internal stimuli.

The most recent research points to serotonin (5-HT), an important and widely found neurotransmitter, as a key mediator of the migraine process. New drugs that selectively stimulate certain types of serotonin receptors are extremely effective at relieving migraine headache in the acute phase. These medications act to both constrict the dilated blood vessels and reduce activity in nerves transmitting pain sensation.

Role of Stress in Migraine

Serotonin Receptors

Migraine sufferers most often find that their headache begins when they try to relax after a stressful event or period. The reason for this is not immediately apparent, but may relate to withdrawal of the fight-or-flight drive and subsequent overcompensation by relaxation and recovery systems, such as the parasympathetic nerves and serotonin pathways. One recent research article found that subjects with migraine had increased sensitivity of a certain serotonin receptor (5-HT1A). This oversensitivity may account for the rebound phenomenon that causes migraines when stress is removed.

Chronic stress and CRH markedly reduce serotonin secretion in the brain and it is feasible that when 'de-stressing', the rise in levels of serotonin and the hypersensitivity of the receptors contribute to the development of a migraine attack.

Mast Cells

There is a well-established connection between stress and the activation of mast cells. Mast cells are found in most tissues, including the brain, best known for their effect in allergy and asthma where their release of histamine and other active chemicals results in tissue inflammation and edema with spasm of the small tubes in the lung. Local neural inflammation and extravasation of fluid from blood vessels into the brain tissue is a vital end-point in migraine and likely responsible for a major component of the pain.

Corticotropin-releasing hormone (CRH), produced by the hypothalamus, is the first hormone in the fight-or-flight cortisol reaction. Its regulation is disrupted in chronic stress, resulting in increased secretion with numerous adverse effects, one of which is the destabilization of mast cells. CRH also has the ability to directly cause degranulation of mast cells, the process by which these cells release their active chemicals to induce inflammation. This has been identified in the lung, skin, and intestine.

Potential Roles of Stress in Migraine
- HPA-axis disruption
- Altered serotonin receptor sensitivity
- Mast cell destabilization and degranulation (via CRH)
- Increased endothelin production
- Low blood sugar

Recently, a similar mechanism has been noted in the brain. One study found CRH to cause massive degranulation of mast cells in the brain tissue of rats. Interestingly, rats pretreated with capsaicin (a natural inhibitor of inflammatory neurotransmitters) showed no such activation of their mast cells, indicating that CRH acts through inflammatory neurotransmitters such as substance-P. This mechanism is thought to be important in the triggering of migraines by stress.

Endothelin

Endothelin levels are also increased during a migraine attack. One study from Finland found levels were significantly elevated during the first 2 hours of a migraine attack and dropped to normal or even below normal by 4 to 6 hours. A recent study in the journal *Brain* found endothelin to be a potent inducer of a neuronal change in rats considered the equivalent of a migrainous aura in humans.

Blood Sugar

Low blood sugar (hypoglycemia) is known to be a common trigger for migraine and may be a factor behind the 'Saturday morning headache' due to a late breakfast, lack of caffeine, and ingestion of alcohol the previous night. Chronic stress induces metabolic changes, including insulin resistance, that exaggerate swings in blood sugar levels. This is likely a further contributing factor of stress to the frequency and severity of migraine attacks.

Other Factors

Additional association between chronic stress and migraine include alterations in immune function with reduced levels of helper T-cells and altered natural killer (NK) cell function. There is also a change in the cycle of prolactin secretion (hormone released from the pituitary under the control of the hypothalamus) with a reduced nocturnal peak. Secretion of melatonin from the pineal gland is also lower, and the nocturnal peak delayed coincident with sleep disturbance.

✔ **STRESS FACT HPA-Axis Disruption**

There is evidence for disruption of the hypothalamus-pituitary-adrenal axis in chronic migraine. The daily cortisol rhythm is altered as in chronic stress with overall increased levels of this hormone. In one study, migraine sufferers were found to have significantly impaired dexamethasone suppression tests, indicating impaired feedback in the HPA axis, a finding common with the chronic stress syndrome.

Stress Management of Migraine

A greater understanding of the mechanisms behind migraine will likely provide better insight into its relationship with stress, which, after all, appears to be the most important trigger. Treatment regimes are already showing how stress management and relaxation can reduce the frequency and severity of headaches.

There are numerous reports supporting the use of stress management and relaxation in the treatment of migraine. The combination of behavioral therapy and medication appears to be synergistic, creating a response greater than either treatment alone.

Treatment Program for Stress-Related Migraine

1. Naturopathic Diet
The naturopathic diet will stabilize blood sugar levels and prevent the onset of hypoglycemic (low sugar) headaches. In addition:
- Do not skip meals.
- Increase water intake.
- Avoid all known food allergens.
- Avoid food triggers, such as chocolate, caffeine, nitrates (preservative-rich foods), food coloring, alcohol, white refined sugar.

2. Cardiovascular Exercise
Any type of exercise is good, but take these precautions:
- Ensure adequate water and electrolyte replacement
- Eat small protein-carbohydrate balanced snacks 30 minutes before and after exercise

3. Physical and Relaxation Therapies
- Deep Breathing
- Acupuncture
- Massage Therapy
- Meditation
- Craniosacral Therapy

4. Stress Supplements
- Milk Peptide
- Calcium-Magnesium
- Vitamin B complex
- 5-HTP

5. Migraine Supplements
- Essential Fatty Acids
- Licorice Root
- CoQ-10

Fibromyalgia and Chronic Fatigue Syndrome

Fibromyalgia and chronic fatigue syndrome (CFS) are conditions characterized by a preponderance of symptoms in the absence of any clear disease process or pathology. In effect, there are illnesses that rely on clinical evaluation rather than positive test results for diagnosis. This may be one reason why these conditions remain somewhat controversial as distinct medical 'diseases', their existence even denied by some practitioners.

Symptoms of Fibromyalgia

Pain
- Widespread pain throughout the body
- Tenderness at specific points (e.g., back of head, upper back, neck)
- 11 of 18 specific points tender on testing
- Persistent for at least 3 months
- Associated with stiffness

Headache
- Chronic headaches and facial pain
- 'Tension' type headaches with neck pain

Fatigue
- Reduced energy
- Non-refreshing sleep

Poor Concentration and Memory
- 'Fibro fog'

Irritable Bowel Syndrome

Depression

Researchers in the field of chronic stress have faced similar hurdles in their attempt to gain recognition for this seemingly ubiquitous condition. However, the past 10 years has seen significant advances in the mechanisms linking stress with both fibromyalgia and chronic fatigue syndrome, which may not only allow a better understanding of these conditions as true illnesses, but could provide exciting possibilities for treatment.

Fibromyalgia and Chronic Fatigue Syndrome Basics

Fibromyalgia is more common than CFS, affecting an estimated 2% to 4% of the population (around 3.7 million Americans), opposed to 0.1% to 0.3% for CFS (half a million Americans). It may be that CFS is purely a subgroup of fibromyalgia sufferers with more extensive and complex symptoms. Both conditions are more common in women and tend to affect those aged 25 to 45 years of age (up to age 60 for fibromyalgia). Children are only rarely diagnosed but teenage girls are considered a risk category. Caucasians are more likely to suffer from these conditions than any other ethnic group.

Diagnosis of both fibromyalgia and CFS relies on the identification of certain patterns of symptoms or complaints by the patient. Unfortunately, due to significant overlap of the symptoms between the two conditions, fibromyalgia and CFS are frequently used interchangeably or even concurrently by medical practitioners.

An infectious disease expert may be more familiar with the chronic fatigue syndrome criteria developed by the CDC (Center for Disease Control and Prevention), whereas a rheumatologist will likely veer toward fibromyalgia and the guidelines of the American College of Rheumatology. Regardless of medical leanings, the diagnosis of either condition carries with it the stigmata of chronicity, disability, psychological upset, and incredibility, combined with unknown etiology and poorly defined treatment regimes.

Causes of Fibromyalgia and Chronic Fatigue Syndrome

No one etiological factor has been found that clearly results in the development of either fibromyalgia or CFS. There are no blood tests or X-rays that can diagnose the condition and no infective organism isolated. The fact that there is no clear 'gold standard' test for diagnosing the existence of either condition means that the subjects evaluated may vary greatly from study to study, further compromising interpretation of results. Current opinion is that the diseases are 'multifactorial', stemming from a number of etiologies occurring simultaneously or consecutively, exceeding the body's ability to cope.

Role of Stress in Fibromyalgia and Chronic Fatigue Syndrome

Hormonal Abnormalities

Abnormalities of HPA-axis function identified in fibromyalgia and CFS are consistent with those seen in chronic stress. Reduced negative feedback of cortisol on the hypothalamus ('cortisol resistance') results in increased CRH activity with subsequent reduction in sex hormones, growth hormone, and thyroid function. As a result, similar disturbances in sexual function, fertility, menstruation, and sleep are seen in CFS and chronic stress. Similarly, the response of both the pituitary and the adrenal glands to stress (either 'true' or artificially on testing with administered CRH) is blunted.

Low-dose cortisol replacement is found to help CFS patients, demonstrating an ability to override the cortisol resistance, thereby dropping CRH activity, which is thought to be at least partially responsible for CFS symptoms. In addition, administered cortisol improves the adrenal response to CRH, a finding that may relate to normalization of the pituitary ACTH release, along with changes in CRH-binding protein levels in the blood.

Overall activity of the sympathetic nervous system appears impaired in CFS much as it is in chronic stress. The 'sit-up test', in which blood pressure is monitored lying down then sitting, is a good indicator of sympathetic function. A normal individual will show a 10 mm/Hg rise on sitting. An individual in the early stages of chronic stress with a hyperactive fight-or-flight system will show a 20 mm/Hg rise. Someone in the resistance phase with 'adrenal exhaustion' will actually show a fall with dizziness or visual disturbance. This last pattern occurs in more than 90% of CFS patients.

Symptoms of Chronic Fatigue Syndrome

Fatigue
- Predominant symptom
- Present for at least 6 months (with no other medical cause)
- Interferes with work, recreation and social interaction
- Does not improve with rest

Impaired Memory and/or Concentration

Immune Disorders
- Persistent sore throat
- Lymph node tenderness

Pain
- Muscle pain
- Multiple joint pain (arthralgia) without inflammation
- Headaches

Non-refreshing Sleep

Post-exertion Malaise
- Lasting more than 24 hours

 STRESS FACT **Fibromyalgia and Chronic Fatigue Syndrome**

The identification of chronic stress as a factor in the development and prolongation of both fibromyalgia and CFS appears to be a valuable diagnostic adhesive, which not only helps link the two conditions, but permits their rationalization, understanding, and treatment.

Immunological Abnormalities

Although there is no clear evidence that fibromyalgia and CFS result directly from dysfunction of the immune system, there is ample research to document abnormalities, many of which are common to chronic stress. For example, reduced natural killer (NK) cell number and activity; impaired neuro-endocrine regulation through impaired response of the hypothalamus and adrenal gland to interleukin-6; reduced levels of cysteine and glutamine (low CG syndrome); and altered T-cell population and activation. Findings are consistent enough for some researchers to consider CFS "a disease of deficient neuroendocrine-immune communication."

Recent research indicates a possible autoimmune factor in CFS, antibodies directed against the body's own tissues, in this case to cholinergic receptors. There was a strong correlation of antibody levels to symptoms in the patients tested. There is good immunological evidence for the involvement of chronic stress and HPA-axis abnormality in the development and progression of other autoimmune conditions, as in arthritis.

The similarities of immune dysfunction in fibromyalgia /CFS and chronic stress are obvious, providing further evidence of a significant link between the two conditions.

Virus Reactivation

Although no infective, contagious, or causal relationship between viral infection and fibromyalgia or CFS has been identified, research has demonstrated reactivation of certain viruses (herpes virus 6, for example) in these patients. Similar to the reactivation seen in chronic stress (the astronauts are a good example), this likely relates to one of the deficiencies in the immune system associated with the conditions. It is unclear whether the reactivation itself results in fibromyalgia /CFS symptoms or whether it is purely an indicator of the immune compromise.

Treating & Preventing Stress-Related Disorders & Diseases

Alterations in Brain Function

Findings of altered neurotransmitter activity in fibromyalgia and CFS are well documented, though often inconsistent between studies. There does seem to be a fairly consistent decrease in noradrenaline activity with an increase in substance-P. The effect of this alteration is to increase the amount of 'noise' the brain receives from incoming sensory stimuli. Rather than 'important' information being isolated from the background information, excessive amounts of data arrive for processing. This results in hypersensitivity, a hallmark of both fibromyalgia and CFS. The effect of raised substance-P was demonstrated in one study in which normal volunteers were injected with this neurotransmitter into the fluid surrounding the brain. They subsequently experienced temporary symptoms of diffuse pain and muscle aching reminiscent of fibromyalgia.

Although some studies show a decrease in the neurotransmitter serotonin, others reveal an increase in activity within the brain and hypersensitivity of certain serotonin receptors. This may explain why drugs that increase serotonin, such as fluoxitine (Prozac), have not been found useful in fibromyalgia and CFS, while serotonin receptor blockers (experimental 5-HT3 antagonist granisetron) significantly reduce symptoms.

Serotonin pathways within the brain are intimately linked to the HPA axis through CRH-containing cells within the hypothalamus, providing the main stimulus to CRH release. While not yet fully elucidated, it is likely the interaction between chronic stress and fibromyalgia/CFS is at least in part based on impaired communication and disruption in these two systems.

Conditions Associated with Fibromyalgia and Chronic Fatigue Syndrome
- Irritable Bowel Syndrome
- Irritable Bladder
- Dry Eyes, Skin, and Mouth
- Painful Menstrual Periods
- Dizziness
- Restless Legs Syndrome
- TMJ (temporomandibular joint) Pain

✔ STRESS FACT Fibromyalgia and CFS

Anecdotally, stress is often related to the onset or exacerbation of both fibromyalgia and CFS. Most information on the two diseases lists 'stress' as an important factor with regards to both causation and progression of symptoms. However, only recently, with the surge of research into the neuro-endocrine effects of stress and development of chronic stress theory, has headway been made into a link between HPA-axis activation and fibromyalgia/CFS etiology.

Stress Management of Fibromyalgia and Chronic Fatigue Syndrome

Of the various treatments available for fibromyalgia and CFS, none has proved 'curative', although many offer improvements in quality of life. Prognosis remains variable and difficult to assess given the tremendous variation in symptoms between patients and within individual patients from day to day.

Probably the most evaluated and successful therapy is graded aerobic exercise, with physical modalities, such as acupuncture and massage therapy, imparting added benefit. Exercise, such as yoga or tai chi, that incorporates both muscular activity and a component of relaxation may prove to be beneficial.

We have found nutritional supplements, such as calcium-magnesium, vitamin B complex, SAMe, and essential fatty acids to be useful, along with an appropriate diet with sufficient protein to avoid large swings in blood sugar. An immune-booster, such as biologically active whey protein (Immunopro/HMS-90), can also be beneficial.

Research has shown cognitive behavior therapy to produce some lasting benefits. It can be used along with stress reduction and relaxation techniques, such as meditation, biofeedback, breathing exercise, and music therapy.

Reduced levels of growth hormone have been found in some investigations of CFS patients, and this has been used as a rationale for treatment with growth hormone replacement therapy. However, low growth hormone is not a consistent feature of CFS or fibromyalgia and treatment results have been unimpressive. Growth hormone cannot currently be recommended as therapy for these conditions.

Treatment Program for Stress-Related Fibromyalgia and Chronic Fatigue Syndrome

1. Education and Counseling
Learning more about the condition is a vital part of therapy in this condition.

2. Aerobic Exercise

3. Physical Therapies
- Massage Therapy
- Acupuncture
- Craniosacral Therapy
- Yoga or Tai Chi

4. Naturopathic Diet
- Increase protein
- Reduce sugar, caffeine, alcohol

5. Natural Supplements
- Calcium-Magnesium
- Antioxidants (vitamins A,C,E and selenium)
- Vitamin B complex
- Ginger Extract
- Essential Fatty Acids
- Immune boosting supplements (Activated Whey Protein, Plant Sterols)
- Capsicum

6. Cognitive Behavioral Therapy

7. Pharmacologic (Drug) Therapy
- Anti-inflammatory Medications
- Antidepressants
- Steroids

Note: Most pharmaceutical drugs used in fibromyalgia/CFS have an unpredictable response, significant side effects, or are experimental.

Anxiety and Depression

No More Panic

Tim was 47 years old when he was promoted at work. Despite being pleased about his promotion, he now faced much more responsibility. Tim began working longer hours, skipped his regular workouts and increased the 'junk food' in his diet. He also began to experience heart palpitations, chest pain, dizziness, and insomnia.

When Tim first saw his general practitioner, he sent him for a complete cardiac workup. With the exception of a little weight gain and slightly elevated systolic blood pressure, Tim was deemed "just fine." His doctor told him he was having panic attacks and that he needed to rest and relax.

At this point, Tim sought alternative therapies to help balance his body again. After dietary alterations to stabilize swings in blood sugar, deep-breathing and meditation exercises to help him relax, and regular exercise, Tim felt much better, though not 100%.

Tim then began regular supplementation with magnolia extract during the day and early evening, with valerian root at night. Within days, he felt much more relaxed. He did not feel his heart pounding in his chest anymore, and his concentration returned to normal. He began to sleep through the nights with ease, which made his workdays much more productive, thereby allowing Tim to get back to the gym.

Tim has now been able to discontinue the valerian root and takes the magnolia only when his workload temporarily increases. This is more of a preventive measure for him, since his breathing exercises, diet, and exercise help him manage his day-to-day stress.

THERE IS INCREASING EVIDENCE that dysfunction of the HPA axis, including altered responsiveness and sensitivity, plays an important role in the development of affective (mood) disorders, such as anxiety and depression. This is not surprising given the integration of pathways controlling the stress response and those associated with mood. They share the same neurotransmitters and interact extensively in the formation of memory, interpretation of stimuli, and perception of stress.

Anxiety and Depression Basics

Anxiety

Anxiety is an outcome of stress. A threatening event triggers the fight-or-flight stress response, initiated in the amygdala and hippocampus, where external events are interpreted in the light of both innate behavior and life experience. The 'set point' of this process is under the influence of the serotonin system, which also controls mood, hunger, sleep, and aggression. The lower the set point, the more reactive the system, and the more likely the stress response is to be triggered. In addition, the emotional memory of the event stored in the amygdala is stronger and carries greater influence when interpreting future events. This is called 'conditioned fear' and is the basis of 'perceived' stress. It allows even the thought of an event or situation to trigger the fight-or-flight response, even though the individual may be nowhere near facing it directly. This perceived input or thought comes from the medial prefrontal cortex, an area exerting direct influence over the amygdala and hippocampus. Fortunately, this area can also be used to control the stress response, providing the basis for behavioral treatment in stress and anxiety.

 STRESS FACT Neuron Loss

The interaction between the HPA axis, cortisol, and the brain is clearly important in anxiety and depression, but recent evidence has indicated an even more profound effect of chronic stress — that of neuron death, shrinkage of certain areas of the brain, and altered function. Chronic stress or prolonged cortisol secretion induces neuron loss within the hippocampus and is associated with impairment of brain functions, including learning and memory. While cortisol has the ability to enhance memory formation in the acute situation, chronic secretion impairs memory formation. In addition, hippocampal atrophy appears to limit the ability of this area of the brain to shut off the stress response, effectively disinhibiting the HPA axis.

Depression

Hyperactivity of the serotonin system in anxiety and underactivity in depression is an attractive theory. Until recently, depression was thought to be primarily due to reduced activity in the serotonin pathways of the brain, a theory supported by the therapeutic benefit of drugs, such as Prozac and other SSRIs (selective serotonin reuptake inhibitors), that increase serotonin activity. In addition, dietary intake of tryptophan (used by the body to make serotonin) influences symptoms in depression. There is also evidence for a genetic abnormality of the serotonin receptor in depressed patients. Recent research has questioned this theory, noting that it takes up to 6 weeks for SSRIs to work and that not all depressed people have genetic predisposition and vice versa.

Role of Stress in Anxiety and Depression

Knowing that cortisol modulates the HPA axis and the integration of data within the amygdala and hippocampus, it is not difficult to conclude that HPA abnormalities, along with cortisol receptor dysfunction, play an important role in the development or progression of mood disorders. One of these factors appears to be dysfunction in the HPA axis. In both depression and post-traumatic stress disorder (PTSD), CRH levels are increased. However, in depression, cortisol levels are generally raised, while in PTSD they are normal or low. In general anxiety disorder (GAD) and panic disorder (PD), there is reduced sensitivity to noradrenaline, and although CRH and cortisol levels are normal, feedback within the HPA axis is blunted.

Brain and HPA-Axis Response

These abnormalities are explained through variations in the responsiveness of the brain and HPA axis to the various hormones, mediated via alterations in receptor number and sensitivity. In depression, for example, there is effective cortisol resistance due to reduced cortisol receptor numbers, a similar scenario to that seen in chronic stress. In PTSD, there are increased receptors and receptor sensitivity, resulting in enhanced negative feedback. Despite chronic high CRH release, ACTH and cortisol thus stay low.

There is also evidence that reduced hippocampus size and function may result from genetic susceptibility and from trauma during childhood. These factors create an 'at-risk' population more likely to have adverse psychological effects from stress as an adult.

The role of cortisol in hippocampal neuron death is currently being elucidated. The finding that hippocampal shrinkage is greatest in subjects with high-cortisol depression alludes to its effect. Cortisol is certainly found to sensitize neurons to potentially damaging insults, such as lack of oxygen and high concentration of glutamine. In addition, chronic stress results in 'down-regulation' of the brain's cortisol receptors.

Cognitive Impairment Associated with HPA Activation

Disease	HPA Disruption	Memory Shrinkage?	Impairment?
Depression	raised CRH, ACTH, cortisol	Yes	Yes
PTSD	raised CRH	Yes	Yes
Alzheimer's	raised ACTH, cortisol	Yes	Yes
Steroid Therapy	raised cortisol	Unknown	Yes

Pharmaceutical Drugs for Anxiety and Depression

Beta-blockers (Inderal, Tenormin)

Block the action of adrenaline to reduce the associated feelings of panic associated with situation-specific anxiety. Used in social anxiety disorder. Not to be used in the presence of asthma, heart failure, artery disease, and hypothyroidism.

Benzodiazepines (Valium, Xanax, Serax)

Enhance the function of GABA within the brain. Used in GAD and panic disorder. May cause drowsiness and depression.

SSRIs (Prozac, Paxil, Zoloft)

Selective serotonin reuptake inhibitors influence serotonin concentration and receptor sensitivity in the brain. Used in GAD, panic disorder, OCD and PTSD. Take 2 to 6 weeks to be effective. Can cause nervousness, nausea, reduced libido.

MAOIs (Eldepryl, Nardil, Parnate)

Monoamine oxidase inhibitors block the action of an enzyme in the brain that breaks down serotonin and noradrenaline, thereby increasing their concentration. Used in PD and PTSD, particularly when other drugs have not been successful. Require dietary controls. Severe drug interactions, affect blood pressure, reduce libido, and cause insomnia.

Tricyclic Antidepressants (Anafranil, Tofranil, Elavil)

Affect serotonin and noradrenaline activity within the brain. Used in PD and PTSD usually as second-line drugs. Take 2 to 6 weeks to be effective. Side effects include dry mouth, constipation, blurred vision, dizziness, and low blood pressure.

Buspirone

A relatively new psychotropic drug with anxiolytic properties. Relieves anxiety without causing sedation. Unlike the benzodiazepines, Buspirone does not act on the GABA receptor, but works through the dopamine and serotonin (5-HT) system.

Panic Attacks

Every year, nearly 2.4 million Americans suffer from panic attacks (also called panic disorder or PD). This amounts to approximately 2% of the adult population between the ages of 18 and 55. It usually first appears before the age of 24 and is twice as common in women as men.

Whether we have experienced the symptoms of a panic attack firsthand or have a friend with panic disorder, most of us are well aware of the debilitating symptoms. Sudden and unexpected intense fear is associated with symptoms such as chest pain, heart palpitations, shortness of breath, dizziness, and abdominal unease. This scenario is often mistaken for a heart attack, and the overlap of symptoms means that a cardiac workup is generally required to rule out other pathology before a diagnosis of panic disorder is made.

Between the acute panic attack episodes, patients usually experience tremendous anxiety and may become phobic about places in which the attacks have occurred. The more places that become associated with attacks, the wider the phobia, eventually leading to a fear of going outside at all, a condition called agoraphobia.

All but the coolest of characters will experience a feeling of intense anxiety under certain circumstances. This could be anything from an oral test during final exams to kicking the deciding penalty goal during the final moments of a soccer game. The fight-or-flight system is activated despite your wishes. Besides making you feel awful, it also has a detrimental effect on your performance. Unfortunately, this sometimes has disastrous consequences. But imagine this same feeling occurring out of the blue with no examiner or net in sight. This is the problem in panic disorder.

Role of Stress in Panic Attack

Panic attacks are essentially an inappropriate fight-or-flight response — inappropriate, that is, from an objective viewpoint. Subjectively, the hypothalamus, the sympathetic nervous system, and the adrenal glands are acting appropriately to a 'threatening' stimulus. It is the minor nature of that stimulus that makes the response inappropriate.

CRH Priming

Persistent low-level stimulation of the amygdala by CRH, insufficient to induce a panic attack, seems to 'prime' the system. A relatively minor stimulus is then able to promote a rapid and exaggerated anxiety reaction.

In addition, several studies have found altered sensitivity of the HPA axis in affected subjects when compared to normal individuals. Given the importance of CRH in the induction of panic attacks, it may well be that reduced adrenal responsiveness and impaired feedback on the hypothalamus results in unchecked release of CRH. This would certainly fit with our understanding of chronic stress and its relationship to

---

✔ STRESS FACT Panic Attack Initiation

CRH has the ability to 'prime' the amygdala-hypothalamus connection, which results in easier triggering of the stress cascade, a factor likely important in the initiation of a panic attack. We know that chronic stress causes an alteration in the regulation of the HPA axis. This same dysfunction is found in patients with panic disorder.

panic disorder. Furthermore, the reduced ability of the hippocampus to shut down the fight-or-flight response will cause exaggerated and prolonged symptoms.

CCK

There is a strong connection between the primitive area of the brain in the temporal lobe called the amygdala and the hypothalamus. The temporal lobe and the amygdala are areas that integrate memory and the interpretation of experienced events. Stimulation of the amygdala reproduces anxiety and panic behavior in animals and can be achieved through administration of CRH or CCK (cholecystokinin), a neurotransmitter that also plays an important role in feedback within the intestines.

The role of CCK remains to be clarified. It is certainly a strong stimulator of the cortisol reaction, causing a large rise in ACTH and cortisol levels in human subjects with associated symptoms of panic or anxiety. In patients with panic disorder, this response is exaggerated. These studies point to a role for CCK in the regulation of the HPA axis and an altered sensitivity in panic disorder patients.

Cortisol Irregularities

Increases in cortisol levels in subjects with panic attacks are subtle. One study examined salivary cortisol levels in people with panic disorder during panic attacks and compared them to levels taken 24 hours later. While cortisol levels were higher during their spontaneous panic attacks, the rise was not tremendous and there was no correlation with the severity of the attack. Another study evaluated cortisol responsiveness in subjects with panic disorder compared to normal control subjects. The panic disorder patients had *lower* initial cortisol levels, but failed to show any reduction in levels during the course of the study. Normal subjects on the other hand demonstrated marked decreases in resting cortisol levels. These irregularities demonstrate not only impaired regulation of the HPA axis, but also a relative reduction in adrenal responsiveness, something also seen in chronic stress.

Autonomic Dysfunction

Autonomic dysfunction — altered reactivity and level of activation of the sympathetic and parasympathetic nervous systems — is implicated in other stress-related or affected disorders, including irritable bowel syndrome, hypertension and asthma. It may also play a role in the development of panic disorder, perhaps by mediating the action of CRH.

Treating & Preventing Stress-Related Disorders & Diseases

Stress Management of Panic Attacks

Treatment for panic disorder involves medication with a type of psychotherapy called cognitive-behavioral therapy. This therapy attempts to reduce stress and anxiety, as well as alter the individual's perception of panic attacks. Combining these two types of treatment significantly reduces the likelihood of symptom recurrence. In a recent study, patients received integrated intervention with medication and cognitive-behavioral psychotherapy; the relapse rate was only 14% compared to nearly 80% in those given medication alone.

Treatment Program for Stress-Related Panic Disorder

1. Naturopathic Diet
The naturopathic diet will stabilize blood sugars to prevent anxiety-inducing hypoglycemia (low blood sugar).
In addition:
- Use chocolate-flavored protein supplements
- Avoid caffeine

2. Cardiovascular Exercise
Try to train for longer, at lower intensity, within the Healthy Heart or Fitness zone.

3. Physical and Relaxation Therapies
- Deep Breathing
- Meditation
- Yoga
- Massage Therapy
- Craniosacral Therapy

4. Stress Supplements
- Lavender Oil (topical)
- Milk Peptide
- Magnolia Bark
- Vitamin B complex

5. Psychotherapy

6. Medications
(May be prescribed by your physician in some cases)
- Benzodiazepines (e.g., Valium, Ativan)
- Tricyclic Antidepressants
- Buspirone

General Anxiety Disorder (GAD)

General anxiety disorder (GAD) has been recognized as a true clinical entity over the past decade. Originally reserved for 'anxious' individuals without panic attacks, obsessive-compulsive behavior, or PTSD, it is now seen as a discreet diagnosis with both clinical and neuro-chemical features. About 5% of people develop GAD, an estimated 4 million Americans at any one time. The rate is 60% higher in women. GAD does not generally resolve without treatment and can become a chronic condition. It is estimated that individuals with GAD have the condition for an average of 7 years before seeking treatment.

The precise cause of GAD remains elusive. There may be a slight genetic predisposition, and some studies have indicated that significant stressful life events pose a significant risk factor to GAD development. Most research points to abnormal functioning of neurotransmitter systems within the brain, particularly gamma-aminobutyric acid (GABA) and serotonin.

Role of Stress in General Anxiety Disorder

GAD has many associations familiar to our discussion of chronic stress, including fatigue, headaches, irritable bowel syndrome, poor sleep and immunity.

GABA and Serotonin

GABA is the brain's calming transmitter, a largely inhibitory neurotransmitter acting through benzodiazepine receptors — the same receptors on which benzodiazepine drugs like Valium exert their effect. GABA neurons comprise 60% to 75% of all neural connections within the central nervous system. Their inhibitory actions on other neurons induce muscle relaxation, sedation (through reduced noradrenaline), and reduction in anxiety, likely by inhibiting serotonin activity. GABA activity is reduced in GAD and (PD), secondary to reduced receptor sensitivity.

The efficacy of benzodiazepine drugs, such as Valium and Xanax, is due to their ability to restimulate these receptors. Noradrenaline activity is increased in GAD/PD subjects, and this likely has a significant impact on their heightened fight-or-flight sensitivity.

The role of serotonin in GAD and PD remains controversial since it acts to increase anxiety in some areas of the brain, while reducing it in others. However, there does appear to be increased serotonin receptor sensitivity, and this dysfunction is likely the underlying problem in anxiety disorders.

Treatment Program for Stress-Related GAD

1. Naturopathic Diet
The naturopathic diet will stabilize blood sugars to prevent anxiety-inducing hypoglycemia (low blood sugar).
In addition:
- Use chocolate-flavored protein supplements
- Avoid caffeine

2. Cardiovascular Exercise
Try to train for longer, at lower intensity, within the Healthy Heart or Fitness zone.

3. Physical & Relaxation Therapies
- Deep Breathing
- Meditation
- Yoga
- Massage Therapy
- Craniosacral Therapy

4. Stress Supplements
- Lavender Oil (topical)
- Milk Peptide
- Magnolia Bark
- Vitamin B complex

5. Psychotherapy

6. Medications
(May be prescribed by your physician in some cases)
- Benzodiazepines (e.g., Valium, Ativan)
- Tricyclic Antidepressants
- Buspirone

Post-Traumatic Stress Disorder (PTSD)

PTSD has gained the media spotlight over the past 10 years, yet, according to many experts, still remains underdiagnosed. Although a reported 13 million Americans suffer from the condition at any one time, this number may in fact be an underestimate.

PTSD is the development of an anxiety disorder stemming from a recent or remote psychological trauma. Originally postulated to involve severe physical trauma or disastrous events, such as war, earthquake, or vehicle crashes, inductive stressors now include childhood abuse, incest, or rape. Sufferers often relive the experience through nightmares and flashbacks, have difficulties sleeping, and become detached from relationships. PTSD is also associated with other psychological conditions such as depression, substance abuse, and memory impairment. It can adversely affect functioning within the family, socially, and at work.

Most people who are exposed to a particularly traumatic event experience mild symptoms of PTSD in the weeks following the event, with 60% of all men and 50% of all women reporting at least one significant traumatic event in their life. Only a very small number go on to develop PTSD. Of these, 8% of men and 20% of women develop clinical

PTSD. And of these, 30% will progress to a chronic form. This number is estimated at 30% for those involved in war.

Risk factors include the severity and unpredictability of the event, although clearly this is very individual. Both genetic and social/environmental factors play a role. Pre-existing anxiety and chronic stress may also impose an influence on whether the condition develops.

Role of Stress in Post-Traumatic Stress Disorder

High CRH levels, low or normal cortisol, enhanced cortisol receptor sensitivity, and shrinkage of the amygdala and hippocampus are well-recognized biologic changes in PTSD. In addition, it appears that an individual's initial response to a traumatic event may be of significance when it comes to the development of PTSD. Studies have indicated that an inadequate cortisol reaction immediately following a stressor puts an individual at higher risk of developing PTSD. This inadequate response may be genetic or possibly acquired. Chronic stress and HPA-axis stimulation leads to adrenal fatigue with impaired ability to mount an adequate cortisol release in the presence of significant trauma.

Future treatment of PTSD may involve the use of CRH or cortisol-receptor blocking drugs to modulate this HPA disruption of hypersensitivity to cortisol and overproduction of CRH.

Treatment Program for Stress-Related PTSD

Treatment regimens are dependent on a number of factors, including type of symptoms, associated psychiatric or medical conditions, and patient age.

1. Psychotherapy
- Exposure Therapy
- Cognitive Therapy
- Anxiety Management

2. Stress Management
- Naturopathic Diet
- Exercise
- Physical Therapies
- Stress Supplements

3. Medications
- SSRIs (Nefazodone, Venlafaxine)
- Tricyclic Antidepressants
- Benzodiazepines (Buspirone)

Glossary

ACTH See adrenocorticotropic hormone.

ADH Antidiuretic Hormone. A hormone released by the posterior pituitary gland. Also called Vasopressin.

ATP See Adenosine Tri-Phosphate.

Absorption The selective taking-in or abstraction of water or other materials from the alimentary canal (digestive tract) into the blood or lymphatic system.

Acidosis An accumulation of hydrogen in body fluids due to increased production as seen in a diabetic coma or failure of normal elimination by the kidney or excessive administration of acids.

Addison Disease A disease characterized by abnormally low or absent cortisol production.

Adenosine Tri-Phosphate (ATP) A compound containing three phosphates that when broken down produces energy and enables muscles and organs to function.

Adipokine Messenger or hormone produced by fat cells, e.g., leptin, resistin.

Adipose Tissue Fatty tissue.

Adrenaline The catecholamine released by the adrenal medulla in response to stress. It is short acting and causes activation of the adrenergic receptors. Responsible for the initial fight-or-flight response.

Adrenal Cortex The outer layer of the adrenal gland that secretes the glucocorticoid hormones, such as cortisol in response to stress. Also releases mineralocorticoids.

Adrenal Fatigue A syndrome whereby the adrenal gland does not respond sufficiently to stress, producing inadequate amounts of cortisol.

Adrenal Glands Two small glands that sit one on top of each kidney. They contain the adrenal medulla and adrenal cortex.

Adrenal Medulla The central portion of the adrenal gland that secretes the catecholamines, such as adrenaline and noradrenaline, in response to stress.

Adrenocorticotropic hormone (ACTH) The hormone produced by the anterior pituitary gland that stimulates the adrenal glands to secrete cortisol.

Afferent Pertaining to the nervous system. A nerve fiber going from a receptor in the body to the spinal cord or brain.

Alarm Reaction The first stage of Hans Selye's general adaption response.

Aldosterone A mineralocorticoid hormone produced by the adrenal cortex that helps to regulate sodium and potassium levels in the body.

Alpha Wave One of the natural electrical rhythms of the brain observed on an EEG (electroencephalogram) — indicative of a relaxed yet awake individual.

Amino Acid An inorganic nitrogen rich acid that forms the basic subunit of protein. Each subunit or amino acid is linked to another though a peptide bond. There are eight essential amino acids (nine for infants) and thirteen (or twelve) non-essential acids for adults and children, respectively.

Amygdala Area of the brain within the temporal lobe. Part of the limbic system. Important in initiation of the stress response.

Androgens The male sex hormones, such as testosterone. These are produced in the testes and adrenal glands in men, and only in the adrenal glands in women.

Anorexia A condition of being without or having lost the appetite for food leading to severe weight loss and associated with amenorrhea, the absence of menstruation, and psychological or physiological issues.

Antibody Protein molecule of the immune system. Produced by lymphocytes and able to bind to foreign material, bacteria, or viruses.

Antioxidant A substance that neutralizes free radicals in the body. This aids the body in faster recovery and promotes stronger, more healthy tissues.

Arteriosclerosis A common blood vessel disorder characterized by calcified yellow plagues, lipids, and debris that line the walls of the arteries.

Atrophy Shrinkage or wasting away.

Autonomic Nervous System The part of the nervous system that is not under conscious or voluntary control. It is responsible for functions such as blood pressure, heart rate, sweating, etc.

Basal Metabolic Rate The rate at which the body expends energy for maintenance activities, such as organ function and breathing.

Basophil A type of white blood cell that produces histamine.

Beta Wave An electrical rhythm of the brain seen on EEG of an individual who is awake, alert, and with open eyes.

Bioavailability The ability of ingested nutrients to pass through the digestive tract into and through the bloodstream to its destination cells to be used.

Biochemical Reactions The chemical activities associated with life as exhibited in humans and other living organisms. These are the reactions that drive all bodily functions.

Bioflavonoid Also known as vitamin P. A group of plant pigments that provide the colors to many plants and flowers. In humans, they play a role in combating pain and inflammation, in absorption of certain nutrients.

Biotin Also known as vitamin H. A necessary vitamin for the body and an essential cofactor in many enzymatic reactions.

Blood Pressure The pressure of the blood measured against the walls of the arteries. Normal is considered 120/80.

Brown Fat Fatty deposits found in particular places on the body, such as between the shoulder blades. This is the type of fat that generates heat, particularly in hibernating animals.

Bulimia Perpetual and voracious appetite for large quantities of food to a morbid degree. It is usually associated with vomiting the food after consumption and psychological issues.

CCK Cholecystokinin. A chemical that acts as a gut hormone and central nervous neurotransmitter.

CFS Chronic Fatigue Syndrome.

COX Cyclooxygenase. An enzyme responsible for generating immune system chemicals, such as prostaglandins and leukotrienes. Blocked by COX-1 or COX-2 anti-inflammatory drugs.

CRH See corticotropin-releasing hormone.

Calcium An essential mineral to the body, necessary for bone strength, cardiac function, muscle regulation, and much more.

Calorie A unit that characterizes the amount of energy available from food.

Carbohydrate An organic compound in nature consisting of carbon, hydrogen, and oxygen that is used by the body as a potential fuel source. This includes starches, sugars, fiber, cellulose, and gums.

Carnitine An amine that is often considered an amino acid that helps to transport fat to the mitochondria to be burned for energy.

Catecholamine A generic term used to describe the stress hormones or neurotransmitters adrenaline and noradrenaline.

Central Nervous System The main part of the nervous system that includes the spinal cord and brain.

Central Obesity The accumulation of fat around the abdominal or trunk area, not over the extremities.

Cerebellum The part of the brain behind the pons that controls fine motor movements of the body.

Cerebral Cortex (CCK) The outer layer of the main frontal part of the brain, the most sophisticated and highly developed area of the brain.

Cholecystokinin A chemical that acts as a gut hormone and central nervous neurotransmitter. Formed in the presence of dietary fat, it stimulates contraction of the gall bladder and induces a sensation of satiation (feeling 'full').

Cholesterol A waxy substance present in all cell membranes that is important for the transportation and absorption of substances in and out of cells. Cholesterol is widely manufactured by the body and many dangers arise when it is produced in excess.

Chromium An essential mineral for the body which helps to stabilize blood sugar levels.

Chronic Fatigue Syndrome (CFS) A syndrome characterized by persistent and debilitating fatigue, muscle weakness, headaches, poor sleep, and emotional disturbances, such as depression or anxiety.

Circadian Rhythm The body's natural wake-sleep cycle controlled via the hormone melatonin.

Coenzyme A substance that must be present with an enzyme to allow that enzyme to function. Coenzymes are necessary for the use of vitamins and minerals in the body.

Collagen Long-chain protein molecule providing strength to many tissues, including cartilage and tendons.

Complex Carbohydrate A carbohydrate that also contains fiber and has a slower release of sugar into the blood stream than a simple carbohydrate.

Conjugated Linoleic Acid An essential fatty acid.

Constipation A condition in which stools are passed infrequently and with difficulty.

Corticotropin-Releasing Hormone (CRH) A hormone that is produced in the hypothalamus in response to stress and stimulates the pituitary to release ACTH.

Cortisol The body's major stress hormone produced in the adrenal glands in response to stimulation by ACTH from the pituitary glands. Responsible for the prolonged phase of the stress response.

Cushing's Disease A disease characterized by high levels of circulating cortisol leading to symptoms, such as trunkal obesity, depression, osteoporosis, sleep disturbance, etc.

Cysteine Amino acid essential for the production of Glutathione.

Cytokines Chemical messengers secreted by white blood cells that regulate the magnitude of the inflammatory response, including interferon, tumor necrosis factor (TNF), interleukins, etc.

Delta Waves A natural wave pattern of the brain observed on the EEG of a sleeping individual.

Dexamethasone A drug that mimics cortisol.

Dexamethasone Suppression Test A test of hypothalamus-pituitary-adrenal (HPA) axis sensitivity and feedback.

Diarrhea The frequent passage of unformed liquid stools.

Diabetes A disorder characterized by the inability to control blood sugar levels, excessive urine excretion, and thirst, with oscillations between hypoglycemia and acidosis.

Diuretic A substance that causes increased urine output by forcing the kidneys to excrete more salt, potassium, and water.

Down-Regulation An decrease in receptor density making a cell less responsive to a hormone.

Edema Fluid retention in the body resulting in swelling and bloating in the skin and other tissues.

Efferent A nerve fiber leaving the brain or spinal cord, going to muscles or glands of the body.

Electroencephalogram (EEG) A recording of the electrical activity of the cerebral cortex.

Electrolytes The ionized salts in the blood. A specific ratio known as the electrolyte balance is essential for proper bodily function.

Endocrine System The collection of glands that produce and secrete hormones and chemical messengers in the body.

Endocrine Glands Organs of the body containing specialized cells that secrete hormones. Includes the pituitary, adrenal, pineal, pancreas, and thyroid.

Endometrium The internal layer of the uterus.

Endorphins Protein molecule that acts as a neurotransmitter in the brain and spinal cord primarily to inhibit pain. Opiate drugs, such as morphine, act on its receptors.

Endothelin Molecule produced by blood vessels. Induces vessel contraction, heart contraction, and blood pressure.

Enkephalins Protein molecule that acts as a neurotransmitter in the brain and spinal cord primarily to inhibit pain. Opiate drugs, such as morphine, act on its receptors.

Enzyme One group of proteins produced in cells that are capable of greatly accelerating chemical reactions in the body without being broken down or consumed itself.

Eosinophils A type of white blood cells that protects against parasitic infections and allergies.

Essential Fatty Acids The good fats used by the body for hormone communication, cholesterol control, reduction of inflammation, and more. They include omega-3, -6, and -9.

Essential Nutrients Substances that the body cannot produce itself and are necessary for survival.

Estrogen A female sex steroidal hormone produced and secreted from the ovaries.

Extracellular Outside the cell.

FSH See Follicle-Stimulating Hormone.

Fat Cell A cell that stores fatty acids for energy.

Fatty Acids Components of fat molecules that can provide energy, but in high quantity can be harmful. These include cholesterol, triglycerides, prostaglandins, lecithin, choline, and others. There are essential fatty acids, which the body cannot manufacture yet requires, and non-essential ones, which it can make on its own.

Fertilization The successful union of the ovum and the sperm.

Fiber Plant compounds that are indigestible to the human digestive tract.

Fibromyalgia A disorder characterized by widespread pain, muscle tenderness, fatigue, and headaches.

Fight-or-Flight Response The series of reactions or events designed to help the body handle acute stress.

Follicle-Stimulating Hormone (FSH) A hormone from the anterior pituitary gland that is responsible for maturation of the sperm and ovum.

Free Radical A highly reactive molecule that is known to injure cell membranes, damage DNA, and contribute to aging and degenerative illnesses.

Free Radical Scavenger A substance, such as antioxidants, that seeks out and destroys free radicals in the body.

Fructose A simple carbohydrate or sugar that comes from fruits and is absorbed and utilized by the body at a slower rate than glucose.

GABA Gamma-aminobutyric Acid. A neurotransmitter.

GAD General Anxiety Disorder.

GH See Human Growth Hormone.

GnRH See Gonadotropin-releasing Hormone.

General Adaptation Syndrome The term used by Hans Selye to describe the three stages of stress — the alarm, resistance and exhaustion phases.

Genistein An isoflavone found in soy products. (See Isoflavone)

Ghrelin Hormone produced in the stomach. Increases hunger and reduces fat utilization.

Glucagon A polypeptide hormone secreted by the pancreas in response to hypoglycemia. It is responsible for raising blood sugar levels when they fall too low.

Glucocorticoids Steroid hormones, including cortisol, that are secreted by the adrenal cortex.

Gluconeogenesis The synthesis of glucose by the liver and kidneys from non-carbohydrate sources, like amino acids and fatty acids.

Glucose A simple carbohydrate or sugar that is the end product of carbohydrate metabolism and is the main energy source for all living organisms.

Glucose Intolerance A sensitivity of the glucose or sugar receptors to glucose, leading to very unstable blood sugar levels and hypoglycemia.

Glutamine An amino acid that has been shown to increase the rate of muscle growth in humans and decrease fat production. Essential for the production of the anti-oxidant Glutathione.

Glutathione The body's most important anti-oxidant. Essential to adequate function of the immune system.

Glycemic Index A scale used to measure the amount of glucose present in different foods.

Glycogen The main storage form of glucose, manufactured by and largely stored in the liver and muscles.

Glyconeogenesis The breakdown of glycogen stores in the liver to produce glucose in response to low blood sugar levels.

Gonadotropin-Releasing Hormone (GnRH) A hormone from the hypothalamus that controls the release of FSH and LH from the pituitary gland.

Growth Hormone A peptide hormone secreted by the anterior pituitary gland. Has widespread affects on growth and metabolism.

Growth Hormone-Releasing Hormone (GHRH) A hormone secreted from the hypothalamus that controls the production and release of growth hormone from the pituitary gland.

Growth Hormone-Inhibiting Hormone (GHIH) A hormone secreted from the hypothalamus that controls the production and release of growth hormone from the pituitary gland.

HCG (hCG) Human Chorionic Gonadotrophin. Hormone that maintains pregnancy.

HGH (hGH) Human Growth Hormone.

HPA Axis Hypothalamus-Pituitary-Adrenal axis. Central hormonal pillar of the stress response.

High-Density Lipoproteins (HDL) Complexes of lipids and proteins that are important in structural and catalytic activities in cell membranes. These are the 'good' lipids that help prevent the 'bad' lipids (LDLs) from building up in the arteries.

Hippocampus Area of the temporal lobe of the brain and part of the limbic system. Central to control of the stress response.

Histamine A substance released from mast cells and basophils that increases inflammation, swelling, redness, and itching.

Homeostasis The steady state of the body where all systems lie balanced within their natural and normal levels.

Hormone A chemical substance formed in one part of the body and transported to a different area, where it has a regulatory effect on different tissues.

Hypercholesterolemia An excess of cholesterol in the blood.

Hyperglycemia An excessive amount of sugar in the blood.

Hyperinsulinemia An excess of insulin secretion, resulting in low blood sugar levels or hypoglycemia.

Hyperlipidemia A condition in which lipids are present in excess in the blood.

Hypertension Persistently high arterial blood pressure, usually diagnosed after three consecutive readings of 140/90 or more on three different dates.

Hypoglycemia Low blood sugar concentration.

Hypothalamus The region of the brain that controls the release of hormones from the pituitary gland. This area of the brain receives signals from almost all other areas of the body. 'Oversees' the stress response.

IBD Inflammatory Bowel Disease.

IBS Irritable Bowel Syndrome.

Immune System The protective system of the body that recognizes and attempts to destroy foreign material, such as bacteria, viruses, tumors, and allergens.

Immunoglobulin Antibody protein molecules that recognize foreign material in the body and help to activate the immune response

Inflammatory Bowel Disease A disease of the bowel or gastrointestinal tract characterized by pain, inflammation, ulceration, and blood and mucus in frequent bowel movements.

Insomnia Inability to sleep well.

Insulin A protein hormone formed and secreted by the pancreas in response to a rise in blood sugar level. It promotes lipid synthesis since it stores the sugar from the blood as fat.

Insulin-Like-Growth Factor 1 A hormone produced in the liver and other tissues in the body that has been proven to increase the growth of cancerous cells.

Insulin Resistance A condition in which the body is insensitive and even resistant to the effects of insulin. In most cases, the body responds by producing even more insulin.

Interleukins Specific substances released during an immune reaction that activate other cells within the immune system.

Irritatable Bowel Syndrome A condition in the bowel characterized by alternating diarrhea and constipation, gas, bloating, and pain without blood.

Isoflavone A type of phytoestrogen found in soy products. (See Phytoestrogen)

Ketone Body An acidic substance produced by the rapid metabolism of fatty acids.

Ketosis The presence of excessive ketone bodies in the tissues usually the result of starvation or diabetes mellitus.

LH See Luteinizing Hormone.

Leptin A hormone produced by the fat that decreases appetite and increases energy expenditure.

Leukotrienes Chemical mediators of inflammation and the immune response.

Limbic System The extensive neuronal circuitry of the brain that controls emotion and behavior and initiates the stress response.

Lipids Fat or fatty substances, including fatty acids, waxes, and steroids.

Lipogenesis The formation of fat and the transformation of non-fat materials into body fat.

Lipoprotein Lipase The enzyme involved in the chemical reaction that stores fat in the body.

Liver The central organ of metabolism of carbohydrates, proteins, and fats. It stores glycogen and takes part in regulating blood sugar levels and other essential substances, such as vitamins. It is also the chief detoxifying organ of the body rendering toxic or foreign substances innocuous.

Low Density Lipoproteins (LDLs) Complexes of lipids and proteins found in the blood that contribute to heart disease and high cholesterol when produced in great concentrations.

Luteinizing Hormone (LH) A hormone secreted from the anterior pituitary gland that is required for the secretion of estrogen and testosterone by the ovaries and testes. LH also controls ovulation.

Lymphocyte A type of white blood cell that is involved in specific immune reactions.

MAOI Mono-amine oxidase inhibitor. Class of antidepressant medication.

Macronutrient The nutrients that are required daily by the body in large amounts, such as ounces and grams. They include protein, carbohydrates, lipids, and water.

Macrophage A type of white blood cell derived from monocytes that engulfs and digests foreign materials.

Magnesium An essential mineral for the body that plays a role in metabolism and muscle maintenance, and is required for many enzymatic reactions in the body.

Melatonin Hormone produced by the pineal gland in the brain.

Metabolic Syndrome (Syndrome-X) A disease complex characterized by central obesity, high blood pressure, insulin resistance, increased cholesterol, and increased risk of heart disease and stroke.

Metabolism The chemical processes of every living cell in which energy is produced, tissues are built up (anabolism), and tissues are degraded (catabolism).

Micronutrient Nutrients that are necessary in the diet in small amounts, generally measured in milligrams or micrograms. They include vitamins, minerals, and herbs.

Mineral An inorganic substance found in the earth obtained through mining.

Mitochondria The cell components that produce the energy required for metabolism. They are also called fat burners or power-house cells.

Monocyte A type of white blood cell that helps to fight infection.

NK Cells Natural Killer Cells.

Natural Killer Cells Cells within the immune system that are responsible for identifying and destroying cancer or virus-infected cells.

Naturopathy Medical practice using clinical nutritional, botanical medicine, homeopathic medicine, Asian medicine, bodywork, and lifestyle counseling to stimulate the body's innate healing response and produce therapeutic effects.

Neuron A nerve cell.

Neuropathy A disease process characterized by the disintegration or destruction of specialized tissue in the nervous system. Resulting symptoms include numbness and tingling, pain, muscle weakness, and visual disturbances.

Neurotransmitter A chemical messenger released by a neuron that activates another neuron or specific receptors on muscle cells or glands to orchestrate an action, emotion, or message.

Neutrophil A white blood cell that, like macrophages, can ingest and destroy bacteria.

Noradrenaline A catecholamine released from the adrenal glands in response to stress.

OTS Overtraining Syndrome.

Obesity An excessive accumulation of fat in the body, mainly deposited in the subcutaneous tissues. It is generally considered 30% above normal body weight.

Ovary The female gonad that contains follicles and secretes estrogen and progesterone.

Ovulation The release of a mature ovum from its follicle.

PD Panic Disorder.

PMS Pre-Menstrual Syndrome.

PTSD Post-Traumatic Stress Disorder.

Pancreas The organ or gland in the body, which secretes insulin and glucagon upon differing metabolic demands to help regulate blood sugar levels.

Parasympathetic Nervous System One of the two major divisions of the autonomic nervous system.

Phosphate A mineral that is essential to the body as it is exists in tissue, blood, bone, and chemical reactions in the body.

Physiological Pertaining to all the reactions and systems in the body and how they connect together to function as a whole.

Phytoestrogen A type of phytosterol that mimics endogenous estrogen in the body. (See Phytosterol)

Phytosterol A plant extract with properties similar to our own estrogen hormones.

Pituitary Gland An endocrine gland that is located below the hypothalamus and secretes six hormones, including ACTH, FSH, LH, TSH, GH and prolactin.

Pons The region of the brainstem that is located between the medulla and the midbrain.

Potassium A mineral that is essential for the body and is found in high concentrations in tissues. It is necessary to maintain proper electrolyte balances in the body through its ionic charge, and is used to excite or enhance action potential reactions.

Progesterone One of the female sex hormones.

Prostaglandins A series of chemicals, structurally similar to fatty acids, that are involved in inflammation, cardiovascular and gastric functioning, uterine contractions, etc.

Protein A compound formed from nitrogen, occurring in every living cell. It is essential for the growth, repair, and maintenance of every part of the body.

Psychology The branch of science/medicine that deals with the mind and all mental processes.

Qi Energy in Chinese medicine.

RDA RDA is the Recommended Daily Allowance of vitamins, minerals, and other nutrients as suggested by the FDA.

REM Rapid Eye Movement.

Rapid Eye Movement (REM) The phase of sleep characterized by desynchronized brain activity and dreaming. This is a paradoxical form of sleep as it is non-restful.

Receptors Membrane-bound molecules with specific sites for other molecules, such as hormones and neurotransmitters, to bind into.

Resistin Messenger molecule produced by fat cells (adipokine). Induces insulin resistance.

SSRI Selective Serotonin Re-uptake Inhibitor. Class of antidepressant medication.

Saturated Fats A fatty acid that has every possible bond filled with hydrogen atoms and is therefore less reactive. They tend to be solid at room temperature and generally have an animal origin.

Serotonin An important and widespread neurotransmitter important in mood and sleep control.

Simple Carbohydrate A simple form of sugar, such as glucose, lactose, and fructose, that is rapidly absorbed into the bloodstream.

Soy A leguminous plant with many medicinal properties.

Starvation A condition induced by continuous lack of sufficient food, causing renal failure, muscle cramping, and fatigue.

Sympathic Nervous System One of two divisions of the autonomic nervous system. Activated during the stress response.

Synapse The junction between two neurons.

Syndrome X See Metabolic Syndrome

TSH Thyroid Stimulating Hormone.

TNF Tumor Necrosis Factor.

Testosterone The main male sex hormone secreted by the testes.

Thalamus Area of the brain responsible for relaying incoming messages.

Theta Waves The low frequency waves seen on an EEG of an individual who is in Stage 1 sleep.

Thymus An organ of the lymph system (within the chest) that produces T-lymphocytes.

Thyroid Gland in the neck producing thyroid hormones.

Thyroid-Stimulating Hormone Hormone produced by the pituitary gland to stimulate the thyroid.

Triglyceride A combination of glycerol and a fatty acid, such as oleic or stearic acid. Most animal and vegetable fats are triglyceride esters and form the majority of ingested fat in the diet. High levels in the blood greatly increase the risk for heart disease.

Tumor Necrosis Factor Cytokine messenger of the immune system.

UC Ulcerative colitis. Type of inflammatory bowel disease.

Up-regulation An increase in receptor density making a cell more responsive to a hormone.

VIP Vasoactive Intestinal Peptide. Gut and central nervous system neurotransmitter/hormone.

Vasoconstriction The narrowing of a blood vessel, which decreases blood flow and increases the pressure within it.

Vasodilation The relaxation or expansion of the blood vessel, which increases blood and decreases blood pressure.

Vasopressin A hormone released by the posterior pituitary gland. Also called Antidiuretic Hormone (ADH).

Vitamin A constituent of the diet other than protein, carbohydrate, fat, and inorganic salts that is necessary for the growth and repair of the body.

Water Soluble Ability to dissolve in water.

White Fat The fat that is subcutaneous and found around the internal organs. This fat changes in size and is the fat lost during weight loss.

References

Abelson JL, Curtis GC, Cameron OG. Hypothalamic-pituitary-adrenal axis activity in panic disorder: Effects of alprazolam on 24h secretion of adrenocorticotropin and cortisol. J Psychiatr Res 1996 Mar-Apr;30(2):79-93.

Abelson JL, Liberzon I. Dose response of adrenocorticotropin and cortisol to the CCK-B agonist pentagastrin. Neuropsychopharmacology 1999 Oct;21(4):485-94.

Abo T, Kawamura T. Immunomodulation by the autonomic nervous system: A therapeutic approach for cancer, collagen diseases, and inflammatory bowel disease. Ther Apher 2002;6(5):348-57.

Akhondzadeh S, Naghavi HR, Vazirian M, Shayeganpour A, Rashidi H, Khani M. Passionflower in the treatment of generalized anxiety: A pilot double-blind randomized controlled trial with oxazepam. J Clin Pharm Ther 2001 Oct;26(5):363-67.

Altemus M, Dale JK, Michelson D, Demitrack MA, Gold PW, Straus SE. Abnormalities in response to vasopressin infusion in chronic fatigue syndrome. Psychoneuroendocrinology 2001 Feb;26(2):175-88.

Amrani A, Verdaguer J, Serra P, Tafuro S, Tan R, Santamaria P. Progression of autoimmune diabetes driven by avidity maturation of a T-cell population. Nature 2000 Aug 17;406(6797):739-42.

Angeli A, Dovio A, Sartori ML. Interactions between glucocorticoids and cytokines in the bone microenvironment. Ann N Y Acad Sci 2002 Jun;966:97-107.

Asakawa A, Inui A, Kaga T, et al. A role of ghrelin in neuroendocrine and behavioral responses to stress in mice. Neuroendocrinology 2001 Sep;74(3):143-47.

Bandelow B, Wedekind D, Pauls J, Broocks A, Hajak G, Ruther E. Salivary cortisol in panic attacks. Am J Psychiatry, 2000 Mar;157(3):454-56.

Banerjee RR, Rangwala SM, Shapiro JS, Rich AS, Rhoades B, Qi Y, Wang J, Rajala MW, Pocai A, Scherer PE, Steppan CM, Ahima RS, Obici S, Rossetti L, Lazar MA. Regulation of fasted blood glucose by resistin. Science 2004 Feb 20;303(5661):1195-98.

Barron JL, Noakes TD, Levy W, et al. Hypothalamic dysfunction in overtrained athletes. J Clin Endocrinol Metab 1985 Apr;60(4):803-06.

Beglinger C, Degen L. Role of thyrotrophin releasing hormone and corticotrophin releasing factor in stress related alterations of gastrointestinal motor function. Gut 2002 Jul;51 (Suppl 1):i45-9.

Bennett EP, Tennant CC, Piesse C, et al. Level of chronic life stress predicts clinical outcome in IBS. Gut 1998;43(2):256-61.

Bennett MP, Zeller JM, Rosenberg L, McCann J. The effect of mirthful laughter on stress and natural killer cell activity. Altern Ther Health Med 2003 Mar-Apr;9(2):38-45.

Berman SM, Naliboff BD, Chang L, et al. Enhanced preattentive central nervous system reactivity in IBS. Am J Gastroenterol 2002 Nov;97(11):2791-97.

Bermond P. Therapy of side effects of oral contraceptive agents with vitamin B-6. Acta Vitaminol enzymol 1982:4(1-2):45-54.

Bernet F, Montel V, Noel B, Dupouy JP. Diazepam-like effects of a fish protein hydrolysate on stress responsiveness of the rat pituitary-adrenal system and sympathoadrenal activity. Psychopharmacology 2000 Mar;149(1):34-40.

Bilia AR, Gallan S, Vincieriff. Kava Kava and anxiety: Growing knowledge about the efficacy and safety. Life Sci 2002;19:70(22):2581-97.

Biondi M, Picardi A. Increased probability of remaining in remission from panic disorder with agoraphobia after drug treatment in patients who received concurrent cognitive-behavioral therapy: A follow-up study. Psychother Psychosom 2003 Jan-Feb;72(1):34-42.

Birketvedt GS, Sunscfjord J, Florholmen JR. Hypothalamic-pituitary-adrenal axis in the night eating syndrome. Am J Physiol Endocrinol Metab 2002 Feb;282(2):E366-69.

Bittman B, Bruhn KT, Stevens C, Westengard J, Umbach PO. Recreational music-making: A cost-effective group interdisciplinary strategy for reducing burnout and improving mood states in long-term care workers. Adv Mind Body Med 2003;Fall-Winter;19(3-4):4-15.

Bjorntorp P, Rosmond R. The metabolic syndrome – a neuroendocrine disorder? British J. Nutrition 2000 Mar;83 Suppl: S49-57.

Bjorntorp P, Holm G, Rosmond R, Folkow B. Hypertension and the metabolic syndrome: Closely related central origin? Blood Pressure 2000; 9(2-3):71-82.

Blumenthal JA, Babyak M, Wei J, O'Connor C, Waugh R, Eisenstein E, Mark D, Sherwood A, Woodley PS, Irwin RJ, Reed G. Usefulness of psychosocial treatment of mental stress-induced myocardial ischemia in men. Am J Cardiol 2002 Jan 15;89(2):164-68.

Blumenthal JA, Jiang W, Babyak MA, Krantz DS, Frid DJ, Coleman RE, Waugh R, Hanson M, Appelbaum M, O'Connor C, Morris JJ. Stress management and exercise training in cardiac patients with myocardial ischemia. Effects on prognosis and evaluation of mechanisms. Arch Intern Med 1997 Oct 27;157(19):2213-23.

Bone K. Kava – a safe herbal treatment for anxiety. British Journal of Phytotherapy 1993-94;3(4):147-53.

Bonner G. Hyperinsulinemia, insulin resistance and hypertension. J Cardio Pharm 1994;24(Suppl.2): S39-49.

Borstein SR, Rutkowski H. The adrenal hormone metabolism in the immune/inflammatory reaction. Edocr Res 2002 Nov;28(4):719-28.

Bourin M, Bougerol T, Guitton B, Broutin E. A combination of plant extracts in the treatment of outpatients with adjustment disorder with anxious mood: Controlled study versus placebo. Fundam Clin Pharmacol 1997;11(2):127-32.

Brody S, Preut R, Schommer K, Schurmeyer TH. A randomized controlled trial of high dose ascorbic acid for reduction of blood pressure, cortisol, and subjective responses to psychological stress. Psychopharmacology 2002;159(3):319-24.

Brun J, Chamba G, Khalfallah Y, Girard P, Boissy I, Bastuji H, Sassolas G, Claustrat B. Effects of modafinil on plasma melatonin, cortisol and growth hormone rhythms, rectal temperature and performance in healthy subjects during 36 hours sleep deprivation. France J Sleep Res 1998 Jun; 7(2):105-14.

Buske-Kirschbaum A, Gierens A, Hollig H, Hellhammer DH. Stress induced immunomodulation is altered in patients with atopic dermatitis. J Neuroimmunol 2002 Aug;129(1-2):161-67.

Buske-Kirschbaum A, Geiben A, Hollig H, et al. Altered responsiveness of the HPA axis and the sympathetic adrenomedulary system to stress in patients with atopic dermatitis. J Clin Endocrinol Metab 2002 Sep;87(9):4245-51.

Buskila D. Fibromyalgia, chronic fatigue syndrome, and myofascial pain syndrome. Curr Opin Rheumatol 2001 Mar;13(2):117-27.

Carels RA, Blumenthal JA, Sherwood A. Emotional responsivity during daily life: Relationship to psychosocial functioning and ambulatory blood pressure. Int J Psychophysiol 2000 Apr;36(1):25-33.

Cassidy EM, Tomkins E, Dinan T, Hardiman O, O'Keane V. Central 5-HT receptor hypersensitivity in migraine without aura. Cephalalgia 2003 Feb;23(1):29-34.

Castejon-Casado, et al. Hormonal response to surgical stress in schoolchildren. European Journal of Paediatric Surgery 2001 Feb;11(1):44-47.

Cetin A, Gokce-Kutsal Y, Celiker R. Predictors of bone mineral density in healthy males. Rheumatol Int 2001 Nov;21(3):85-88.

Christensen NJ, Jensen EW. Sympathoadrenal activity and psychosocial stress: The significance of aging, long term smoking and stress models. Ann NY Acad Sci 1995 Dec;771:640-47.

Cleare AJ, Miell J, Heap E, Sookdeo S, Young L, Malhi GS, O'Keane V. Hypothalamo-pituitary-adrenal axis dysfunction in chronic fatigue syndrome, and the effects of low-dose hydrocortisone therapy. J Clin Endocrinol Metab 2001 Aug;86(8):3545-54.

Colgan SM, Faragher EB, Whorwell PJ. Controlled trial of hypnotherapy in relapse prevention in duodenal ulceration. Lancet 1988 Jun;1(8598): 1299-300.

Cott JM. In vitro receptor binding and enzyme inhibition of Hypericum perforatum extract. Pharmacopsychiatry 1997;30(Suppl 2):108-112.

Crompton R, Clifton VL, Bisits AT, et al. Corticotropin-releasing hormone causes vasodilation in human skin via mast cell-dependent pathways. J Clin Endocrinol Metab 2003;88(11): 5427-32.

Cutolo M, Foppiani L, Minuto F. Hypothalamic-pituitary-adrenal axis impairment in the pathogenesis of rheumatoid arthritis and polymyalgia rheumatica. J Endocrinol Invest 2002;25(10 Suppl):19-23.

Dallman MF, Pecoraro N, Akana SF, la Fleur SE, Gomez F, Houshyar H, Bell ME, Bhatnagar S, Laugero KD, Manalo S. Chronic stress and obesity: A new view of "comfort food." PNAS 2003:100(20);11696-11701.

Davis MC, Matthews KA, McGrath CE. Hostile attitudes predict elevated vascular resistance during interpersonal stress in men and women. Psychosom Med 2000;62:17-25.

Diego MA, Jones NA, Field T, Hernandez-Reif M, Schanberg S, Kuhn C, McAdam V, Galamaga R, Galamaga M. Aromatherapy positively affects mood, EEG patterns of alertness and math computations. Int J Neurosci 1998; 96(3-4):217-24.

Dobson H, Smith RF. What is stress, and how does it affect reproduction? Animal Reprod Sci 2000 July; 60-61:743-52.

Dreier JP, Kleeberg J, Petzold G, et al. Endothelin-1 potently induces Leao's cortical spreading depression in vivo in the rat: A model for an endothelial trigger of migrainous aura? Brain 2002 Jan;125(Pt 1):102-12.

Droge W, Holm E. Role of cysteine and glutathione in HIV infection and other diseases associated with muscle wasting and immunological dysfunction. FASEB J 1997 Nov;11(13):1077-89.

Duclos M, Gouarne C, Bonnemaison D. Acute and chronic effects of exercise on tissue sensitivity to glucocorticoids. J Appl Physiol 2002 Oct.

Elenkov IJ, Wilder RL, Bakalov VK, et al. IL-12, TNF-alpha and hormonal changes during late pregnancy and early postpartum: Implications for autoimmune disease activity during these times. J Clin Endocrinol Metab 2001 Oct;86(10):4933-38.

Elsenbruch S, Orr WC. Diarrhea- and constipation-predominant IBS patients differ in postprandial autonomic and cortisol responses. Am J Gastroenterol 2001 Feb;96(2):460-66.

Epel E, Lapidus R, McEwen B, Brownell K. Stress may add bite to appetite in women: A laboratory study of stress-induced cortisol and eating behaviour. Psychoneuroendocrinology 2001 Jan;26(1):37-49.

Fassoulaki A, Paraskeva A, Patris K, Pourgiezi T, Kostopanagiotou G. Pressure applied on the extra 1 acupuncture point reduces bispectral index values and stress in volunteers. Anesth Analg 2003: 96(3)885-90.

Field T, Henteleff T, Hernandez-Reif M, Martinez E, Mavunda K, Kuhn C, Schanberg S. Children with asthma have improved pulmonary function after massage therapy. J Pediatr 1998;132(5):854-58.

Field T, Ironson G, Scafidi F, Nawrocki T, Goncalves A, Burman I, Pickens J, Fox N, Schanberg S, Kuhn C. Massage therapy reduces anxiety and enhances EEG paterns of alertness and math computations. Int J Neurosci 1996;86(3-4): 197-205.

Field T, Schanberg S, Kuhn C, Field T, Fierro K, Henteleff T, Meuller C, Yando R, Shaw S, Burman I. Bulimic adolescents benefit from massage therapy. Adolescence 1998;33(131):555-63.

Filaretova LP, Bagaeva TR, Podvigina TT, Morozova O. Deficit of glucocorticoid production in rats aggravates ulcerogenic effects of stimuli of various modality and intensity. Ross Fiziol Zh Im I M Sechenova 2002 May;88(5):602-11.

Frei B, England L, Ames BN. Ascorbate is an outstanding antioxidant in human blood plasma. Proc Natl Acad Sci 1994;86, 6377-81.

Friede M, Henneike von Zepelin HH, Freudenstein J. Differential therapy of mild to moderate depressive episodes (ICD-10 F 32.0: F32.1) with St John's wort. Pharmacopsychiatry 2001;34 (Suppl 1):38-41.

Fukudo S, Nomura T, Hongo M. Impact of corticotropin-releasing hormone on gastrointestinal motility and adrenocorticotropic hormone in normal controls and patients with irritable bowel syndrome. Gut 1998 Jun;42(6): 845-49.

Gebner B, Cnota P. Extracts of Kava-Kava rhizome in comparison with diazepam and placebo. Zeitschrift fur Phytother 1994;15:30-37.

Gianoulakis C, Dai X, Brown T. Effects of chronic alcohol consumption on the activity of the hypothalamic-pituitary-adrenal axis and pituitary beta-endorphin as a function of alcohol intake, age and gender. Alcohol Clin Exp Res 2003; 27(3):410-23.

Goldstone AP, Howard JK, Lord GM, et al. Leptin prevents the fall in plasma osteocalcin during starvation in male mice. Biochem Biophys Res Commun 2002 Jul;295(2):475-81.

Goleman D. Emotional Intelligence: Why It Can Matter More Than IQ? New York: Bantam Publishing, 2000.

Golub MS. The adrenal gland and the metabolic syndrome. Current Hypertension Reports 2001 Apr;3(2):117-20.

Golf SW, Happel O, Graef V, Seim KE. Plasma aldosterone, cortisol and electrolyte concentrations in physical exercise after magnesium supplementation. J Clin Chem Clin Biochem 1984 Nov;22(11):717-21.

Gonzales Ortiz M, Marinez Abundis C, Balcazar Munoz BR, Pascoe Gonzales S. Effects of sleep deprivation on insulin and cortisol concentrations in healthy subjects. Diabetes, Nutrition and Metabolism – Clinical and Experimental Diabetes 2000 Apr;13(2):80-83.

Goode HF, Burns E, and Walker BE. Vitamin C depletion and pressure sores. Lancet 1974;ii, 544-46.

Grassi G, Kiowski W. Is the autonomic dysfunction the missing link between panic disorder, hypertension and cardiovascular disease? J Hypertens 2002 Dec;20(12):2347-49.

Groop L. Pathogenesis of type 2 diabetes: The relative contribution of insulin resistance and impaired insulin secretion. International Journal of Clinical Practice 2000 Oct; Suppl. (113):3-13.

Guyatt G, Mitchell A, Irvine EJ, et al. A new measure of health status for clinical trials in IBD. Gastroenterology 1989;96(3):804-10.

Gupta V, Sheffield D, Verne GN. Evidence for autonomic dysregulation in the irritable bowel syndrome. Dig Dis Sci 2002 Aug;47(8):1716-22.

Hadjidakis D, Tsagarakis S, Roboti C. Does subclinical hypercortisolism adversely affect the bone mineral density of patients with adrenal incidentalomas? Clin Endocrinol 2003 Jan;58(1):72-77.

Hamel WJ. The effects of music intervention on anxiety in the patient waiting for cardiac catheterization. Intensive Crit Care Nurs 2001;17(5):279-85.

Hammarqvist F, Ejesson B, Wernerman J. Stress hormones initiate prolonged changes in the muscle amino acid pattern. Clinical Physiology 2001 Jan;21(1):44-50.

Han KS. The effect of an integrated stress management program on the psychologic and physiologic stress reactions of peptic ulcer in Korea. J Holist Nurs 2002 Mar;20(1):61-80.

Heinrichs SC, Tache Y. Therapeutic potential of CRF receptor antagonists: A gut-brain perspective. Expert Opin Investig Drugs 2001 Apr;10(4):647-59.

Heitkemper M, Jarrett M, Cain K, et al. Increased urine catecholamines and cortisol in women with IBS Am J Gastroenterol 1996 May;91(5):906-13.

Henry M, de Rivera JL, Gonzalez-Martin IJ, Abreu J. Improvement of respiratory function in chronic asthmatic patients with autogenic therapy. J Psychosom Res 1993 Apr;37(3):265-70.

Hockemeyer J, Smyth J. Evaluating the feasibility and efficacy of a self-administered manual-based stress management intervention for individuals with asthma: Results from a controlled study. Behav Med 2002 Winter;27(4):161-72.

Hurwitz EL, Morgenstern H. Immediate and long-term effects of immune stimulation: Hypothesis linking the immune response to subsequent physical and psychological well-being. Med Hypotheses 2001 Jun;56(6):620-24.

Ierusalimschy R, Moreira Filho PF. Precipitating factors of migraine in patients with migraine without aura. Arq Neuropsiquiatr 2002 Sep;60 (3-A):609-13.

Imrich R. The role of the neuroendocrine system in the pathogenesis of rheumatic diseases. Endocr Regul 2002 Jun;36(2):95-106.

Ironson G, Field T, Scafidi F, Hashimoto M, Kumar M, Kumar A, Price A, Goncalves A, Burman I, Tetenman C, Patarca, R, Fletcher MA. Massage therapy is associated with enhancement of the immune system's cytotoxic capacity. Int J Neurosci 1996;84(1-4):205-17.

Jefferies WM. Cortisol and immunity. Med. Hypotheses 1991 Mar;34(3):198-208.

Jenkins DJ, Axelsen M, Kendall CW, Augustin LS, Vuksan V, Smith U. Dietary fibre, lente carbohydrates and the insulin-resistant diseases. British Journal of Nutrition 2000 Mar;83 Suppl 1:S157-63.

Johannsson G, Bengtsson BA. Growth hormone and metabolic syndrome. Journal of Endocrinological Investigation 1999;22(5 Suppl):41-46.

Johnston CS, Martin LJ, Cia X. Antihistamine effect of supplemental ascorbic acid and neutrophil chemotaxis. J Am Coll Nutr 1992;11:172-76.

Jones JE, et al. Disinhibition of female sexual behaviour by a CRH receptor antagonist in Syrian hamsters. Am J Physiol Regul Integr Comp Physiol 2002 Sep;283(3):R591-97.

Kahn RS, Westenberg HG. L-5-hydroxytrytophan in the treatment of anxiety disorders. J Affect Disord 1985:8(2):197-200.

Kahn RS, Westenberg HG, Verhoeven WM, Gispen-de Wied CC, Kamerbeek WD. Effects of a serotonin precursor and uptake inhibitor in anxiety disorders: A double-blind comparison of 5-hydroxytrytophan, clomipramine and placebo. Int Clin Psychopharmacol 1987;2(1):33-45.

Kakuda T, Nozawa A, Unno T, Okamura N, Okai O. Inhibiting effects of theanine on caffeine stimulation evaluated by EEG in the rat. Biosci Biotechnol Biochem 2000;64(2):287-93.

Kallela M, Farkkila M, Saijonmaa O, Fyhrquist F. Endothelin in migraine patients. Cephalalgia 1998 Jul-Aug;18(6):329-32.

Kaltsas GA, Korbonitis M, Isidori AM, Webb JA, Trainer PJ, Monson JP, Besser GM, Grossman AB. How common are polycystic ovaries and the polycystic ovarian syndrome in women with Cushing's syndrome. Clin Endocrinol 2000:53(4):493-500.

Kamei T, Toriumi Y, Kimura H, Ohno S, Kumano H, Kimura K. Decrease in serum cortisol during yoga exercise is correlated with alpha wave activation. Japan 2000; 90(3 pt 1): 1027-32.

Karush A, Daniels GE, O'Connor JF, et al. The response to psychotherapy in chronic UC. Psychosom Med 1969;31(3):201-26.

Kato K, Asai S, Murai I, et al. Melatonin's gastroprotective and antistress roles involve both central and peripheral effects. J Gastroenterol 2001 Feb;36(2):91-95.

Kavelaars A, Kuis W, Knook L, Sinnema G, Heijnen CJ. Disturbed neuroendocrine-immune interactions in chronic fatigue syndrome. J Clin Endocrinol Metab. 2000 Feb;85(2):692-96.

Keefer L, Blanchard EB. A one year follow-up of relaxation response meditation as a treatment for irritable bowel syndrome. Behav Res Ther 2002 May;40(5):541-46.

Kemler MA, Barendse GA, VanKleef M. Relapsing UC associated with spinal cord stimulation. Gastroenterology 1999 Jul;117(1):215-17.

Kentta G, Hassmen P, Raglin JS. Training practices and overtraining syndrome in Swedish age-group athletes. Int J Sports Med 2001 Aug;22(6):460-65.

Kilpelainen M, Koskenvuo M, Helenius H, Terho EO. Stressful life events promote the manifestations of asthma and atopic diseases. Clin Exp Allergy 2002 Feb;32(2):256-62.

Kim CK, Bartholomew BA, Mastin ST, et al. Detection and reproducibility of mental stress-induced myocardial ischemia with Tc-99m sestamibi SPECT in normal and coronary artery disease populations. J Nucl Cardiol 2003 Jan-Feb;10(1):56-62.

Kim MS, Cho KS, Woo H, Kim JH. Effects of hand massage on anxiety in cataract surgery using local anesthesia. Korea J Cataract Refract Surg 2001;27(6):884-90.

Kimyai-Asadi A, Usman A. The role of psychological stress in skin disease. J Cutan Med Surg 2001 Mar-Apr;5(2):140-45.

Knight WE, Rickard NS. Relaxing music prevents stress-induced increases in subjective anxiety, systolic blood pressure and heart rate in healthy males and females. J Music Ther 2001;38(4):254-72.

Kondwani KA, Lollis CM. Is there a role for stress management in reducing hypertension in African Americans? Ethn Dis 2001 Fall;11(4):788-92.

Kretzschmar R, Meyer H. Comparative experiments on the anticonvulsant efficacy of Piper methysticum pyrone bonds. Arch Int Pharmacodyn 1967;177:261-77.

Krook A, Holm I, Pettersson S, Wallberg-Henriksson H. Reduction of risk factors following lifestyle modification programme in subjects with type 2 (non-insulin dependent) diabetes mellitus. Clin Physiol Funct Imaging 2003 Jan;23(1):21-30.

Krsek M, Silha JV, Jezkova J, Hana V, Marek J, Weiss V, Stepan JJ, Murphy LJ. Adipokine levels in Cushing's syndrome; elevated resistin levels in female patients with Cushing's syndrome. Clin Endocrinol (Oxf). 2004 Mar;60(3):350-57.

Kuiper, NA, Martin, RA. (1993). Humor and self-concept. Humor: International Journal of Humor Research 1993;6,251-70.

Kuipers H. Training and overtraining: An introduction. Med Sci Sports Exerc, 1998 Jul;30 (7):1137-39.

Kumar V, Singh PN, Bhattacharya SK. Anti-stress activity of Indian Hypericum perforatum L. Indian J Exp Biol 2000;39(4):344-49.

Kuribara H, Kishi E, Hattori N, Yuzurihara M, Maruyama Y. Application of the elevated plus-maze in mice for evaluation of the content of honokiol in water extracts of magnolia. Phytother Res 1999;13(7):593-96.

Lake AE 3rd. Behavioral and non-pharmacologic treatments of headache. Med Clin North Am 2001 Jul;85(4):1055-75.

Lane JD, Pieper CF, Phillips-Bute BG, Bryant JE, Kuhn CM. Caffeine affects cardiovascular and neuroendocrine activation at work and home. Psychosom Med 2002;64(4):595-603.

Laube BL, Curbow BA, Costello RW, Fitzgerald ST. A pilot study examining the relationship between stress and serum cortisol concentrations in women with asthma. Respir Med 2002 Oct;96(10):823-28.

Lehmann M, Foster C, Dickhuth HH, Gastmann U. Autonomic imbalance hypothesis of overtraining syndrome. Med Sci Sports Exerc 1998 Jul; 7:1140-45.

Lehman M, Jakob E, Gastmann U. Unaccustomed high mileage vs. high intensity training related performance and neuromuscular responses in distance runners. Eur J Appl Physiol 1995;70:457-61.

Lehman MJ, Lormes W, Opitz-gress A, et al Training and overtraining: An overview and experimental results in endurance sports. J Sports Med Phys Fitness 1997;37:7-17.

Lehrer P, Feldman J, Giardino N, et al. Psychological aspects of asthma. J Consult Clin Psychol 2002 Jun;70(3):691-711.

Lemstra M, Stewart B, Olszyski WP. Effectiveness of multidisciplinary intervention in the treatment of migraine: A randomized clinical trial. Headache 2002 Oct;42(9):845-54.

Levenstein S. The very model of a modern etiology: A biopsychosocial view of peptic ulcer. Psychosom Med 2000 Apr;62(2):176-85.

Levenstein S, Ackerman S, Kiecolt-Glaser JK, Dubois A. Stress and peptic ulcer disease. JAMA 1999 Jan;281(1):10-11.

Levenstein S, Prantera C, Varvo V, et al. Stress and exacerbation in UC: A prospective study of patients enrolled in remission. Am.J.Gastroenterol 2000; 95(5):1213-20.

Linden W, Lenz JW, Con AH. Individualized stress management for primary hypertension: A randomized trial. Arch Intern Med 2001 Apr 23;161(8):1071-80.

Liu S, Manson JE. Dietary carbohydrates, physical inactivity , obesity and the "metabolic syndrome" as predictors of coronary heart disease. Current Opinion in Lipidology 2001 Aug;12(4):395-404.

Louis M, Kowalski SD. Use of aromatherapy with hospice patients to decrease pain, anxiety, and depression and to promote an increased sense of well-being. Am J Hosp Palliat Care 2002; 19(6):381-86.

Luo L, Nong Wang J, Kong LD, Jiang QG, Tan RX. Antidepressant effects of Banxia Houpu decoction, a traditional Chinese medicinal empirical formula. J Ethnopharmacol 2000;73(1-2):277-81.

Lydiard RB. Irritable bowel syndrome, anxiety and depression: What are the links? J Clin Psychiatry 2001;62 (Suppl 8):38-45.

MacKinnon LT. Special feature for the Olympics: Effects of exercise on the immune system. Immunol Cell Biol 2000 Oct;78(5):502-09.

Makrigiannakis A, Zoumakis E, Kalataridou S, Chrousos G, Gravanis A. Uterine and embryonic trophoblast CRH promotes implantation and maintenance of early pregnancy. Ann NY Acad Sci 2003997:85-92 .

Mangiafico RA. Malatino LS, Attina T, et al. Exaggerated endothelin release in response to acute mental stress in patients with intermittent claudication. Angiology 2002 Jul-Aug;53(4):383-90.

Marckmann P. Dietary treatment of thrombogenic disorders related to the metabolic syndrome. British Journal of Nutrition 2000;83(Suppl 1):S121-6.

Martignoni E, Facchinetti F, Rossi F, et al. Neuroendocrine evidence of deranged noradrenergic activity in chronic migraine. Psychoneuroendocrinology 1989;14(5):357-63.

Martin R A. Humour as therapeutic play: Stress-moderating effects of sense of humour. Journal of Leisurability 1996;23(4).

Martynov AI, Ostroumova OD, Mamaev VI, Novinskii AA. Correction of sleep disorders and efficacy of antihypertensive monotherapy in elderly patients: Use of ivadal. Ter Arkh 2001; 73(10):77-79.

Masi AT, Bijlsma JW, Chikanza IC, et al. Neuroendocrine, immunologic, and microvascular systems interactions in rheumatoid arthritis: Physiopathogenetic and therapeutic perspectives. Semin Arthritis Rheum 1999 Oct;29(2):65-81.

Mastorakos G, Ilias L. Maternal hypothalamic-pituitary-adrenal axis in pregnancy and the postpartum period. Postpartum related disorders. Ann N Y Acad Sci 2000;900:95-106.

McCarty MF. High-dose pyridoxine as an "anti-stress" strategy. Med Hypotheseses 2000;54(5):803-07.

McEwan BS with Lasley EN. The end of stress as we know it. Washington, DC: Joseph Henry Press, 2002.

Milde AM, Murison R. A study of the effects of restraint stress on colitis induced by dextran sulphate sodium in singly housed rats. Integr Physiol Behav Sci 2002 Apr-Jun;37(2):140-50.

Miller DB, O'Callaghan JP. Neuroendocrine aspects of the response to stress. Metabolism 2002 Jun;51(6 Pt 2):5-10.

Miller GE, Cohen S, Ritchey AK. Chronic psychological stress and the regulation of pro-inflammatory cytokines: A glucocorticoid resistance model. Health Psychol 2002 Nov;21(6):531-41.

Milne B, Joachim G, Niedhardt J. A stress management programme for IBD patients. J Adv Nurs 1986 Sep;11(5):561-67.

Muller WE. Current St. John's wort research from mode of action to clinical efficacy. Pharmacol Res 2003 Feb;47(2):101-09.

Muller-Wieland D, Kotzka J, Knebel B, Krone W. Metabolic syndrome and hypertension: Pathpysiology and molecular basis of insulin resistance. Basic Research in Cardiology 1998;93 (Suppl 2):131-34.

Munck A, Guyre PM, Holbrook NJ. Physiological functions of glucocorticoids in stress and their relation to pharmacological actions. Endocr Rev 1984 Winter;5(1):25-44.

Nandi J, Meguid MM, Inui A. Central mechanisms involved with catabolism. Curr Opin Clin Nutr Metab Care 2002 Jul;5(4):407-18.

Neeck G. Pathogenic mechanisms of fibromyalgia. Aging Res Rev 2002 Apr;1(2):243-55.

Neeck G, Crofford LJ. Neuroendocrine perturbations in fibromyalgia and chronic fatigue syndrome. Rheum Dis Clin North Am 2000 Nov;26(4):989-1002.

Nemeroff CB. New directions in the development of antidepressants: The interface of neurobiology and psychiatry. Hum Psychopharmacol 2002 Jun;17 (Suppl 1):S13-16.

Okabe N. The pathogenesis of Crohn's disease. Digestion 2001;63 (Suppl 1):52-59.

Pang X, Alexacos N, Letourneau R, et al. A neurotensin receptor antagonist inhibits acute immobilization stress-induced cardiac mast cell degranulation, a CRH-dependent process. Pharmacology and Experimental Therapeutics 1998:287(1);307-14.

Paolisso G, Sgambato S, Gambardella A, et al. Daily magnesium supplements improve glucose handling in elderly subjects. Am J Clin Nutr 1992;55:1161-67.

Palkhivala A. Can stress keep you from making babies? Webmd;Article 16/1728 83745.htm.

Papadelis C, Kourtidoiu-Papadeli, et al. Effects of mental work load and caffeine on catecholamines and blood pressure compared to performance variations Brain Cogn 2003;51(1):143-54.

Patacchioli FR, Angelucci L, Dellerba G, Monnazzi P, Leri O. Actual stress, psychopathology and salivary cortisol levels in the irritable bowel syndrome. J Endocrinol Invest Mar;24(3):173-77.

Patarca R. Cytokines and chronic fatigue syndrome. Ann N Y Acad Sci. 2001 Mar;933:185-200.

Path G, Scherbaum WA, Bornstein SR. The role of interleukin-6 in the human adrenal gland. Eur.J.Clin.Invest. 2000 Dec;30 Suppl 3:91-95.

Peres MF, Sanchez del Rio M, Seabra M. Hypothalamic involvement in chronic migraine. J Neurol Neurosurg Psychiatry 2001 Dec;71(6): 747-51.

Peters EM, Anderson R, Nieman DC, Fickl H, Jogessar V. Vitamin C supplementation attenuates the increases in circulating cortisol, adrenaline and anti-inflammatory polypeptides following ultramarathon running. Int J Sports Med 2001:22(7):537-43.

Pittler MH, Ernst E. Kava extract for the treatment of anxiety. Cochraine Database Systems Review (United Kingdom) 2002;2:CD003383.

Porges SW, Doussard-Roosevelt JA, Portales AL, Greenspan SI. Infant regulation of the vagal 'brake' predicts child behavior problems: A psychobiological model of social behavior. Dev Psychobiol 1996; 29:697-712.

Prinz PN, Bailey SL, Wood DL. Sleep impairments in healthy seniors. Chronobiology Internat 2000 May 17;(3):391-404.

Prinz P, Baily S, Moe K., Wilkinson C, Scanlan J. Urinary free cortisol and sleep under baseline and stressed conditions in healthy senior women: Effects of estrogen replacement therapy. Journal of Sleep Research 2001 Mar;10(1):19-26.

Raber J. Detrimental effects of chronic hypothalamic-pituitary-adrenal axis activation. Molecular Neurobiology 1998;18(1):1-22.

Rakugi H, Kamide K, Ogihara T. Vascular signaling pathways in the metabolic syndrome. Current Hypertension Reports 2002;4(2):105-11.

Rex A, Morgenstern E, Fink H. Anxiolytic-like effects of Kava-Kava in the elevated plus maze test – a comparison with diazepam. Prog Neuropsychopharmacol Biol Psychiatry 2002;26(5):855-60.

Richter, R. Stress hormones may contribute to breast cancer deaths. Breast CA 2000 Jun;628.

Riedel W, Schlapp U, Leck S, Netter P, Neeck G. Blunted ACTH and cortisol responses to systemic injection of corticotropin-releasing hormone (CRH) in fibromyalgia: Role of somatostatin and CRH-binding protein. Ann N Y Acad Sci 2002 Jun;966:483-90.

Root, J Martin. Stress zaps your immune system. Prescription for Healthy Living 2002;1-2.

Rosmond R, Bjorntorp P. Occupational status: Cortisol secretion pattern and visceral obesity in middle-aged men. Obesity Research 2000 Sep.8;(6):445-50

Ross MC, Bohannon AS, Davis DC, Gurchiek L. The effects of a short-term exercise program on movement, pain and mood in the elderly: Results of a pilot study. J Holist Nurs 1999;17(2):139-47.

Sajdyk TJ, Schober DA, Gehlert DR, Shehar A. Role of corticotropin releasing factor and urocortin within the basolateral amygdala of rats in anxiety and panic responses. Behav Brain Res 1999 Apr;100(1-2):207-15.

Sasaki N, Kusano E, Ando N, et al. Changes in osteoprotegerin and markers of bone metabolism during glucocorticoid treatment in patients with chronic glomerulonephritis. Bone 2002 Jun;30(6):853-58.

Schell FJ, Allolio B, Schonecke OW. Physiological and psychological effects of Hatha-Yoga exercise in healthy women. Int J Psychosom 1994;41(1-4):46-52.

Schreiber W, Lauer CJ, Krumrey K, et al. Dysregulation of the hypothalamus-pituitary-adrenocortical system in panic disorder. Neuropsychopharmacology 1996 Jul;15(1):7-15.

Schulz H, Jobert M. Effects of hypericum extract on the sleep EEG in older volunteers. Journal of Geriatric Psychiatry and Neurology, 1994;7(suppl 1):39-43.

Scott LV, Medbak S, Dinan TG. Blunted adrenocorticotropin and cortisol responses to corticotropin-releasing hormone stimulation in chronic fatigue syndrome. Acta Psychiatr Scand 1998 Jun;97(6):450-57.

Seelig MS. Consequences of magnesium deficiency on the enhancement of stress reactions; preventive and therapeutic implications (a review). J Am Coll Nutr 1994 Oct;13(5):429-46.

Shephard RJ. Cytokine responses to physical activity, with particular reference to IL-6: Sources, actions, and clinical implications. Crit Rev Immunol 2002;22(3):165-82.

Sheps DS, McMahon RP, Becker L. Mental stress-induced ischemia and all-cause mortality in patients with coronary artery disease: Results from the Psychophysiological Investigations of Myocardial Ischemia study. Circulation 2002 Apr 16;105(15):1780-84.

Shin TY, Kim DK, Chae BS, Lee EJ. Antiallergic action of Magnolia officinalis on immediate hypersensitivity reaction. Arch Pharm Res 2001;24(3):249-55.

Simon JA. Vitamin C and cardiovascular disease: A review. J Am Coll Nutr 1992;1:107-25.

Singh LK, Pang X, Alexacos N, Letourneau R, Theoharides TC. Acute immobilization stress triggers skin mast cell degranulation via corticotropin releasing hormone, neurotensin, and substance P: A link to neurogenic skin disorders. Brain Behav Immun 1999 Sep;13(3):225-39.

Skowera A, Cleare A, Blair D, Bevis L, Wessely SC, Peakman M. High levels of type 2 cytokine-producing cells in chronic fatigue syndrome. Clin Exp Immunol 2004 Feb;135(2):294-302.

Smith LL. Cytokine hypothesis of overtraining: A physiological adaptation to excessive stress. Med Sci Sports Exerc 2000 Feb; 32(2):317-31.

Smolen D, Topp R, Singer L. The effect of self-selected music during colonoscopy on anxiety, heart rate and blood pressure. Appl Nurs Res 2002;15(3):126-36.

Smyth JM, Stone AA, Hurewitz A, Kaell A. Effects of writing about stressful experiences on symptom reduction in patients with asthma or rheumatoid arthritis: A randomized trial. JAMA 1999 Apr;281(14):1304-09.

Speroni E, Minghetti A. Neuropharmacological activity of extracts from Passiflora incarnata. Planta Med 1988 Dec;54(6):488-91.

Spieker LE, Hurlimann D, Ruschitzka F. Mental stress induces prolonged endothelial dysfunction via endothelin-A receptors. Circulation 2002 Jun;105(24):2817-20.

Spierings EL, Ranke AH, Honkoop PC. Precipitating and aggravating factors of migraine versus tension-type headache. Headache 2001 Jun;41(6):554-58.

Stones A, Groome D, Perry D, Hucklebridge F, Evans P. The effects of stress on salivary cortisol in panic disorder patients. J Affect Disord 1999 Jan-Mar;52(1-3):197-201.

Stowe RP, Pierson DL, Barrett AD. Elevated stress hormone levels relate to Epstein-Barr virus reactivation in astronauts. Psychosom Med 2001;63(6):891-95.

Stowe RP, Mehta SK, Ferrando AA, Feeback DL, Pierson DL. Immune responses and latent herpesvirus reactivation in spaceflight. Aviat Space Environ Med 2001;72(10):884-91.

Straub RH, Cutolo M. Involvement of the hypothalamic-pituitary-adrenal/gonadal axis and the peripheral nervous system in rheumatoid arthritis: Viewpoint based on a systemic pathogenetic role. Arthritis Rheum 2001 Mar;44(3):493-507.

Straub RH, Herfarth H, Falk W, et al. Uncoupling of the sympathetic nervous system and the HPA axis in IBD? J Neuroimmunol 2002 May;126(1-2):116-25.

Straub RH, Kittner JM, Heijnen C. Infusion of epinephrine decreases serum levels of cortisol and 17-OHP in patients with rheumatoid arthritis. J Rheumatol 2002 Aug;29(8):1659-64.

Straub RH, Paimela L, Peltomaa R, et al. Inadequately low levels of steroid hormones in relation to IL-6 and TNF in untreated patients with early rheumatoid arthritis and reactive arthritis. Arthritis Rheum 2002 Mar;46(3):654-62.

Strohle A, Holsboer F, Rupprecht R. Increased ACTH concentrations associated with cholecystokinin tetrapeptide-induced panic attacks in patients with panic disorder. Neuropsychopharmacology 2000;22(3):251-56.

Stromberg E, Edebo A Svennerholm AM, Lindholm C. Decreased epithelial cytokine response in the duodenal mucosa of H. pylori-infected duodenal ulcer patients. Clin Diagn Lab Immunol 2003 Jan;10(1):116-24.

Surwit RS, van Tilburg MA, Zucker N, et al. Stress management improves long-term glycemic control in type 2 diabetes. Diabetes Care 2002;25(1):30-34.

Svedlund J. Functional gastrointestinal diseases. Psychotherapy is an efficient complement to drug therapy. Lakartidningen 2002 Jan;99(3):172-74.

Tachikawa E, Takahashi M, Kashimoto T. Effects of extract and ingredients isolated from Magnolia obovota thunberg on catecholamine secretion from bovine adrenal chromaffin cells. Biochem Pharmacol 2000;60(3):433-40.

Tanaka S, Kuratsune H, Hidaka Y, et al. Autoantibodies against muscarinic cholinergic receptor in chronic fatigue syndrome. Int J Mol Med 2003 Aug;12(2):225-30.

Theoharides TC, Spanos C, Pang X. Stress-induced mast cell degranulation: Corticotropin-releasing hormone-mediated effect. Endocrinology 1995 Dec;136(12):5745-50.

Timar O, Sestiet F, Levy E. Metabolic Syndrome X. Canadian Journal of Cardiology 2000 Jun;16(6):779-89.

Treiber FA, Kapuku GK, Davis H, et al. Plasma endothelin-1 release during acute stress: Role of ethnicity and sex. Psychosom Med 2002 Sep-Oct;64(5):707-13.

Unger RH. Lipotoxic diseases. Ann Rev Medicine 2002;53:319-36.

Urhausen A, Kindermann W. Diagnosis of Overtraining: What tools do we have? Sports Med 2002 32(2):95-102.

Vanitallie TB. Stress: A risk factor for serious illness. Metabolism 2002 Jun;51(6 Pt 2):40-45.

Vergely N, Lafage-Proust MH, Caillot-Augusseau A, et al. Hypercorticism blunts circadian variations of osteocalcin regardless of nutritional status. Bone 2002 Feb;30(2):428-35.

Volz HP, Murck H, Kasper S, Moller HJ. St John's Wort extract (LI 160) in somatoform disorders: Results of a placebo-controlled trial. Psychopharmacology, 2002;164(3):294-300.

Wagner JD, Kaplan JR, Burkman RT. Reproductive hormones and cardiovascular disease mechanism of action and clinical implications. Obstet Gynecol Clin North Am 2002 Sep;29(3):475-93.

Walker BR. Steroid metabolism in metabolic syndrome X. Research Clinical Endocrinology and Metabolism 2001 Mar;15(1):111-22.

Wang Y, Ohtsuka-Isoya M, Shao P, et al. Effects of methylprednisolone on bone formation and resorption in rats. Jpn J Pharmacol 2002 Nov;90(3):236-46.

Webster EL, Barrientos RM, Contoreggi C, Isaac MG, Ligier S, Gabry KE, Chrousos GP, McCarthy EF, Rice KC, Gold PW, Sternberg EM. Corticotropin releasing hormone (CRH) antagonist attenuates adjuvant induced arthritis: Role of CRH in peripheral inflammation. J Rheumatol 2002 Jun;29(6):1252-61.

Wilder RL. Neuroimmunoendocrinology of the rheumatic diseases: Past, present and future. Ann N Y Acad Sci 2002 Jun;966:13-19.

Williams JE, Paton SC, Siegler ML, et al. Anger proneness predicts coronary heart disease risk: Prospective analysis from the atherosclerosis risk in Communities (ARIC) study. Circulation 2000;101:2034-39.

Xiao E, Xai-Zhang L, Ferin M. Inadequate luteal function is the initial clinical cyclic defect in a 12-day stress model that includes a psychogenic component in the rhesus monkey. J Clin Endocrinol Metab 2002 May;87(5):2232-37.

Ziegler DK, Hassanein RS, Kodanaz A, Meek JC. Circadian rhythms of plasma cortisol in migraine. J Neurol Neurosurg Psychiatry 1979 Aug;42(8):741-48.

Index

A

abdominal exercises, 117
absorption, 39, 90, 190, 208, 223, 265
acid production, 199-200
acidophilus (probiotic), 101
acidosis, 87, 265
ACTH. *See* adrenocorticotropic hormone
activated whey protein, 102, 209
active stretching, 108
acupuncture, 132-134
acute stress response, 8
Addison disease, 44, 265
adenosine tri-phosphate (ATP), 88, 265
ADH. *See* antidiuretic hormone
adipokine, 60, 61, 63, 223, 265
adipose tissue, 59, 265
adrenal cortex, 27, 33, 34, 37, 265
adrenal cortisol secretion, 8-9
adrenal fatigue, 41, 42, 45, 47
adrenal glands
  and adrenal fatigue, 42
  and alcohol, 78
  and autonomic nervous system, 21
  combating overactive, 80
  and daily cortisol cycle, 36
  defined, 34, 265
  and diet, 55, 56
  and fight-or-flight response, 37, 39
  and hypothalamus, 31
  and hypothalamus-pituitary-adrenal axis, 35
  location of, 24
  and pituitary gland, 32, 33
  and stress response, 8, 17, 43
  and their hormones, 26-27
adrenal medulla, 33-34, 37, 88, 265
adrenaline, 6-8, 17, 26, 33-34, 37-38, 40, 265
adrenocorticotropic hormone (ACTH), 24-27, 29, 31-32, 35-37, 39-43, 265
aerobic zone, 120
afferent, 265
affirmation, positive, 151
alarm reaction, 45, 180, 265
alcohol, and stress, 78
aldosterone, 26, 27, 33, 34, 45, 181, 182, 265
allergic reactions, type 1, 212
allergic response, 212-216
allergies, 127, 202-216
allostatic load, 46

alpha waves, 96, 97, 106, 241, 265
amino acids
  defined, 82, 265
  and diet, 53, 54, 56, 61, 66
  and fight-or-flight response, 27, 38
  and glutamine therapy, 199
  and immune impairment, 208-210, 219
  and immune system supplements, 102
  and vitamin C, 86, 87
amputations, and diabetes, 175
amygdala, 57, 59, 61, 256, 257, 259, 260, 265
amygdala hijack, 44
anaphylaxis, 213
androgens, 265
anorexia, 32, 62, 154, 222, 223, 234, 266
antalarmin, 155
anti-chart, 74-75
anti-stress diet, 50-79
anti-stress exercise therapies, 104-122
anti-stress hormone, 39
anti-stress natural supplements, 80-103
anti-stress physical therapies, 123-140
antianxiety medication, 155
antibodies, 205, 206, 213, 215, 252, 266
antidepressants, 93-94, 155
antidiuretic hormone (ADH), 26, 78, 265
antioxidants, 86, 202, 209-211, 216-217, 219, 221, 229, 254, 266
antiviral activity of vitamin C, 87-88
anxiety, 9, 10, 255-264
appetite, 58
arm exercises, 115
aromatherapy, 130
arteries, hardening of, 185
arteriosclerosis, 266
arthritis, 224-227
assertiveness, 141, 150
astressin, 155
atopy, 213-214
ATP. *See* adenosine tri-phosphate
atrophy, 256
attitudes toward stress, 10
autonomic imbalance, 219
autonomic nervous system, 17, 20-21, 31, 33, 37, 190, 194
  defined, 266
  and inflammatory bowel disease, 195
  and irritable bowel syndrome, 191-192
  and role of stress in allergies, 214

  and role of stress in arthritis, 226
autonomic role, 20

B

B-cells, 206
back exercises, 114
ballistic stretching, 109
basal metabolic rate, 266
basophil, 204, 213, 214, 215, 216
behavioral therapy, 153
benzodiazepines, 91, 92, 98, 156, 258, 261-264
beta-blockers, 156, 258
beta wave, 204, 266
bioavailability, 266
biochemical reactions, 82, 266
bioflavonoid, 102, 266
biotin, 266
blindness, and diabetes, 175
blood pressure
  and anxiety and depression, 255, 258
  and attitudes toward stress, 10
  and bodywork, 127, 137, 140
  and cardiovascular disease, 179-185, 187-188
  and chronic pain disorders, 251
  and chronic stress, 44-46
  controlling, 183
  and cortisol, 181
  defined, 266
  and diabetes, 175
  dynamics of rising, 180
  and exercise therapies, 104, 118, 120
  high. *See* high blood pressure
  lowering, 179
  and medications, 156
  and mental therapies, 142, 145, 148, 150
  and metabolic syndrome, 9
  and musculoskeletal disorders, 219
  and natural supplements, 84-86, 88-90, 95, 97-99
  and nutrition, 51, 62-64, 77
  and sleep disorders, 243
  and stress-related diseases and disorders, 11
  and stress response, 9, 37, 38
  and stress solution, 170
  and stress systems, 20, 21, 27
blood sugar, 6, 8, 9, 11, 37-39, 45
body fat levels, 70
body mass index, 68-69
body system messengers, 23
bodywork, 123-140, 163, 166, 169, 171. *See also* physical therapies
bone marrow, 203

bowel disorder supplements, 101
brain, 17, 18
breathing, 7-9, 141, 142, 145
breathing exercises, 138-139, 142
brown fat, 52, 266
bulimia, 154, 266

C

cabbage, 101
caffeine, 76-77
calcium, 27, 82, 88-92, 181, 221, 223-224, 237, 266
calmness, 143
calorie, 51-53, 58-59, 65, 67, 77, 105, 120, 221, 223, 266
cancer, 209-210
capsicum, 103
carbohydrate abuse, 54
carbohydrate fatigue, 55
carbohydrate index, 70-71
carbohydrates, 53-55
  complex, 53, 267
  defined, 266
  glycemic index of common, 71
  reintroducing, 73
  restricted, 72
  simple, 53, 65, 174, 273
cardiovascular disease, 179-188
cardiovascular exercise, 118-122, 161, 163, 165, 168-169, 171
  benefits of, 118
  components of, 118-120
  program for beginners, 121
  program for intermediates, 121
  stages of, 120
  for stress-related arthritis, 227
  for stress-related diabetes, 178
  for stress-related general anxiety disorder, 263
  for stress-related heart attack, 186
  for stress-related hypertension, 184
  for stress-related inflammatory bowel disease, 196
  for stress-related irritable bowel syndrome, 193
  for stress-related low back pain, 229
  for stress-related migraines, 249
  for stress-related panic attacks, 261
  for stress-related peptic ulceration, 201
carnitine, 266
catecholamine, 33, 37, 77, 88, 90, 91, 267
CCK. *See* cholecystokinin

CCK hormone, 52
CD. *See* Crohn's disease
CD8 cells, 206
cellular immunity, 208
cellular processes, 8
central nervous system, 77, 93, 96, 140, 190-191, 196, 211, 262, 267
central obesity, 60, 267
central sensitization, 228
central stress response, 43-44
cerebellum, 17, 18, 267
cerebral cortex (CCK), 29, 52, 190, 267
CFS. *See* chronic fatigue syndrome
chest exercises, 114
cholecystokinin (CCK), 29, 52, 157, 190, 260, 266, 267
cholesterol, 5, 9, 11, 13, 44, 46, 62, 64, 65, 70, 182, 184, 185, 267
chrelin excess, 60
chromium, 82, 174, 178, 267
chronic fatigue syndrome (CFS), 11, 191, 209, 245, 249-254, 267
chronic pain disorders, 245-254
chronic stimulation, 7
chronic stress, 40-47, 210-211
chronic stress response, 8-9
circadian rhythm, 24, 36, 267
citrus aurantium, 103
coenzymes, 82, 83, 85, 87, 267
cognitive therapy, 154
colds, recurrent, 10
collagen, 86, 87, 211, 221, 227, 267
comfort food, 61
complex carbohydrates, 53, 267
conjugated linoleic acid, 103, 267
constipation, 77, 82, 94, 106, 156, 191, 258, 267
cool-down, 118
corticotrophin-releasing hormone (CRH), 25, 26, 31, 59, 106, 233, 245, 247, 267. *See also* CRH-receptor blockers
adverse effects of, 42
defined, 267
and inflammatory conditions, 186
and role of stress in allergies, 215
cortisol, 6, 8, 9, 17, 33
and anorexia, 62
and blood pressure, 181
daily cycle, 36
defined, 267
effects of, 37, 210, 223
and insulin, 181-182
levels of, 40-41, 244
rhythm disruption, 36
and role of stress in allergies, 214
and role of stress in arthritis, 225

and role of stress in peptic ulcer disease, 198-199
cortisol activity, 56
cortisol resistance, 9, 42-43
cortisol response, 219
cortisol secretion, 9
counseling, 150-154
COX. *See* cyclooxygenase
craniosacral therapy, 136
CRH. *See* corticotrophin-releasing hormone
CRH-receptor blockers, 155, 157, 158
Crohn's disease (CD), 194
cry wolf response, 9
Cushing's disease, 222, 223, 234, 267
cyclooxygenase (COX), 205, 208, 266
cysteine, 86, 102, 208, 209, 210, 219, 221, 251, 267
cytokine action, 206
cytokine hypothesis, 220
cytokines, 22-23, 194, 205-208, 210-211, 213, 219-220, 222
defined, 267
typical, 29

D

daily routine, 143
danger, perception of, 9
deep-tissue massage, 128
delta waves, 240, 241, 267
dental disease, and diabetes, 176
depression, 8, 9, 255-264
detoxification, 236
dexamethasone, 42, 63, 248, 267
dexamethasone suppression test, 42, 248, 267
diabetes, 9, 10, 174-178
age onset of, 177
basics of, 174-177
causes of, 177
complications of, 175-176
defined, 268
pre-, 177
preventing, 174, 175
prevention of, 178
role of stress in, 177-178
supplements for stress-related, 178
treatment of, 178
types of, 176
diarrhea, 79, 87, 189, 191, 192, 193, 213, 267
diet, 9, 50-79
diet trends, 64-66
dietary balance, 75
dietary preventions and treatment of stress, 63
digestive enzymes, 101
disease, and stress, 64
diseases, 11, 174-264
disorders, 11, 174-264
diuretic, 26, 78, 83, 268
down-regulation, 28, 30, 42, 209, 257, 268
dream interpretation, 152
duodenal ulcers. *See* peptic ulcers
dynamic stretching, 108

E

edema, 247, 268
EEG. *See* electroencephalogram
EFAs. *See* essential fatty acids
efferent, 268
effleurage massage, 128
8-week stress solution program, 159-172
eldepryl, 156, 258
electroencephalogram (EEG), 93-96, 126, 145, 240, 268
electrolytes, 88, 268
endocrine glands, 23, 246
defined, 268
and hormones, 26-27
major, 24, 26
endocrine system, 16-17, 21-30, 47, 106, 207
controls, 23
daily cycles, 24
defined, 268
feedback, 25
receptor number, 28
sensitivity, 28
endometrium, 157, 268
endorphins, 78, 106, 118, 126, 132, 268
endothelin, 182-183, 185, 247, 248, 268
energy (Qi), 132, 133, 140, 272
enkephalins, 29, 106, 126, 268
enzymes, 11, 52, 58, 65, 83-84, 87-88, 97, 99, 193, 195-198, 201
defined, 82, 268
digestive, 101
eosinophils, 203, 204, 208, 210, 215, 268
essential fatty acids (EFAs), 51, 99-101
balancing, 100-101
defined, 82, 268
types of, 100
essential nutrients, 268
essential oils, aromatherapy, 130
estrogen, 26-27, 84, 92, 187, 224, 232-233, 236-238, 240
defined, 268
and role of stress in osteoporosis, 223
exercise
for arthritis, 227
basics of, 104-106
basics of strength-training, 113
cardiovascular, 118-122
components of, 105-106
hormonal changes induced by, 106
for low back pain, 229
pace of, 107
for stress-related chronic fatigue syndrome, 254
for stress-related fibromyalgia, 254
for stress-related sleep disorders, 244
exercise options, 106

exercise therapies, 104-122
exercises
meditation, 146-147
strength-training, 113-117
stretching, 107-112
extracellular, 268

F

fat cell, 23, 37, 52, 57-60, 66, 223, 268
fat levels, 70
fatigue, carbohydrate, 55
fatigue, 10
fats, 51-52
fatty acids, 13, 37, 39, 51, 56, 82, 84, 193, 196, 268
feedback controls, faulty, 42
feedback impairment, 207
fertility, 7, 236
fertilization, 232, 268
fiber, 17, 53, 103, 126, 128, 140, 192, 221, 227-228, 268
fibromyalgia, 4, 11, 228, 245, 249-254, 268
fight-or-flight, triggers, 19
fight-or-flight response, 6, 8-9, 36-39
fitness zone, of heart zone training, 120
5-HTP, 98-99
follicle-stimulating hormone (FSH), 26-27, 31-32, 231-238, 268
foods, limited in naturopathic diet, 72
forebrain, 17, 18
free association, 152
free radical, 83, 86, 97, 127, 202, 210, 266, 269
free radical scavenger, 83, 87, 219, 269
friction massage, 128
fructose, 73, 268, 273
FSH. *See* follicle-stimulating hormone

G

GABA. *See* gamma-amniobutyric acid
GAD. *See* general anxiety disorder
gamma-amniobutyric acid (GABA), 84, 92-94, 97-98, 156, 258, 262, 269
garcinia cambogia, 103
GAS. *See* general adaptation syndrome
gastrointestinal disorders, 189-201
general adaptation syndrome (GAS), 45, 269
general anxiety disorder (GAD), 42, 156, 257, 258, 261, 262
defined, 269
treatment for stress-related, 263
genistein 269. *See also* isofavone
Gestalt therapy, 152-153
gestational diabetes, 176
GH. *See* growth hormone
GHIH. *See* growth hormone-inhibiting hormone

ghrelin, 23, 59-60, 63, 269
GHRH. *See* growth
  hormone-releasing
  hormone
glucagon, 26, 37, 39, 54, 56,
  70, 269
glucocorticoids, 174, 181,
  276
gluconeogenesis, 54, 269
glucose, 27, 37-39, 45, 53-57,
  60-61, 67, 70-71, 73, 84,
  88-99, 157, 174, 177, 269
glucose intolerance, 269
glutamine, 29, 37-38, 86,
  257, 269
glutamine therapy, 199
glutathione, 83, 86, 87, 102,
  209, 210, 219, 267, 269
glycemic index, 61, 70-71,
  73, 269
glycogen, 39, 54, 55, 57, 84,
  269
glyconeogenesis, 269
GnRH. *See* gonadotropin-
  releasing hormone
gonadotropin-releasing
  hormone (GnRH), 26, 31,
  58, 223, 231, 233-236, 269
granulocytes, 204
green tea, 96-97
growth hormone (GH), 24,
  26-27, 31-32, 50, 57-62,
  137, 161, 200, 240, 243,
  251, 254
  defined, 269
  and exercise-induced
    hormonal changes, 106
growth hormone-inhibiting
  hormone (GHIH), 26, 31,
  269
growth hormone-releasing
  hormone (GHRH), 31,
  32, 57, 269

H

H. pylori, and peptic ulcers,
  198
hamstring exercises, 115-116
HCG (hCG). *See* human
  chorionic gonadotrophin
HDLs. *See* high-density
  lipoproteins
healing, 7, 200
heart, in acupuncture
  treatment, 133
heart attack, 9, 184-188
heart disease, and diabetes,
  175
heart rate, 7, 8, 9, 119
heart zone training, 120
helper T-cells, 205
herbs, 82, 90-96
HGH (hGH). *See* human
  growth hormone
high blood pressure, 9-11,
  44-46, 51, 62-64, 100,
  175, 179-180, 182-185.
  See also hypertension
high-carbohydrate diets,
  65
high-density lipoproteins
  (HDLs), 65, 269
high-protein diets, 66
high-turnover osteoporosis,
  222

hippocampus, 19-20, 39, 43,
  57, 59, 245, 256-257, 260,
  264, 270
histamine, 86, 91, 102, 192,
  204, 212, 214-215, 246,
  270
HMS-90, 102
homeostasis, 16, 36, 39, 47,
  67, 105, 159, 270
hops, 92
hormonal imbalance, 7
hormone actions, 25
hormone feedback loop, 28
hormones, 23, 106
  and massage therapy,
    126-127
  and pituitary gland, 32
HPA axis. *See*
  hypothalamus-pituitary-
  adrenal axis
human chorionic
  gonadotrophin
  (HCG/hCG), 232, 269
human growth hormone
  (HGH/hGH), 269
humanistic therapy, 153-154
hypercholesterolemia, 270
hyperglycemia, 54, 174, 181,
  270
hyperinsulinemia, 55, 60,
  62, 73, 76, 181, 182
  defined, 270
  signs of, 74-75
hyperlipidemia, 270
hypertension, 88, 175, 184,
  260
  basics of, 180
  defined, 270
  role of stress in, 180-183
  stress management of,
    183-184
  supplements for stress-
    related, 184
  treatment of, 181, 184
hypertension stress cascade,
  182
hypoglycemia, 60, 160, 162,
  164, 167, 244, 248, 261,
  263, 270
hypoglycemia-
  hyperglycemia
  connection, 54-55
hypothalamus, 17-19, 20-26,
  29-32, 34-37, 39, 41-43,
  47
  defined, 270
  neuropeptide hormones
    released by, 31
hypothalamus-pituitary-
  adrenal axis (HPA axis),
  34-35, 41-42, 45-46
  defined, 269
  and irritable bowel
    syndrome, 191
hypothalamus-pituitary-
  adrenal interactions,
  30-34

I

IBD. *See* inflammatory
  bowel disease
IBS. *See* irritable bowel
  syndrome
IgE, 213
illness, 8, 9

immune feedback, 210-211
immune impairment, 207,
  219
immune reaction, 207, 208
immune system, 23, 27, 29,
  38, 70, 84, 86, 94, 217
  and adrenal gland
    interaction, 206
  defined, 270
  direct effects of cortisol on,
    210
  effects of stress on, 207
  and massage therapy, 127
  mediators in, 205
immune system activity,
  and irritable bowel
  disease, 194-195
immune system organs, 203
immune system
  supplements, 102
ImmunePro, 102
immunity, 7, 199, 202, 211
immunity disorders, 203-211
immunoglobulin, 29, 91,
  205, 206, 212, 252, 270
inderal, 156, 258
infections, 8, 9, 201-205
infertility, 230-236
inflammation, and massage
  therapy, 127
inflammatory bowel disease
  (IBD), 11, 101, 157-158,
  207, 211, 215, 257
  basics of, 194
  defined, 270
  idiopathic forms of, 194
  role of stress in, 194-196
  treatment for stress-
    related, 196
insomnia, 11, 154, 243, 255,
  258, 270
insulin, 26, 37-38, 44, 46,
  176-178
  and cortisol, 181-182
  defined, 270
insulin levels, 9
insulin-like-growth factor 1,
  270
insulin resistance, 9, 37-38,
  44, 46, 55, 57, 60-64, 75,
  174, 178, 270
interleukins, 29, 205, 270
irritable bowel syndrome
  (IBS), 11, 47, 101,
  109-111, 250, 253,
  260, 262
  basics of, 190-191
  defined, 270
  role of stress in, 191-192
  stress factors affecting, 195
  stress management of, 192,
    196
  supplements for stress-
    related, 193
  symptoms of, 191
  treatment of, 192-193
isoflavone, 238, 270
isometric stretching, 109

J

journaling, 151

K

kava kava, 94-95
ketone body, 270

ketosis, 66, 70, 270
kidney disease, and diabetes,
  175
kidneys, in acupuncture
  treatment, 133

L

L-theanine. *See* theanine
laughter therapy, 149
lavender, 95-96
LDLs. *See* low density
  lipoproteins
leptin, 58-59, 223, 270
leptin resistance, 59
leukocytes. *See* white blood
  cells
leukotrienes, 205, 208,
  271
LH. *See* luteinizing
  hormone, 23, 31, 231,
  271
lifestyle, 9, 150-151
limbic system, 17, 19-20, 22,
  30, 34, 39, 57, 59, 228,
  245, 271
linoleic acid, conjugated,
  103
lipids, 271
lipogenesis, 52, 271
lipoprotein lipase, 65,
  271
liver, 27, 37-39, 53-54, 56-58,
  83-84, 95, 99, 101, 182,
  193, 271
low back pain, 217, 227-229
low-calorie diets, 65
low CG syndrome, 208-209
low density lipoproteins
  (LDLs), 271
low-fat diets, 65
low-turnover osteoporosis,
  222
luteinizing hormone
  (LH), 23, 26-27, 31-32,
  231-238, 271
lymph nodes, 203
lymphocytes, 29, 84,
  203-206, 208, 210,
  215, 219, 271

M

macronutrient, 271
macrophage, 29, 203, 204,
  205, 206, 210, 271
magnesium, 88-89, 271
magnolia bark, 90-91
MAOIs. *See* monoamine
  oxidase inhibitors
marshmallow, 101
massage holding patterns,
  129
massage therapy, 126-129
mast cells, 186, 213
McEwan, Bruce, 46
medications, 155-158
meditation, 144-147
melatonin, 26, 98, 103, 198,
  200, 244, 248
  defined, 271
  and role of stress in peptic
    ulcer disease, 200
  and stress-related sleep
    disorders, 244
menopause, 237-238
menstruation, 236-237

mental disorders, medication for stress-related, 156
mental stress, 183, 229
mental therapies, 141-154
metabolic balance, and weight maintenance, 73-76
metabolic disruption, 57
metabolic imbalance, 7
metabolic retraining, in stage one of naturopathic diet, 67-72
metabolic syndrome, 7, 9, 44, 45, 62, 271
metabolism, 7, 8, 27, 38, 39, 44, 46, 51, 58, 61, 64, 67, 68, 75, 174, 181, 271
micronutrient, 271
microphages, 204
midbrain, 17, 18
migraines, 246-249
milk peptide hydrolysate, 97-98
mind, bodywork for, 123
minerals, 82, 88-90, 271
mitochondria, 55, 83, 271
monoamine oxidase inhibitors (MAOIs), 94, 156, 258, 271
monocytes, 203, 204, 208, 210, 215, 271
mood change, and overtraining syndrome, 219
mood disorders, medication for stress-related, 156
multitasking, 150
muscles, 8, 9
musculoskeletal disorders, 217-229
music therapy, 148-149

N
Nardil, 156, 258
natural biological therapies, 11
natural killer cells (NK cells), 29, 199, 206, 208, 210, 271
natural supplements, 80-103, 160, 163, 165, 168, 171
naturopathic diet, 64-76, 160, 162, 164, 167-168, 170
    principles of, 66-67
    stages of, 67-76
    for stress-related allergic response, 216
    for stress-related arthritis, 227
    for stress-related chronic fatigue syndrome, 254
    for stress-related diabetes, 176
    for stress-related fibromyalgia, 254
    for stress-related general anxiety disorder, 263
    for stress-related heart attack, 186
    for stress-related hypertension, 184

    for stress-related immunity disorders, 211
    for stress-related inflammatory bowel disease, 196
    for stress-related irritable bowel syndrome, 193
    for stress-related low back pain, 229
    for stress-related migraines, 249
    for stress-related overtraining syndrome, 221
    for stress-related panic attacks, 261
    for stress-related peptic ulceration, 201
naturopathy, 271
negative feedback, 39
nerve stimulation, 132-133
nervous system, 17-21
nervous system disease, and diabetes, 175
neurons, 23, 28, 29, 256, 257, 262, 271
neuropathy, 177, 271
neuropeptide hormones, 31
neurotransmitters, 11, 22-23, 28-29, 61, 83-85, 92-93, 97-98, 155, 157, 272
neutrophil, 204, 208, 210, 215, 272
NK cells. See natural killer cells
noradrenaline, 26, 33-34, 37-38, 42, 77, 272
normal stress, 40
nutrition, 51-55, 59

O
obesity, 9, 11, 44, 46, 51, 58-60, 62-64, 70, 157, 177-178, 272
olive leaf extract, 102
Omega-3 essential fatty acids, 100
Omega-6 essential fatty acids, 100
Omega-7/9 essential fatty acids, 100
oregano oil, 102
osteocalcin, 222-223
osteoporosis, 221-224
osteoprotegerin, 222
OTS. See overtraining syndrome
ovary, 27, 131, 233, 234, 272
overnutrition, 59
overstimulation, 8
overtraining syndrome (OTS), 7, 217-221, 272
overweight, 8-10
ovulation, 231-237, 246, 272

P
pain, 113
pain relief, through massage therapy, 126-127
pain supplements, 103
pancreas, 23-24, 26, 54, 57-58, 101, 131, 174, 176-177, 272

panic attacks, 258-261
panic disorder (PD), 42, 257, 258, 262, 272
parasympathetic nervous system, 21, 145, 260, 272
parasympathetic overactivity, 214
passionflower, 91-92
passive stretching, 109
Paxil, 99, 156, 258
PD. See panic disorder
peptic ulcers, 197-201
pet therapy, 149
petrissage, 128
peyer's patches, 203
phosphate, 84, 221, 272
physical therapies, 161, 163, 166, 169, 171. See also bodywork
    anti-stress, 123-140
    for stress-related allergic response, 216
    for stress-related arthritis, 227
    for stress-related chronic fatigue syndrome, 254
    for stress-related diabetes, 178
    for stress-related fibromyalgia, 254
    for stress-related general anxiety disorder, 263
    for stress-related heart attack, 186
    for stress-related hypertension, 184
    for stress-related immunity disorders, 211
    for stress-related inflammatory bowel disease, 196
    for stress-related irritable bowel syndrome, 193
    for stress-related low back pain, 229
    for stress-related migraines, 249
    for stress-related overtraining syndrome, 221
    for stress-related panic attacks, 261
    for stress-related peptic ulceration, 201
physiological, 11, 78, 127, 137, 148, 242, 272
physiological changes, during meditation, 145
phytoestrogen, 270, 272
phytosterol, 272
pituitary gland, 17, 19, 22, 24, 30-34, 36-37, 39, 43, 272
PMS. See pre-menstrual syndrome
PNF. See propioceptive neuromuscular facilitation stretching
pons, 17, 272
positive affirmation, 151
post-traumatic stress disorder (PTSD), 42, 43, 156, 257, 258, 261, 263-264, 272

potassium, 27, 82, 89, 90, 272
pre-diabetes, 177
pre-menstrual syndrome (PMS), 237, 272
pregnancy, 176, 226
pressure, 8
prevention, of stress-related disorders and diseases, 174-264
progesterone, 26-27, 232-233, 236-238, 272
proprioceptive neuromuscular facilitation (PNF) stretching, 109
prostaglandins, 51, 99, 197, 199, 204-205, 208, 219, 235, 272
proteins, 52-53, 272
    activated whey, 102, 209
    deficiency, 53
protein catabolism, 55
protein sources, common, 70
Prozac, 91, 99, 156, 192, 253, 256, 258
psychoanalysis, 151-152
psychological factors, 183, 195-196
psychological stress, 183, 229
psychology, 221, 272
psychosocial stress, 215
PTSD. See post-traumatic stress disorder

Q
Qi (energy), 132, 133, 140, 272
quadricep exercises, 115-116
quercitin, 102

R
rage, 7
rapid eye movement (REM), 240, 241, 272
RDA. See recommended daily allowance
receptors, 25, 28, 30, 42-43, 272
recommended daily allowance (RDA), 272
recurrent back pain, and stress, 228-229
reflexology, 130-131
Rei-Ki, 135
relaxation
    aromatherapy essential oils for, 130
    music therapy for, 149
    through acupuncture, 133
relaxation techniques, 142-150, 161, 163, 166, 169, 172
relaxation therapy
    for stress-related allergic response, 216
    for stress-related arthritis, 227
    for stress-related diabetes, 178
    for stress-related general anxiety disorder, 263
    for stress-related heart attack, 186

for stress-related hypertension, 184
for stress-related immunity disorders, 211
for stress-related inflammatory bowel disease, 196
for stress-related irritable bowel syndrome, 193
for stress-related low back pain, 229
for stress-related migraines, 249
for stress-related overtraining syndrome, 221
for stress-related panic attacks, 261
for stress-related peptic ulceration, 201
REM. *See* rapid eye movement
renin-angiotensin, 182
rep (repetition), 113
reproductive disorders, 230-238
resistance, 113
resistin, 60, 63, 272

S
saturated fats, 51, 273
selective serotonin reuptake inhibitors (SSRIs), 94, 99, 156, 256, 258, 262, 264, 272
Selye, Hans, 45
Serax, 156, 258
serotonin, 61-62, 273
set, 113
set point, 8-9
shiatsu, 135-136
simple carbohydrates, 53, 65, 174, 273
skin rashes, 10
sleep deprivation, 8, 9
sleep disorders, 239-244
sleep supplements, 103
slippery elm, 101
soy, 72, 100, 238, 273
spleen, 203
SSRIs. *See* selective serotonin reuptake inhibitors
St. John's wort, 93-94
starvation, 58, 59, 60, 65, 70, 223, 273
static stretching, 108
stomach ulcers. *See* peptic ulceration
strength-training, 113-117
stress
  beating, 202
  and cancer, 209-210
  controlling levels of, 189
  and diet, 55-64
  and disease, 64
  effects of, 7
  and low back pain, 217
  lowering, 50, 179
  and viral infections, 209
  and weight, 63, 64
stress checklist, 11
stress emergencies, 143

stress hormones, 6, 126-127, 218
stress problem, 16-47
stress-relief, exercise for, 104
stress response, 16-17, 22, 35-39, 43-44
stress solution program, 8-week, 159-172
stress solutions, 9-13, 49-173
stress symptom journal, 12
stress systems, 16-34
stressors, avoiding, 150
stretching, benefits of, 107-112
stretching exercises, 107-112, 138-139
stroke, 9, 175
sugar lows, 61
supplements
  anti-stress natural, 80-103
  basic terms for, 82
  quality of, 81
  safety of, 81
  selecting and combining, 81-82
  for stress-related allergic response, 216
  for stress-related arthritis, 227
  for stress-related chronic fatigue syndrome, 254
  for stress-related diabetes, 178
  for stress-related fibromyalgia, 254
  for stress-related general anxiety disorder, 263
  for stress-related heart attack, 186
  for stress-related hypertension, 184
  for stress-related immunity disorders, 211
  for stress-related infertility, 236
  for stress-related inflammatory bowel disease, 196
  for stress-related irritable bowel syndrome, 193
  for stress-related low back pain, 229
  for stress-related menopause symptoms, 238
  for stress-related migraines, 249
  for stress-related osteoporosis, 224
  for stress-related overtraining syndrome, 221
  for stress-related panic attacks, 261
  for stress-related peptic ulceration, 201
sweat, 7
Swedish massage, 128
sympathetic nervous system, 8, 9, 21, 37, 211
sympathic nervous system, 273

synapse, 29, 273
syndrome-X. *See* metabolic syndrome

T
Tai Chi, 140
tapotement, 128
Tenormin, 156, 258
testosterone, and role of stress in osteoporosis, 223
testosterone, 27, 219, 223, 235, 273
thalamus, 17, 19, 20, 273
theanine, 96-97
therapy, 148-149
theta waves, 241, 244, 273
thinking about stress, 16
threat, 8
thymus, 203, 273
thyroid, 23-24, 26-27, 50, 70, 131, 235, 251, 273
thyroid-stimulating hormone (TSH), 26, 27, 31, 32, 58, 273
TNF. *See* tumor necrosis factor
treating stress-related disorders and diseases, 174-264
treatment program
  for stress-related allergic response, 216
  for stress-related arthritis, 227
  for stress-related chronic fatigue syndrome, 254
  for stress-related diabetes, 178
  for stress-related fibromyalgia, 254
  for stress-related general anxiety disorder, 263
  for stress-related heart attack, 186
  for stress-related hypertension, 184
  for stress-related immunity disorders, 211
  for stress-related infertility, 236
  for stress-related inflammatory bowel disease, 196
  for stress-related irritable bowel syndrome, 193
  for stress-related low back pain, 229
  for stress-related menopause, 238
  for stress-related migraines, 249
  for stress-related osteoporosis, 224
  for stress-related overtraining syndrome, 221
  for stress-related panic attacks, 261
  for stress-related peptic ulceration, 201
  for stress-related post-traumatic stress disorder, 264

for stress-related sleep disorders, 244
trigger point therapy, 128
triglyceride, 39, 65, 273
TSH. *See* thyroid-stimulating hormone
tumor cells, 206
tumor necrosis factor (TNF), 29, 91, 202, 205-208, 210, 225, 226, 273
type 1 allergic reactions, 212
Type 1 diabetes, 176, 177-178
Type 2 diabetes, 176, 178

U
ulcerative colitis (UC), 193, 194, 196, 273
ulcers, 10, 197-201
unsaturated fats, 51
up-regulation, 273

V
vagal brake, 187
vagus nerve, 186, 186-187
valerian, 92-93
valium, 91, 92, 156, 258, 261, 262, 263
vasoactive intestinal peptide (VIP), 190, 273
vasoconstriction, 273
vasodilation, 182, 273
vasopressin, 78, 273
VIP. *See* vasoactive intestinal peptide
viral infections, 208, 209
viruses, 206-207
visualization, 144
vitamin B-1, 83
vitamin B-2, 83
vitamin B-3, 84
vitamin B-6, 84-85
vitamin B-12, 85
vitamin C, 85-88
vitamins, 82, 83-88, 273

W
warm-up, 118
water soluble, 83, 85, 87, 273
weekly weight and anti-stress chart, 74-75
weight, 7, 50, 56, 61, 63, 64, 67-76
weight chart, 74-75
weight-management supplements, 103
whey protein, activated, 102, 209
white blood cells, 204
white fat, 52, 273
work, absence from, 7

X
Xanax, 156, 258, 262

Y
yoga, 136-139

Z
zinc, 102
Zoloft, 99, 156, 258